Also by Suzanne Somers
available from Random House Large Print

Suzanne Somers' Slim and Sexy Forever
The Sexy Years

SUZANNE SOMERS

AGELESS

The Naked Truth About
Bioidentical Hormones

R A N D O M H O U S E
L A R G E P R I N T

This book contains general information and is not intended to be, nor should be, used as a substitute for specific medical advice.

Published in the United States of America by Random House Large Print in association with Crown Publishers, New York.
Distributed by Random House, Inc., New York.

Library of Congress Cataloging-in-Publication Data
Somers, Suzanne, 1946–
Ageless: the naked truth behind bioidentical hormones / by Suzanne Somers.—1st large print ed.
p. cm.
Originally published: New York: Crown Publishers, c2006.
ISBN-13: 978-0-7393-2588-9
ISBN-10: 0-7393-2588-4
1. Longevity. 2. Menopause—Hormone therapy.
3. Middle-aged women—Health and hygiene.
4. Middle-aged men—Health and hygiene.
5. Large type books. I. Title.
RA776.75.S68 2006b
618.1'7506—dc22
2006029000

www.randomlargeprint.com

FIRST LARGE PRINT EDITION

10 9 8 7 6 5 4 3 2 1

This Large Print edition published in accord with the standards of the N.A.V.H.

To my granddaughters,
Camelia, Daisy, and Violet
This is for you . . .

When the time comes
this passage will be easier

And for my grandsons,
you, too, will have
an easier time of it

ACKNOWLEDGMENTS

WRITING THIS BOOK was like getting my PhD with the world's greatest professors. What a thrill. Obtaining this cutting-edge information has been empowering. Understanding how our bodies work allows each of us to make better choices for a longer, healthier life. I am deeply indebted to all the people and professionals who gave me their time and knowledge.

First of all, my editors. Kristin Kiser, Editorial Director for Crown Publishers, has guided me through eleven books to date. As usual, her advice, enthusiasm, and steering of this project were superb. She never bugs me, just gently prods.

Maggie Greenwood Robinson, my editor, was excellent at shuffling this vast array of information. I am very grateful for your assistance.

Marsha Yanchuck, my assistant of thirty years, devoted excellent work to the resources and bibliography. Thank you for the hours spent putting this together for me, and for making sure I came off grammatically correct.

My new agent, David Vigliano: I look forward to years of working together.

Marc Chamlin (The Closer), my lawyer for the last eleven books—I couldn't get it going without you.

Sandi Mendelson, my publicist, has chosen to carry on under the most adverse conditions and continues to excel. I thank you and admire you.

Caroline Somers, my daughter-in-law and ace. After the book was written, it was Caroline who helped me write and hone the introduction.

Bruce Somers, my son, gave me his usual excellent insight in his interview on periandropause.

Thanks to Gloria, for her honesty; Wendy Fitzgerald, for her candor and appreciation of her new healthy life; and Larry G., for the remarkable turnaround in his health (and for the compliments).

And now, the doctors—each one of them amazing people doing the most incredible work to thwart the onslaught of the environment and the devastating and misunderstood passage of hormone loss.

Dr. Michael Galitzer, my doctor and friend, thanks for writing the foreword and for your dedication to health and wellness and energy.

Dr. Larry Webster continually supplied me with cutting-edge information and spent hours working on the glossary. I am deeply appreciative.

Thank you to Dr. Eugene Shippen, for his passion; Dr. Julie Taguchi, for her bravery; Dr. Marc Darrow, for his intelligence; Dr. Joe Filbeck, for his incredible work; Dr. Prudence Hall, for her dedication; Dr. Herb Slavin, for his savvy; Dr. Randy Randolph, for his caring; Dr. Erika Schwartz, for her insight; Dr. Daniela Paunesky, for her passion and sincerity; Dr. Philip Lee Miller, for his breakthrough work; Dr. Robert Greene, for his dedication and passion; Dr. Paul Savage, for his amazing comprehension; Dr. Gordon Reynolds, for his wisdom; Dr. Ron Rothenberg, for his cutting-edge understanding; and Dr. Peter Hanson, my friend and teacher.

Thanks to Julie Carmen, who has brought me into the beautiful world of yoga, and special thanks to Paul Schulick, master herbalist and dear friend.

Thank you to Jeff Katz and his team. What a cover! Every time we work together it gets better and better. I never thought you could top the last one, but you did. You know you are my favorite photographer.

And Jeff's team: Stuart Gow, Gabriel Hutchison, and Andrew Strauss.

A huge thank you to T. S. Wiley, who gave and gave and gave. It's been a crash course in molecular biology and a real eye-opener. The bonus is that along the way we became friends.

Special thanks to Dr. Joe Sugarman and Dr. Soram Khalsa.

Thanks to Julie Turkel in my office—you are the best. And to Lindsay Orman, Kristin Kiser's assistant.

And then there's Mooney . . . my darling friend and hairdresser and fellow health-crazed person. You are so special to me.

Barbara Farman, my makeup artist, who took a very tired Suzanne and put life back into her face.

Laurie Baer and Claire Harbo for your styling—it's always the perfect rose.

And Brently Lemons, my computer guy, for helping me make sense of Word.

My team at Crown, for the past thirteen books. What a fantastic group to work with. Most of all, I cherish the laughs we have had together along the way. This is an amazing relationship. You are all wonderful: Jenny Frost, President and Publisher; Steve Ross, Publisher; Philip Patrick, Director of Marketing; Tina Constable, Executive Director of Publicity; and Tammy Blake, Director of Publicity. And to the behind-the-scenes team, who have been with me on many books and are invaluable: Amy Boorstein, Managing Editor; Camille Smith, Production Editor; Leta Evanthes, Production Supervisor; Lauren Dong, Interior Designer; and Dan Rembert, Jacket Designer.

Thanks also to Sona Vogel, my fantastic copy editor, who has an awesome grasp of structure and flow.

And last but never least, thanks to my husband, Alan Hamel, who is supportive, enthusiastic, and a true visionary, who loves me and thinks I am wonderful. With that kind of support, I feel I am capable of anything. I love you with all my heart.

CONTENTS

Contents

THOUGHTS ON AGING

Do you realize that the only time in our lives when we like to get old is when we're kids? If you're less than ten years old, you're so excited about aging that you think in fractions.

How old are you? "I'm four and a half!" You're never thirty-six and a half. You're four and a half going on five! That's the key.

You get into your teens; now they can't hold you back. You jump to the next number or even a few weeks ahead.

How old are you? "I'm gonna be sixteen!" You could be thirteen, but hey, you're gonna be sixteen! And the greatest day of your life . . . you become twenty-one. Even the words sound like a ceremony: You **become** twenty-one. **Yessss!!**

But then you turn thirty. Oooohh, what happened there? Makes you sound like bad milk! He **turned;** we had to throw him out. There's no fun now; you're just a sour dumpling. What's wrong? What's changed?

You **become** twenty-one, you **turn** thirty, then you're **pushing** forty. Whoa! Put on the brakes. It's all slipping away. Before you know it, you **reach** fifty.

And your dreams are gone.

But wait!! You **make it** to sixty. You didn't think you would!

So you **become** twenty-one, **turn** thirty, **push** fifty, and **make it** to sixty.

You've built up so much speed that you **hit** seventy! After that, it's a day-by-day thing. You **hit** Wednesday!

You get into your eighties, and every day is a complete cycle. You **hit** lunch; you **get** to 4:30; you **reach** bedtime. And it doesn't end there. Into the nineties, you start going backward: "I was **just** ninety-two."

Then a strange thing happens. If you make it over one hundred, you become a little kid again. "I'm one hundred and a half!!"*

---

*Attributed to George Carlin, but when I called him he said the first half was written by Larry Miller and the second half is anonymous.

FOREWORD

GOD BLESS SUZANNE SOMERS. She is truly a health hero, one who wants the best for all of us. She writes and lectures with one thing in mind: How can I help people optimize their health, and thus their lives? If she were to write a short dialogue of what is possible in the area of antiaging medicine, it might look like this:

> **Attention, this is your brain. I have exciting news for your body. Muscle mass is up and much more active. Body fat is in the ideal zone. Stress is down. Energy is way up. Hormone levels indicate that you are thirty-five years old. I'll be turning up anabolic activity, sex drive, mental clarity, respiratory efficiency, energy production, and immunity. The guys in the mood department are working overtime, making a perfect balance of all four major neurotransmitters, guaranteed to convince you that you are young again.**

In 1982 I had the privilege to be among the first one hundred MDs in the United States to become board-certified in emergency medicine. In my fifteen years of ER medicine, I treated thousands of patients with pharmaceutical drugs that saved lives. But there is a big difference between acute critical care medicine and antiaging medicine. Why aren't we healthy? It's not the fault of orthodox medicine. Nor is it the fault of the pharmaceutical industry. Who is responsible for our health?

The story starts when Mommy got pregnant with Johnny. The doctor delivered Johnny. During the first day of Johnny's life, he had a vaccination, and he was seen by a pediatrician who performed a well-baby examination. Mommy periodically took Johnny to see his doctor for subsequent vaccinations to prevent him from getting certain childhood illnesses. Also, every time Johnny got sick, he went to the doctor to receive the necessary treatment to get better. As he got older, Johnny finally figured out that the doctor was responsible for his health; it wasn't his own responsibility.

Suzanne Somers wants you to take charge of your body, your nutrition, your fitness, and your need for detoxification. Suzanne wants you to understand what you need to eat to lower your insulin levels; what to take and how to exercise so that the cells of your body become more sensitive to insulin; when to ask your doctor for thyroid supplementation; how to determine that your adrenals are tired, and what you can do about it; and when to see a doctor for bio-identical estrogen, progesterone, and testosterone.

Orthodox medicine frequently views health as being the absence of disease. Antiaging medicine views optimal health as being physically, emotionally, mentally, and spiritually in flow, with the organs and hormonal glands functioning at maximal efficiency.

Antiaging medicine feels that disease is a condition precipitated by a toxin-filled, nutritionally deficient, and stress-dominated system, which will ultimately result in changes in enzyme production and hormone production. This will, in turn, gradually produce a biochemical change with attendant signs and symptoms. Suppressing symptoms and not removing their underlying cause will allow the embers of an illness to smolder quietly, only to erupt with increased intensity at a later date.

Orthodox medicine is based upon the treatment of symptoms, whereas antiaging medicine identifies the source of the symptoms and balances their energetic causes. Orthodox medicine analyzes illness on a physical and chemical level. Physical tests include physical examination, X-rays, mammograms, CAT scans, MRIs, and biopsies. Chemical evaluations involve the analysis of blood tests. If these tests are normal, then the patient is told that he is free of disease and is healthy. Orthodox medicine does very little analysis on the electrical or energetic level, except for the EKG, EEG, and EMG. It does not analyze the electrical liver, kidney, pancreas, adrenal glands, and so on. If one is angry, his ultrasound (physical) of the liver will be unaffected, and his liver function studies (chemical) will also be unaffected. But his electrical (energetic) liver is very much affected, resulting in symptoms such as insomnia and migraines. Just as the electrical QRS complex of an EKG precedes the physical heartbeat, the electrical (or energetic) changes in the organs always precede chemical and physical abnormalities.

Orthodox medicine continues to develop at a rapid rate, becoming ever more technical and specialized. Depending upon what type of headache you have, you may visit an internist who may, in turn, refer you to a neurologist, an ophthalmologist, or even a psychiatrist. In this traditional form of medicine, the different symptoms are viewed as different body parts being ill, but what if all these symptoms are interrelated? What if your headache, skin rash, constipation, stomach ulcer, insomnia, and muscle spasms are all symptoms of the same underlying problem? Most symptoms are the body's way of trying to get rid of toxins and regain homeostasis and balance. Therefore, most diseases should be treated not by suppressing your body's defense mechanisms, but by cooperating with these systems.

Antiaging medicine seeks to identify the root cause of one's symptoms, so if A causes B, instead of treating B (as does orthodox medicine), antiaging medicine will treat A. The ideal therapy for any condition is something that is effective and tolerated by your body. Most drugs are effective but are not well tolerated, causing side effects. Antiaging medicine addresses the cellular or energetic level long before deeper damage takes place and is, thus, truly preventive. The patient's progress can be measured by laboratory tests, clinical observation by the practitioner, and the patient's own feeling of well-being.

There are additional diagnostic tests that are utilized in antiaging medicine. Blood values must be in the optimal range, not the reference range. As an example, we like to see a TSH value (thyroid-stimulating hormone) of less than 2.0, which indicates a healthy thyroid gland, as opposed to the reference range of 0.0 to 5.0. Antiaging medicine measures additional fluids such as saliva and urine for hormone levels and products of metabolism and defines metabolism as the biochemical changes in the living cells by which energy is produced for vital processes and activities. Antiaging medicine utilizes unique tests such as bioimpedance to measure cellular health and integrity of cell membranes; heart rate variability to measure the responsiveness of the autonomic nervous system; and bioelectronic terrain, which measures pH, electron levels, and mineral levels in blood, urine, and saliva, in order to analyze the terrain of your body. This test, developed by the Germans in the early 1970s, was used by NASA to monitor Apollo series astronauts on flights to the moon.

Researchers have long known that one of the mechanisms involved in the aging process is the decline in naturally occurring hormones in the body, first manifesting in our thirties and then accelerating as we enter our fifties, sixties, and beyond. Since hormones affect virtually every bodily process, low levels of certain hormones and impaired communication within the endocrine system create havoc with all other body systems, including the immune, cardiovascular, detoxification, and gastrointestinal systems. Chronic illness is also frequently associated with the body's decline in hormone production. Recent research suggests that proper replacement of bioidentical hormones holds great promise in slowing the aging process, and as a treatment for age-related diseases.

Regulation, which is a cardinal feature of optimal health, is the ability of an organ or tissue to respond appropriately to a stimulus. The systems that have the most profound effect on regulation are the autonomic nervous system and the endocrine system. The autonomic nervous system functions rapidly, making adjustments within seconds. The endocrine system acts more slowly, its effects taking from minutes to hours to develop. Each system has an effect on the other. The main link between the nervous system and the endocrine system is the hypothalamus, a small gland in the brain that acts as the hormone control center. Messages from the brain are sent to the hypothalamus, which in turn releases hormonal messages to the pituitary gland, located just below the hypothalamus. The pituitary gland then produces hormones that stimulate target glands (such as adrenal, thyroid, and ovary) to secrete their hormones.

The word **hormone** means to arouse or excite. Hormones are chemical messengers that are usually secreted from endocrine glands into the bloodstream. Hormones then bind with appropriate receptors, which are selectively present in the cell membranes of their target organs (like a key and a lock), producing the desired effects on both the metabolism and function of the target organs. The most important hormones in antiaging are thyroid, DHEA, cortisol, insulin, growth hormone, testosterone, estrogen, and progesterone.

Nutritional deficiencies, lack of exercise, and exposure to toxins can all result in diminished hormone production and, ultimately, to diminished biological functioning. Chronic stress can also seriously impact hormone production. Other factors include malnutrition, sleep disorders, exposure to electromagnetic fields (EMFs), lack of sunlight, and the long-term use of over-the-counter and prescription medications.

A loss of hormonal balance, as occurs with aging, plays a large role in mental and emotional symptoms, and in all illness. **We age because our hormones decline; our hormones don't decline because we age.** The hormonal system is what most correlates to the emotional person. It is clear that the hormonal system responds to our outlook on the world. Restoration of this balance is ideally achieved through bio-identical hormone replacement therapy (BHRT).

Bioidentical estrogen and progesterone are bio-engineered from natural plant products and contain the exact same chemical structure as natural female sex hormones. They do not mimic female hormones, but instead augment a woman's natural hormone production. In contrast synthetic hormones are produced by altering the natural structure of the hormone in order to obtain a patent. This changes not only its structure but also its effect on the body. It's a chemical with a certain level of toxicity, which is indigenous to all chemicals. Premarin does not contain the same estrogen as that which naturally exists in the body. Premarin contains fifty different forms of estrogen, among which only three are known to occur naturally in humans.

"The times, they are a-changing." Embracing antiaging medicine requires a change in one's consciousness. Consciousness is the sum total of our feelings, thoughts, beliefs, attitudes, and intentions. You need to realize that brain cells can regenerate. It's all about energy, energy that can be both felt and measured. Life should not be defined by age, but by energy. Aging equates to disease. Energy equates to health.

The general state of our health is directly related to our consciousness. A change in our health, either for better or for worse, involves a change in our consciousness. Our bodies are constantly renewing themselves. Our consciousness and beliefs can affect the regeneration of cells and organs positively or negatively. The very cells that are causing distress or disease in our bodies are constantly replacing themselves—and the goal of antiaging medicine is to have those replacement cells be healthy ones.

A change in consciousness always involves a change in focus. What excites you? What are you grateful for? When we continually focus on purpose, passion, and gratitude, we feel whole and happy. Don't we all wish we could jump out of bed every morning with a lust and love for life? I bet Suzanne Somers does. See yourself as healthy and know that this healthy state of being is your natural state. Remember what Hippocrates said: "Let food be your medicine, and let medicine be your food."

So let me offer a few suggestions for an extended, happier, and healthier life. Do what you love; health and healing will follow. Surround yourself with people who make you feel good. Heal your relationship with your parents. Make fun and relaxation a daily priority. Learn to love yourself, really. Once you learn to forgive yourself, it's easy to forgive others. Remember that life is for-giving.

Your home is your sanctuary. Fill it with things that support and nurture you. Enjoy sex as a loving and sacred communion. Make decisions that give you the greatest peace of mind. Do the best that you can, and don't judge others. Connect with your source as often as you can. You may call it God, inner guides, love, higher self. Tap into it as often as possible, for it is a source of knowledge, inspiration, and guidance.

Treat the earth well. Get out into nature as often as possible. Once you decide that "out there" is your friend, everything else flows much more easily. Go barefoot in the damp grass for fifteen minutes at sunset or right before sleep to discharge the excess positive charge that builds up in the body as a result of stress. Walk the beach to inhale the energizing negative ions.

Antiaging medicine will definitely succeed despite the possible hostile attitude of some who will, in the end, be forced to reconsider. It is my sincere desire that the ideas contained here and in the rest of this wonderful book will help to unite medicine and create the level of health that is truly possible for all of us.

Michael Galitzer, MD

AGELESS

INTRODUCTION

So here's a new concept: Forget your age . . . and ask the question, How young is your energy?

It is now possible to recapture your youthful energy by taking advantage of today's "new medicine" that understands the limitations of drugs. As a society, we are not well. The way we are taking care of ourselves at present is not working. This book introduces you to the most forward approaches of maintaining quality of life without drugs. Don't you want to live a long, healthy life without illness and disability? Don't you want energy, youthful vitality, balanced hormones, and a fantastic sex life? Read on and you can have it.

You see, I don't want to "turn," "push," or "hit" anything. I've decided to get over thinking about any number relative to my age. I have embraced being "ageless."

I have always considered myself a healthy person—someone who ate right, exercised regularly in moderation, and had regular doctor's visits with good checkups. Sure, I would encounter the typical colds, flu, or sore throats of the season, particularly when I was very run-down after touring my act on the road, flying in and out of airports, and spending countless nights in hotel rooms. A trip to the doctor and a prescription for an antibiotic would knock out whatever was ailing me. At times I was worried that I was too sick to sing and perform so I would ask my doctor for the occasional cortisone shot. Not something you want to do frequently, but the show must go on. It got to be a vicious cycle—more infections, more antibiotics, more drugs.

Like most people, I defended my doctors. I believed in and trusted them. They knew what was best, and they were managing my care. I knew people who were seeing different types of doctors—doctors who used other methods. That wasn't for me. **My** doctors knew best. They treated lots of high-powered people in my industry and came highly recommended. I just needed to slow down and take better care of myself. Still, I had friends and family members who were concerned.

My son, Bruce, and his wife, Caroline, had been seeing an antiaging doctor, Dr. David R. Allen in Beverly Hills, California, for several years. Bruce and Caroline each took a handful of vitamins morning and evening. I felt it was overkill, bogus, too "granola" for me; they probably just peed it all out anyway. It didn't seem like "real medicine." Nonetheless, they kept trying to convince me to give this type of medicine a try, because supposedly it could build my immune system and make me stronger. My son's allergies had gone away, and his wife had stopped being so susceptible to colds and flu. Even so, I was resistant. I had my routine. I had a relationship with my doctor. He knew my history. He knew what was best for me. Looking back, I now ask myself: What is it about our human nature that we feel the need to defend the choices we've made when it comes to our medical treatment? Without a basis for comparison, how do we know we have the **best** doctors? How do we know we are getting the **best** treatment? How do we know we are giving ourselves the **best** shot at a healthy future?

Then something serendipitous happened. During one of my cycles of being on antibiotics, my trusted ear, nose, and throat doctor was unavailable, so I was referred to another physician, Dr. Sugarman, who wisely offered to send me to a specialist rather than give me another antibiotic. Dr. Sugarman wanted me to talk to a doctor who would treat me by building up my immune system rather than tearing it down with a drug. So he sent me to Dr. Soram Khalsa in Beverly Hills, a Western-trained internist who specializes in preventing illness by treating the cause rather than the symptoms of illness. In fact, he practices medicine in a similar fashion to that of my grown children's antiaging doctor, Dr. Allen. This was my introduction to a whole new world of medicine that would change the course of my life and my health forever. I had come full circle. To this day, I thank Dr. Sugarman for sending me in another direction, and I thank Dr. Khalsa for guiding me through this new medicine. Both doctors realized I was on an unhealthy cycle that needed to be stopped.

For the last decade, I have become immersed in antiaging medicine. Dr. Michael Galitzer, who wrote the foreword for this book, has introduced me to new ways of restoring my youthful energy, strengthening my weakest organs and glands, and bringing hormonal function to perfect balance, among other measures. Antiaging medicine is exciting. I had no idea there were Western-trained doctors—not quacks—who play such an important role in today's health care and who are there to help us live up to our body's ageless potential. These are real doctors who share a different philosophy on how to treat patients to **stay** healthy by dealing with the **cause** of the problem rather than treating the symptoms of illness.

The better I felt, the more passionate I became about researching this branch of medicine. I found there were hundreds of doctors and books sharing the same philosophy. It's about building the immune system, maintaining balance, and increasing your chances for a long and healthy life. It didn't take me long to get on the road to health. Antibiotics are a thing of the past for me. It's the rare case that I have needed one in the last ten years. Today, my treatment is a regimen of vitamins, herbs, and supplements that have completely turned my health around. I know what you're thinking—sounds too "granola," right?

It's not as though I walk into a vitamin store and randomly grab things off the shelf. I am taking supplements based upon my blood work. After my blood is drawn and analyzed, my doctor shows me where the optimal range should be for a variety of vitamins and minerals. If my panel shows I am low in iron, my doctor will prescribe iron to get me within optimal range. If my calcium is low, he'll put me on calcium supplements to make sure my bones are strong and healthy. This is not guesswork. It's all in the blood work, which doesn't lie.

My colds and flu have become a thing of the past. Even with my high-stress lifestyle, I find I am warding off illness and have more energy than ever before. I'm constantly amazed . . . how can I be getting older when I am feeling better than I did in my thirties? How could my hormone and nutrient levels be higher now than they were when I was younger? By following this new regimen, I am combating stress (which breaks down the immune system, the body's built-in defense for staying healthy and strong), avoiding environmental toxins and prescription drugs as much as I can, and following a healthy lifestyle of eating amazing meals made with organic foods, which taste so much better. I have also discovered yoga, which has reshaped my body and calmed me down, and finally, I truly understand the importance of sleep.

By adding back to my system what stress and toxins have depleted, I am reversing the aging process by making myself younger on the inside. I am staving off disease so that even while growing older chronologically, I am restoring and preserving internal youth and energy. The number of my age has become irrelevant. It's about having young energy. I have it . . . you can, too!

Ageless, that's the promise. We have a number of years for our age, but our internal organs, physiology, and hormones also have an age—and that age does not have to equal the number of years we've been alive. What could be better than having your doctor tell you your bones are those of a twenty-year-old? What could be better than having a doctor tell you your heart is that of a thirty-year-old? What could be better than having a doctor tell you your brain is as youthful as that of a twenty-five-year-old? What could be better than having youthful energy all day long?

This new approach to medicine as outlined in this book can do this for you. You go to the doctor when you are **well!** In doing so, you rebuild your system to reverse the normal process of aging. You can stay strong, healthy, and vital, with youthful energy and excitement to greet each day.

If this new medicine is so wonderful, why aren't more people practicing it? Why aren't more of us going to these Western-trained doctors? Why aren't more of us reading the books put out by these specialists? Why aren't we taking control of our health? One reason is that we live in a world that supports conventional medicine. Our medical schools predominantly teach conventional medicine. We see hundreds and hundreds of advertisements for prescription drugs to treat every ailment, from depression to sexual dysfunction to heart disease. I am not anti–conventional medicine. It has its place and its purpose. I want conventional medicine for the times when drugs are called for, as in situations where there is pain or infection or mental illness. For me, it's a backup. My first course of action is to keep myself healthy.

The purpose of this book is for myself, and the doctors whom I've interviewed, to act as a conduit for you to this new approach to medicine. I am here to do for you what Dr. Sugarman and other doctors did for me. I am here to invite you to investigate a branch of Western medicine that wants to treat you to be healthy—not to wait until you are too sick to provide treatment. I am writing this book to use my voice to open a door for you. You will find that these new doctors are not practicing voodoo, it's not hippie treatment, it's not "granola"—it's cutting-edge. It's modern medicine and ancient forms of treatment all in one. It's the key to the fountain of youth for internal health and external beauty.

This book also examines menopause in depth. Menopause is a crisis passage for most women and we are at our wits' end trying to find doctors who "get it." When menopause arrived in my life it hit me like a Mack truck! Why didn't someone warn me? As

I went from doctor to doctor, I realized I was on my own. No doctor seemed to understand this passage. I knew I did not want conventional treatment. I did not want to take what was being offered to me: prescription synthetic so-called hormone drugs to alleviate my hot flashes and a general decline in my quality of life. I wanted a natural, effective way to deal with this passage; I wanted menopause to be a positive experience. I mean, there's no avoiding it, so how could I find a way to enjoy this inevitable passage? I knew eating wild yams and taking black cohosh was not the answer, and then I found the solution—a cutting-edge endocrinologist/antiaging doctor, who prescribed a treatment of bioidentical hormones. Wow! What a difference in my life. I was sleeping again. I was happy again. I stopped itching, and bitching, and crying, and, best of all, getting fat. This became and remains a huge passion for me: to let women know there is a safe, effective, and glorious treatment that is not based on drugs. I can't say enough about it. This is the best I have ever felt in my whole life; by taking bioidentical hormones in perfect balance individualized just for me, I believe I am, for the first time **ever,** hormonally balanced and I am loving this passage of menopause. I wake up every day feeling glorious and frisky. You can have this.

I detailed menopause in my book **The Sexy Years.** This book goes further. More and more doctors are "getting it," and I have found them for you. As with every new science, the information keeps growing.

The purpose of this book is to take you beyond **The Sexy Years.** Bioidentical hormone replacement is the **only** answer to ward off illness, weight gain, and other symptoms associated with hormonal decline. We have come to expect that getting fat and listless is part of aging and there is nothing that can be done about it. Not so; with bioidentical hormone replacement you can regain youthful energy, a youthful body, and your youthful sex drive. You get to feel good again and have clear thinking . . . good-bye to "senior moments." Gratefully I am no longer forgetful, and I can sleep through the nights beautifully without drugs. That is a blessing in itself. Women all over the globe are padding around their houses at night because without hormones you cannot sleep, period! It is impossible. You can't function without sleep, which puts your days out of whack. With balanced hormones the symptoms go away. Your skin won't itch any longer, and your mood is downright cheerful. Balanced, bioidentical hormones are the key. You must replace your declining hormones with **real hormones,** not synthetic drugs created by pharmaceutical companies.

If bioidentical hormones are the answer, why aren't the pharmaceutical companies selling them in individualized doses? Because bioidenticals are a natural substance and cannot be patented; therefore, there is no money to be made from selling the best solution for menopausal women. Instead, our doctors recommend drugs that are pharmaceuticalized from a pregnant mare's urine, even though the testing on these so-called hormones in the Women's Health Initiative study of 2002 showed such dangers to women that the study was called off prematurely to protect the participants! Yet as I write, these harmful drugs are still on the market and are widely prescribed! It boggles the mind.

Ageless is the next level of understanding on the hormone front. Hormones are our life force; the decline of hormones is the hallmark of aging. Now you can "put back" these life-giving hormones by working with a qualified doctor. As hormone production sags, the body begins to slow down in its rejuvenation and repair of tissues and organs; that's when resistance to disease begins and aging accelerates. In fact, the level of hormones in your body is one of the most telling biomarkers of aging.

In this book you will learn the importance of achieving hormonal balance beyond our sex hormones, estrogen, progesterone, and testosterone. This is such exciting medicine. Through hormone replacement and new antiaging measures, you can actually slow down and in some cases reverse the aging process. I know this because I have reversed bone loss along with so many other great advantages of BHRT. I have embraced this medicine because I see and feel results, and I can tell you that I have never felt stronger, healthier, or more vital than I do today.

I believe it is possible to experience aging without illness, which is the big dream for all of us. We don't fear getting older; we fear getting sick, really sick. In today's world, the majority of older and aging people are suffering from one or more of the three major killers—cancer, heart disease, and Alzheimer's—and we have come to accept this as normal: Older people get sick; that's just the way it is. As a young society, we have not realized the full impact of our bad lifestyle and dietary habits. We truly do not realize the aging effects of the chemicals that are part of our everyday world: trans fats, hydrogenated oils, birth control pills, synthetic drugs, recreational drugs, environmental pollution, plastics, and more. If a food or drug is FDA approved, we feel it is safe, but the ramifications of chemical buildup in our systems are killing us. We nonchalantly down our over-the-counter drugs as though they are harmless. We socialize in smoke-filled rooms without thought to the deadly consequences to our precious lungs. We spray our homes and offices with poisons to get rid of pests, not understanding the damage being done to our livers.

The environment and our unhealthy lifestyles have certainly taken their toll on all of us, but with a few simple changes in the way you approach your health and lifestyle, you can expect a longer and healthier quality of life. Wouldn't you want that?

Bioidentical hormone replacement is a big part of this change. Nutrition and lifestyle habits are the others. It's important to understand the dangers of our habits and the changes we need to make to undo this damage in order to enjoy good health and longevity. It requires understanding that as we live longer, it is up to each one of us to make changes in the way we approach our health to have quality of life, a better life, a disease-free life. The fountain of youth exists; that secret elixir we've been looking for is available if you are willing to make some simple life changes. It is about stopping the clock, and it's the new way.

I have interviewed the most forward-thinking doctors in America so you can have a "one-on-one office visit" with them through the pages of this book. I have asked the questions I believe we all would like answered. The doctors in this book are cutting-edge and Western-trained physicians. They have come to realize that as the sickest people on the planet (right here in the United States), we have been handling our declining years in ways that are not working. By restoring your hormones to optimal youthful levels, by strengthening the weakest organs and glands, by restoring your energy, you can be rejuvenated inside and out. The antiaging benefits of hormone replacement are rapid and dramatic. Most people I have spoken with regarding bioidentical hormone replacement regimens say they "wouldn't dream of going back to the way they used to feel."

What you will learn about hormones and health from these medical professionals is life-changing. I'm talking about minor hormones, which are key to our well-being: estrogen, progesterone, testosterone,

DHEA, and others. You'll also understand the crucial importance of strengthening your major hormones: adrenaline, thyroid, insulin, cortisol, and others. You'll see that this new medicine these doctors are practicing works to build up our biochemicals and strengthen our weakest organs and glands.

You will learn about the importance of detoxification to rid our bodies of chemicals and heavy metals from the air and water we drink. This information will help you to understand the importance of having a strong, clean liver, which is the clearinghouse of the body. With a healthy liver, you get the full effect of the nutrients from the food, hormones, and supplements you take. You will realize more than ever before the crucial role diet plays in health. Once you really get this, you will think twice before you eat that preservative, chemical-filled nonfood you have grown so accustomed to tasting. Nutrition is crucial to antiaging. There is no hormone or pill that will be able to reverse bad eating habits and an unhealthy lifestyle. This is a total program. You can be the winner. The more you put into it, the better the outcome.

This is fantastic new Western medicine, but unfortunately the medical establishment (including our medical schools) is slow to jump on this new, fast-moving train. That is why I have gathered together these doctors for you. Most likely there is not a doctor like these doctors in your community . . . yet. It is worth a trip to another city to be a patient of one of these fine professionals, because after an initial visit, most of the follow-up you will be doing with him or her will be through blood work and phone calls.

You can't imagine the change one of these doctors can make in your life. But you must remember this: It is up to you to be an informed patient. This book will give you that information. You must know your stuff, and you must have questions ready that you want answered when you are with your doctor. We are living in a new and changed world; we **are** on our own. Your beloved doctor, whom you have been seeing all your life, can still be your doctor, but if you want to be internally young and healthy, it is important to read every interview in this book and truly grasp what these cutting-edge doctors are teaching. If any one of these physicians appeals to you, look up his or her information at the back of this book and try to schedule an appointment. I have asked all of these doctors that if they cannot see you to please recommend another doctor like themselves who can.

I believe in the near future the mainstream medical establishment will catch up. I am seeing evidence of it. It takes curiosity and a release of ego on the part of a doctor to admit that possibly there is a better way. Fortunately, all over the country doctors are realizing that Western medicine's "standard of care" has for the most part become inadequate and outdated relative to our daily modern lives. We live in a different world. The medical protocols of fifty years ago no longer apply; we did not have the stresses, the pollution, or the technology of today.

Yet sadly (for the most part) the medical establishment has neither been taught nor understands the major health improvements and quality of life that can result from bioidentical (natural) hormone replacement. Today's world is a pharmaceutical society. We have an ailment, we go to our doctor and he or she gives us a drug. But we are part of the problem. We want a prescription when we go to the doctor's office, or else we don't feel we got our money's worth. Did you know in parts of Asia, the only time you pay your doctor is when you are well? If you get sick, it means the doctor did not do his or her job, and there is no charge for the treatment.

As a rule, drugs don't heal; they simply abate. Yet often we are put on certain drugs for life. Drugs make us feel better; and, of course, it's important not to abuse prescription drugs—they have their purpose and are godsends for pain, infection, and mental illness. These conditions are legitimate reasons to take drugs. I would not want to live in a world without pharmaceuticals. But each drug has its consequence. Often we need to take another drug to eliminate the consequence of the last drug, and so on and so on.

Up until now, aging has been a downhill process. Even our doctors tell us gently, "Well, what do you expect? You're getting older, these things happen." I'm here to tell you, "Not so!"

This new medicine substantially slows down or reverses the aging process. You don't have to die sick! It is possible to live a long life with good health, but you have got to start now. The earlier you embrace this type of medicine, the easier time you will have of it. Aging is happening earlier and earlier. Young men and women are experiencing hormonal loss in their twenties, thirties, and forties owing to environmental pollution and stress. This coming generation will be in poorer health than the present one, and that is hard to believe. Did you know that we are the sickest nation on the planet? Women of my generation in this country are ill from years of excessive chemicalization. Wait until you read about the consequences of the high-dose birth control pills we were given and how they are now thought to be connected with the skyrocketing rate of breast cancer. We have been chemicalized for decades, but we now have the opportunity to reverse the damage that has unknowingly been done to us.

It is never too early and it's never too late for women and men of all ages; I did not start this process until I reached my fifties, but at this time I have substantially reversed the aging process in my body. Hey, it's true, cells die. There is nothing any of us can do about that. Even so, the possibility of keeping these cells healthy and restoring vitality, vigor, sexuality, and creative thinking is pretty exciting.

Until now, women in their seventies and eighties

have felt that once they are on the other side of menopause, there is nothing that can be done. They accept their weak hearts, high blood pressure, diabetes, osteoporosis, dementia, inertia, and total loss of a sex drive as part of the deal. Their doctors have told them so. These women have bodies that have adjusted to their hormonal loss, and because they are no longer suffering from the most obvious symptoms, they think they are okay. Because these women are no longer plagued with hot flashes, they don't realize that internally they are experiencing complete body failure due to hormonal decline. That's why we get sick as we age. Hormones have a powerful influence on your body and on how you look and feel. They are the body's way of communicating chemically among the cells, effectively telling them what to do. Your hormones affect virtually every function in your body. Without hormones you cannot sleep, you can't think clearly, your health deteriorates, your weight goes out of control, your sexuality diminishes, your skin gets sallow and dry, your hair loses its luster, your eyesight diminishes, your body temperature becomes impossible to regulate, and on and on and on. Without hormones you slowly die, and the picture is not pretty. As a society, we have accepted sleeplessness at night as part of aging. We have accepted dry skin, thinning hair, wrinkling, bone loss, foggy thinking, heart problems, and cancer as normal when we get older. In essence, hormones affect everything we do. From the minute we are born, our hormones play a major role in how we grow, age, and die.

But guess what? The second half of your life can be better than your first half. A better life, a healthier life, a life of youthful energy, comes from embracing this new medicine, and bioidentical hormone replacement is a big component. Remember, I'm not talking about the dangerous synthetic hormones, which I will discuss at length in this book.

The second half of life can be wonderful. I know it because I am living it. This new approach to health gives you back your lean body, shining hair, and thick skin, provided you are eating correctly and exercising in moderation. This new medicine allows your brain to work perfectly and offers the greatest defense against cancer, heart attack, and Alzheimer's disease. Don't you want that?

Life is supposed to be enjoyed. This book is about accepting the coming years, but without sickness. Why should you care? you ask. After all, we live, we get old, we get sick, and then we die, right? What's the big deal? It's been going on forever. Aging is just something that happens to all of us, right? Well, now there are two ways to age—the old way and the new way.

The old way is obvious, and it is clear that it is not working. We don't need to have a virtual pharmacy in our medicine cabinets to keep us hanging on to life. What kind of life is it if you are living in a wheelchair with tubes up your nose? What kind of life is it if you can't remember anything because of severe hormonal loss? What kind of life is it if you are riddled with heart disease, PMS, osteoporosis, thyroid disease, sexual dysfunction, a heart that no longer works, a brain that has become foggy, or one of the many cancers that most of us can expect to have at some point?

Recently, I was talking with a physician about the alarming statistics relative to breast cancer. Those statistics have recently been readjusted and show that one woman in eight will contract this disease. She said most women feel it is not a matter of "if" but "when" a woman would get this dreaded disease. That's a pretty sad statement—indicating that women are starting to think that this disease is inevitable, and with good reason. Did you know that at the turn of the century, the statistics were that one in ninety-one females would get breast cancer? What has changed?

First, we are living longer, the environment is wreaking havoc on our health, and our lifestyle habits are bad. Most people know that you don't put inferior product into the gas tank or engine of your car. Why don't we realize the damage we incur from the chemicals, drugs, trans fats, and other poisons we are putting into our bodies? What are we thinking? Everything we put into our bodies is some sort of fuel. Would you willingly put the cheapest inferior fuel into your body if you realized that the results of this poor product you are feeding yourself is the reason you are in such bad health? I am not talking just about junk food and sugar, I am also referring to the chemicals, drugs, and the poisons that are part of our everyday lives.

As a result, new diseases are cropping up everywhere. Who heard of lupus thirty years ago? Now just about everyone you talk with knows someone with lupus (an autoimmune disease). There are now strange skin conditions, such as flesh-eating disease, and diseases due to bad lifestyle and eating habits. How long is it going to take us to understand that our bodies need better care? For the most part, most of us do take better care of our cars than we do ourselves!

The new approach to health and aging is to balance our lost hormones with bioidentical hormones, strengthen our major hormones, and detoxify our livers and glands from the outside environmental pollution that is making us sick. Eliminating stress, valuing a good night's sleep, and supplementation with vitamins and herbs to make up for the lost nutrients in our food due to acid rain, chemicals, and overworked soil are also important components of antiaging.

Once you embrace this new approach, you won't believe how great you can feel when the symphony of a well-working body is in concert. Your body should sing. Yet most of us live in internal discordance. We don't have our priorities straight. We live in an environment of constant stress, and we medicate ourselves with sleeping pills and antidepressants to make us feel well enough to carry on our sorry existences.

You don't want to die sick, do you? You don't want to get fat, shrink, lose your energy, your sex drive, and your brain, or contract any of the diseases that seem to be part and parcel of aging, right? You don't want to end up with bones too feeble to hold up your body. You don't want to walk around with an oxygen tank attached permanently to your back because of the choices you made as a young adult. Nor do you want to contract one of the new mystery diseases like antitrypsin deficiency, an incurable emphysemalike condition that is fatal, which is caused by unknowingly breathing in chemicals that are in the environment. I just lost my literary agent to that one. You don't want to lose your energy, lose your sexuality, or be put out to pasture by your family much the same way they do old horses because you are in the beginning or advanced stages of Alzheimer's, do you?

Your best defense to prevent this from happening is to take charge of your health **now!** This gradual decline we all will experience is preventable for the most part by making a few simple changes in the way we take care of ourselves.

This book will help you become internally young, healthy, and energetic. This book will help you achieve agelessness on the outside with vibrant beauty. Here is what to expect.

Part 1—**Keeping Your Insides "Young"**—you will learn about all the hormones that are key to your well-being. You will learn what happens with decline in each transition of your life, from perimenopause (one of the most misunderstood passages) to menopause and beyond.

You will learn how to achieve hormonal balance. You want the right amount—not too much, not too little. You don't want the hormone levels that are normal for a person your age—a person your age is in hormonal decline. The goal is a more youthful body, inside and out!

You will learn about various life transitions, including the dangers of perimenopause and what can be done about it. Perimenopause is generally not understood by the women going through it, nor is it understood by the doctors who are treating them. Perimenopause is a dangerous passage, and this book will explain why. This is very important information. This is life-changing information.

Part 2—**Men and Their Hormones**—turns our attention to men and the antiaging issues they face. Men are the biggest offenders in terms of disregarding the importance of putting back lost hormones. Somehow they think it's not macho. Those who do understand get to live a long, healthy, vital life. Lost hormones are not only the domain of women. Men, and those who love them, are going to find this section and its interviews fascinating.

In part 3—**The Three S's: Sex, Sleep, and**

Stress—you will learn how to restore your sexuality, how to sleep better through hormonal balance, and the importance of sleep in restoring your healing hormones. You will also learn how to assess what stress is doing to your life and ways you can get back the youthful energy you once had.

In part 4—**Detoxification and the Effects of the Environment on Your Health**—you will see how exposure to environmental chemicals and other poisons leads to premature aging—and what to do about it. Chemicals and toxins can come from a multitude of places: mercury in our food supply and our teeth, chemicals inside our homes and offices, poisons in the air, polluted water, and "pesticide enriched" foods.

In part 5—**Ageless Living**—we will look into simple, doable lifestyle changes, from nutrition to supplementation to exercise, that will begin reversing the aging process. This information will give you an edge relative to health and beauty. If you keep yourself young on the inside, it will manifest on the outside.

Being ageless takes a little work. There is no free lunch, but the rewards of this outweigh all the money in the world. You don't need to be rich to take advantage of this new information, either. So get an edge. Stay young and healthy while you age. Learn from these doctors. This can be the best phase of your life!

I embrace bioidentical hormone replacement and

antiaging medicine. I gladly take my supplements, vitamins, herbs, hormones, human growth hormone injections, and vitamin B injections, and follow a healthy lifestyle and diet. I embrace my exercise and yoga programs. I take my new doctors seriously, and I work **with** them. This is true integrated medicine. I have never felt better or been happier in my life. I love my age. I don't dread my next birthday, because I feel great on the outside and inside. Good health brings joy, balanced hormones bring joy, a well-running body brings joy, and emotional health brings joy.

This book holds within it the medical answers to fight the damage we have done to our planet that is affecting each one of us personally. This book gives you the key to unlock the answer to the ravages of aging that we are seeing all around us.

I want to live a long and healthy life and die healthy. What about you? You are never too young to start. So if you are between the ages of twenty and a hundred, man or woman, this book is for you. Enjoy.

CHAPTER 1

TAKING CHARGE OF
YOUR OWN HEALTH

To remain oblivious to the hidden
regenerative processes inside your body
will cause you to die unnecessarily
young.

Ray Kurzweil and Terry Grossman, MD,
–Fantastic Voyage

Five years have passed, and as of this writing I have now been happily pronounced cancer-free. What a relief. No longer does each ache and pain trigger a fear in me of "Oh God, is that 'it' coming back again?"

Cancer does that to you. It's an inner nagging, a constant reminder that there could be something bigger than yourself lurking out there in the shadows, sitting back, like a predator, deciding when and if it cares to strike again. Now, finally, I can release that fear. The predator has been locked up, in prison, hopefully never to be let out again.

Along the way in this war I have been fighting have come the blessings. I am truly loved by those who mean the most to me. They showed me this over and over during this time. Through it all, I learned about my own strength and courage. I didn't know I had it in me to buck the system by choosing unconventional therapies and doing it my way. But you see, I was never able to wrap my arms around the "standard of care" set forth by Western medicine as the way to treat cancer.

When I was diagnosed with cancer, I needed to be emotionally strong to fight the battle. To help with that, I needed to be hormonally in balance. It is hard to be in a fighting mood when you are hormonally depressed. Balanced hormones keep your emotions in check and I believe (based upon my research) are the most effective way to prevent cell proliferation (cancer). Unfortunately, Western medicine's "standard of care" believes that taking away all hormones prevents disease. I believed differently, so I didn't want to go off my bioidentical hormones.

Nor did I want to undergo chemotherapy. You see, I do not believe in the "poison" theory of using chemotherapy. It is my belief that an environment of balanced hormones prevents disease. This is reinforced by many of the doctors interviewed in this book. For one thing, it ablates, or takes away, hormones. Chemotherapy does kill cancer cells, but it also kills the immune system. Without a strong immune system, cancer has a perfect opportunity to recur. We need a strong immune system and balanced hormones to prevent disease. So it didn't make sense to me to "take away" hormones as a means to kill cancer.

As I now see it, there are two ways to fight cancer: build up or destroy. Western medicine's standard of care is to destroy. Well-meaning though it may be, the idea of chemicalizing myself, destroying everything, and hoping my health would come back, coupled with the instructions to give up my hormone therapy, was not appealing.

I decided to approach cancer by "building up." This took courage, because it is daunting to go against the course recommended by one's doctor. But because of the books I write and my understanding of the hormonal connection to health, I had a lot of information. I understood that hormonal balance is key to health and vitality. My decision to go against the standard of care was probably easier for me than it would be for other women not armed with the same information. I approached my cancer through balanced bioidentical hormone replacement and complemented this replacement with Iscador, an anthroposophic medicine whose function is to strengthen and build **up** the immune system so that disease cannot attack and invade.

I believe this was the best decision of my life. Aside from the discomfort of injecting myself with Iscador every other day for these five years, my health has never been better. I have not had so much as a cold during this time; upon my last checkup, my immune system was so high that my doctor was ecstatic. He said he had never seen an immune system this strong in any of his adult patients. That information was able to put all my fears to rest. How could a life-threatening illness get past an immune system this strong? Great. I had done it. I beat it. I did it my way, with my body almost intact.

So you can imagine my surprise (five years and one month after my initial diagnosis) when my gynecologist told me that I had a **pre**-precancerous condition (not cancer, not even precancer) growing in my uterus and that in order to prevent possible severe problems down the road, I would need to have my uterus removed.

Why was the sleeping giant trying to rear its ugly head again? Luckily we caught this before it became cancer, yet it was serious enough to force the removal of an organ. I do not take the removal of any body part lightly. What was wrong? I have thought about this a lot. As a teenage mother, I was given my first major chemical, a shot to dry up my milk, and was encouraged to feed my baby Similac formula. In chapter 5 I will discuss at length the protective aspects of breast-feeding and prolactin production. Second, at age eighteen I was put on the early high-dose birth control pills and stayed on them for twenty-two years. Unknowingly, like so many women of my generation, these chemicals put me into a false menopause. All those years of chemicalization were dangerous to my health. Add to this scenario stress and environmental assault and a brutal childhood and you have a recipe for disaster.

The ninth year of bioidentical hormone replacement, things started going wonky. I had breakthrough bleeding, and then after a while I was bleeding continuously. Something was wrong, obviously.

Because I was bleeding constantly, I was not ovulating. Thus I was not a reproductive person (according to my brain). The object of bioidentical hormone replacement therapy is to fool the body into thinking I can still make a baby, even though I have no eggs left. Bleeding, severe hyperplasia, and adenomyosis (leaks in my uterine lining) made my quality of life unbearable. This excessive bleeding and hyperplasia created a perfect scenario for cancer, so I had no choice but to remove my uterus, thus removing my problem.

Maybe if I had not been chemicalized by the "dry-up" shot and if I had not been on strong birth control pills for so many years, this problem might not have occurred. Several of the doctors I interviewed for this book have also embraced this theory.

Losing my uterus caused me to do a lot of searching. For years, I was unknowingly hormonally imbalanced, not just as a perimenopausal and menopausal woman, but also as a young woman. Unfortunately, I never realized hormonal imbalance was the problem.

Without hormones or imbalanced hormones, we lose any grip on feeling "normal." Without hormones life quality is greatly diminished. Without hormones a woman is at her weakest physically. Without hormones disease can proliferate because the brain perceives the body as no longer reproductive; therefore, nature wants to "eliminate" you to make way for those who are healthy and reproductive.

Loss of hormones is not to be taken lightly. Having no hormones is like having bad premenstrual syndrome (PMS) every day of your life. You are not in control of your emotions, nor are you in control of the cruel physical manifestations of the loss of hormones. Couple this with the stress of having and fighting cancer, and (to me) it doesn't make sense to be without hormones.

According to T. S. Wiley, "We may have changed with the passing of time, but the biology inside us has not. Nature has a job to do, and the brain was hardwired at the begining of time and doesn't know anything else." A healthy woman is hormonally balanced. We can't "outthink" nature. This never works, no matter how hard we try to come up with something better.

Women remain confused about hormones and in some cases terrified of hormone replacement; one day, headlines in the newspapers praise hormone replacement therapy (HRT); the next day, the headlines are screaming that HRT will kill us.

The truth is, despite the widespread use of synthetic hormone brands such as Premarin, Provera, and Prempro these drugs have always been associated with cancer. The first cancer linked with synthetic hormone replacement was cancer of the uterus lining (endometrium).

The most recent resurfacing of the negatives associated with synthetic hormones and cancer came from a government-sponsored study titled the Women's Health Initiative. This study was supposed to last 8.5 years, but it was stopped after only 5.2 years because the risks of using synthetic hormones outweighed the benefits. Breast cancer was just one of the increased risks discovered. Additionally, the study concluded that synthetic hormone replacement therapy protects neither your bones nor your heart. Ironically, bone and heart protection were two of the primary benefits once used by doctors as selling points to get women to fill their prescriptions for these drugs.

The Women's Health Initiative study hoped to show decreases in

- breast cancer
- stroke
- pulmonary embolism
- colorectal cancer
- endometrial cancer
- hip fracture
- death due to any cause

The actual outcome results were shocking:

- 29 percent increase in coronary heart disease
- 41 percent increase in strokes
- 22 percent increase in cardiovascular disease
- 2,100 percent (yes, this is correct) increase in pulmonary embolism (lung blood clots)
- 26 percent increase in breast cancer

So much for synthetic hormones! These statistics alone should convince you right away of the negative effects of synthetic hormones.

Those of us who were on the original birth control pills for any length of time were actually on synthetic hormones—strong synthetic hormones. Any wonder why women of our generation are under siege from an epidemic of breast and ovarian cancers? There is a link, and you'll learn more about it in this book.

See if you relate to my scenario. For twenty-two years, I was on synthetic birth control pills, the original ones that were very strong. I even manipulated my periods with them, if I didn't want to have a period on a particular weekend. Because of this I hold no one to blame—we just didn't know. I also didn't realize what was in those birth control pills, nor did I understand the dangers of messing with nature.

I did not realize that having only a two-day bleed meant that I was not ovulating fully. At the time, I thought it was great to have such a light period. I did not realize that the importance of ovulation in the human female body is to let the brain know I was well, healthy, and reproductive. As far as my brain was concerned, I was not reproductive because I was not fully ovulating, which is a dangerous assumption for the brain to make. If the brain perceives us as unable to reproduce, its job, biologically speaking, is to try to eliminate us to make room for the reproductive ones. This is the **nature** in us. This is the template that was programmed in us from ancient times. This hormonal imbalance I unknowingly put myself in was creating a backdrop for cancer. We all have cancer in us; if we become hormonally **imbalanced,** this signals to the brain that the reproductive system is no longer in working order, and it is in this scenario that the cancer has a chance to come into being.

This is why I believe that Western medicine's standard of care, well-meaning as it is, is treating us incorrectly. It needs updating. Western medicine is looking at everything except the obvious. Western medicine is trying to poison the cancer out of us, further wreaking havoc with our hormonal systems.

Then, to prevent recurrence, we are given hormone targeting drugs such as tamoxifen or Femara, which interfere with the body's ability to read the hormones in some parts of the body. Plus, for many women these drugs cause horrible side effects. To me, it doesn't make sense to take any drug that prevents new hormones from being made in our bodies or to kill off any of the little bit of hormones we might have left. Why has Western medicine been trying to outthink nature? We are given fake hormones that don't replicate exactly what our bodies make naturally, and doctors are expecting them to work in the same way or better. It hasn't worked. Look around. Are the women you know doing well from midlife on? Most everyone has complaints, from mild to severe. No wonder women are in such bad shape.

Once you understand the importance of your brain perceiving the body as reproductive, it will be easier for you to make decisions for yourself. We assume that the professionals who are taking care of us know what they are doing. But they can't know what they haven't been taught, and unless you find yourself a doctor such as the ones I have found for you in this book, you could very well be brought down a path of no return. Remember, your doctor is doing his or her best. This is what they know at the moment, so you can't hold it against them. However, no one is ever going to care about you as much as you care about yourself—so it is up to you to do the research. I will tell you this again and again in this book: You are on your own. When it comes to breast cancer, I believe the answer has been in front of our noses all along. **Just replicate nature!**

That's what bioidentical hormone replacement does. If technology hadn't figured out how to keep us alive longer than human beings have ever lived in the history of mankind, this would not be an issue. But we will live long, long lives. Without hormone replacement, we will end up mere shells of our former selves. There is no quality of life without hormones for men, women, or children.

Thinking back, I realize the birth control pill brought us freedoms and put off childbirth and breast-feeding but harmed us in the process. We did not even realize the importance of breast-feeding. We did not know that lactation builds not only our immune systems, but also that of our babies, and that the more children we have, the longer we breast-feed, the stronger our immune system will be. In most cases, this natural part of giving birth and raising children sets us up for life to protect us against disease. But the acts of delaying childbirth and breast-feeding or, worse, negating breast-feeding chemically with the dry-up shot, coupled with the harmful effects of taking the pill, help set us up for disease, infertility, and probably loss of organs and early aging.

Incidentally, there is a new birth control pill that gives women only **four periods a year.** And another form of birth control that involves getting shots that stop periods for **years.** In my estimation, any woman who goes this route is going to wind up very unhealthy. When are we going to stop trying to out-think nature? Four periods a year! Stopping periods! Crazy! I heard young women on a television program

waxing poetic about this wonderful new convenience. Imagine what chaos this is going to create in
the template for ovulation.

As I said, through my research I now believe that
the effect of those pills on me and women of my generation was to put us into false menopause, which
created severe hormonal imbalance in our young
bodies. By the way, those original birth control pills
we took are the same synthetic hormones that the
Women's Health Initiative 2002 warned us to stop
taking.

Not only didn't I realize the harmful effects of taking birth control pills, but I also didn't realize the severe consequences of taking other prescription drugs
unless absolutely necessary. I remember being given
thyroid pills in my twenties. I never asked why. I figured my doctor knew what he was doing. Turns out
it wasn't a thyroid problem but a consequence of being hormonally imbalanced. Thank God I couldn't
afford to continue taking them at the time. The thyroid is not to be played around with. Every drug has
a consequence. I just never took those proposed side
effects and consequences seriously. I was young and
invincible, or at least I thought so, until I was diagnosed with cancer five years ago.

Since that diagnosis I have taken better care of myself than ever before. Suddenly realizing you are not
invincible and can no longer fool around with your
health is one of the many blessings of this dreadful
disease.

Today breast cancer is not the death sentence it once was. Through early detection, we are finding tumors that are very small and are thus increasing survival rates. Nonetheless, cancer in my breast was the first alarm bell in my life. It rang loudly in my ear: Figure out what you have been doing all of your life to give this to yourself, and correct those habits and behaviors, much as you would approach therapy.

Precancer in my uterus was another opportunity to research deeper. As women we have become informed about our bodies. We cannot turn over life decisions to our doctors. So often conditions in women are misunderstood by standard Western medicine. To make matters worse, often the treatment we are given is antiquated and ego-driven by a medical community that doesn't like to be perceived as "wrong." It's as though they would rather keep feeding us pharmaceuticals than go back and study the latest breakthroughs. The exceptions are represented by the doctors in this book and others I haven't yet discovered.

It was a logical conclusion for me to realize that if I was unknowingly hormonally imbalanced in my youth, then my body was a perfect breeding ground for cancer. The same conclusions are coming from doctors around the country trying to be heard, who feel that bioidentical hormone replacement, exactly as it happens in nature, is the best defense against disease.

As you read further in this book, you will have a

clear understanding of static dosing and rhythmic cycling, which will enable you to choose the way you want to go. This is updated information from **The Sexy Years.** When I wrote that book, I did not know about rhythmic cycling as an option. As medicine progresses, new information keeps coming forth.

Once you fully understand new concepts such as rhythmic cycling, then you can choose what's best for you and decide for yourself what feels right. In order to make an informed choice, you must understand the ramifications of every option offered to women. Those options are the following:

1. Synthetic hormones, which are drugs and not really hormones.
2. Natural aging, which means not taking anything and allowing for the gradual shutdown of your body, accelerated aging, and the diseases that go with it.
3. Nutritional supplements, which are important to antiaging but do **nothing** to replace the hormones lost in aging.
4. Bioidentical hormone replacement on a static dose, explained in chapter 5.
5. Bioidentical hormone replacement dosed in rhythmic cycling, also explained in chapter 5.

To be informed, you must understand each premise or you are doing yourself a disservice. You can choose whatever route you want to go, but at least you will have a complete understanding of the ramifications of each one. This book will help guide you.

I believe there are two ways to approach aging: the right way and the wrong way; the wrong way is taking drugs or doing nothing at all, the right way is to replace the hormones you've lost with bioidenticals, supported by proper diet, supplementation, exercise, sleep, and stress management. They all work together.

It is my opinion, after speaking with so many informed Western-trained doctors, that putting real hormones back is definitely the right way. Bioidentical hormone replacement therapy will allow you to have a happy, healthy, vital life. Without balanced hormones through this natural form of therapy, you can expect extreme discomfort within your own body, a diminished quality of life, and the potential for the diseases of aging.

If this information resonates with you, you will be motivated to find a doctor to prescribe BHRT the right way. Your compounding pharmacist is a good place to be directed to a qualified doctor. You can guide your doctor yourself and take your hormonal health into your own hands safely. A lot of women are now doing exactly that. You will hear from them in this book. The testimonials from women and men who found BHRT are emotional as they explain how it has changed the quality of their lives for the better.

The doctors interviewed for this book are endocrinologists, antiaging endocrinologists, molecular biologists, oncologists, doctors who specialize in male hormones, gynecologists, and internists specializing in Western, Eastern, and holistic medicine. These professionals are excited about the work they are doing in antiaging and in bioidentical hormone replacement. These doctors love their practices because they are putting people back together again, day in and day out. Restoring a person to prime hormonal health is very rewarding. Their attitudes are addictive.

With this knowledge, you will no longer be at the mercy of a doctor who knows nothing about real hormone replacement and is too lazy to find out. We women (and men) must do this. This is our life. If our doctors are not as passionate as we are about finding a solution to these passages of aging, then there is no choice but to become informed and take our health and quality of life into our own hands.

It has been sad for me to find out that the biggest obstacle in finding a solution to age-related illnesses and conditions has been most doctors in our country. I love my doctors, but I go out of my way to seek out cutting-edge doctors who have moved forward in their knowledge and thinking. It takes a youthful spirit and curiosity to be one of these doctors.

In medical school the students receive very little instruction in endocrinology and only four hours in how to prescribe hormones. If a doctor isn't curious, then his or her information comes primarily from the drug companies themselves. It doesn't take a rocket scientist to figure out that the information doctors get in a monthly throwaway magazine from the pharmaceutical companies would most likely be slanted; it is, after all, a business, and you can't really blame the drug companies for wanting to be profitable.

But at this stage of our lives, our primary interest is not what is profitable for the drug companies, but what is healthy for us! Yes, I'm happy they bring us all the wonderful drugs that are essential to keeping us alive in some cases, and nothing is better than Western pharmaceuticals for relieving pain. I do not want to live in a world without the advantage of pharmaceuticals. When you need them, they can be a miracle. But when it comes to hormone replacement, remember this: **There is no hormone drug that is as good as what your body makes, and bioidentical hormones are an exact replica of what your body makes.**

Recently, a younger person said to me, "I hope I look like you when I'm your age," and I said, "Well, you'd better start right now."

The good news is that for those of us who pursue antiaging later in life, it is not too late; the moment you begin living a healthful life, you see and feel the results. The longer you wait to take your health seriously, the more damage you will incur from the aging process. Had I known then what I know now, I would have reconsidered everything I ever put into my body. I would have embraced organic food. I would have realized the importance of sleep. I would have had an understanding of the importance of hormones. I would have started earlier by having hormone panels done to keep a baseline, so I could notice from year to year if there were detectable hormonal declines, among other things. Because I didn't know that optimal health was an option I could **choose,** I did the best I could with the information I had at the time.

Most of us who have embraced health and antiaging started rather late in life. That should be hopeful and encouraging for younger people who are reading this. Keep in mind, too, that good health on the inside manifests on the outside, so taking care of yourself is a true win, win.

PART ONE

KEEPING YOUR INSIDES "YOUNG"

**Getting Old Is Not for Sissies!
I feel like my body has gotten totally
out of shape. So I got my doctor's
permission to join a fitness club and
started exercising. . . . I decided to
take an aerobics class for seniors. I
bent, twisted, gyrated, jumped up and
down, and perspired for an hour. But
by the time I got my leotards on, the
class was over.**

CHAPTER 2

WHY WE AGE

The first indication of aging is the loss of hormones. You don't see it at first. It's happening inside, lurking about, waiting for the reproductive passage of "who you are" to finish. It's almost as though the hormones have grown impatient, sitting inside, tapping their fingers, and waiting to complete their job so they can take time off for good. Once that happens, the trouble inside "you" begins.

Hormonal loss is a very difficult passage for everyone. At forty years old or earlier, you will start to notice either a slight weight gain or an alarming amount of weight gain. Many women report going up as much as two dress sizes. Your bleeding cycle becomes irregular. What was once like clockwork now appears seemingly whenever it wants. Sometimes you skip a month or two.

Hot flashes come without warning. Suddenly heat rises up in you that is like nothing else you have ever experienced. Sleeping—which was once a given, something you didn't even think about—becomes difficult. You now get into bed and pray for a full night of uninterrupted sleep. Mood swings are also part of the equation.

We can visibly see hormonal decline in the mirror. God forbid you have one of those horrible magnifying mirrors, which most of us do, as our eyes betray and no longer work with the clarity they once had. We see the lines and wrinkles, and the skin on the neck and body becomes looser, less firm. As we get older, changes in cellular behavior lead to changes in hormone levels that cause the skin to become thinner. The barrier function of the skin, which attracts and retains moisture, also becomes less effective, making skin drier as well.

Here's the deal: Sooner or later, you are going to start experiencing these symptoms. All women and men go through hormonal decline. Symptoms are part of nature. Symptoms are your body's way of talking to you. With each hot flash or night sweat, your body is screaming for you to do something. The good news is that now you can. You will not have to suffer in silence like your mother or grandmother. To enjoy a satisfying life, hormones must be replaced, but only with bioidentical hormones. As you will read in chapter 5, there are different ways to take them, but taking bioidentical hormones is not negotiable. There is no other or better way to replace hormones and nothing else that your body will respond to like bioidenticals. Because the body recognizes them, it does not reject them. Quite the opposite— it welcomes them.

WHAT EXACTLY IS A HORMONE?

According to Dr. Gary London, OB/GYN, in his book **Thank You, Suzanne Somers** (can you believe it?), a "hormone is a substance produced by a gland and transported in the bloodstream throughout the body, transferring information and instructions between cells. Hormones are molecules that are synthesized and secreted by several glands throughout the body, collectively known as the endocrine system. Each gland produces its own unique hormones and each of those hormones serves as a molecular messenger to deliver very specific information to specific cells or organs in the body. Almost like a key opening a lock, these hormones have the ability to turn certain cells in the body known as target cells (for example, there are specific target cells in the breast and uterus that will respond to estrogen) and each target cell is genetically programmed to respond to particular hormones in a certain way. All aspects of cellular function, including repair and replication, are influenced by one or more hormones."

With the exception of prescribing supplemental estrogen (usually in synthetic form), the conventional medical community considers age-related hormonal decline to be normal and, therefore, takes little action to correct it. Low levels of other hormones such as DHEA, thyroid, testosterone, and growth hormone are not treated unless, or until, a full-blown condition such as adrenal failure, hypothyroidism, or pituitary disease is diagnosed.

Many antiaging doctors take exception to not treating age-related hormonal loss. According to Dr. Philip Lee Miller: "It doesn't matter to me whether that deficiency is the normal condition of the aging human. When we can improve health and function by restoring hormone levels to optimal levels, it makes sense to do so. This is the essence of functional medicine, the goal of which is to restore function and not necessarily to treat disease."

If you are thinking of taking hormones to treat aging, it is important to understand that we once all had optimal levels. To combat aging, you must try to restore those optimal levels in order to mimic your healthiest prime, and in doing so you give your body the greatest gift it has ever received. In the following sections you'll learn about the key hormones you need to balance to start reversing the aging process.

Take the time to read each of the next sections thoroughly. It is important that you understand the functions of each hormone. By doing so, the interviews with the doctors that follow will make complete sense.

Hormone	Site of Production	Function
Estrogen (includes estradiol, estrone, and estriol)	Ovaries, adrenal glands, fat cells, placenta (during pregnancy only)	• Regulates a woman's passage through menstruation, fertility, and menopause • Supports the growth and regeneration of female reproductive tissues • Develops secondary sex characteristics such as body hair, breasts, and distribution of body fat • Keeps the uterus, urinary tract, breasts, and blood vessels toned and flexible
Proges-terone	Ovaries, adrenal glands (women and men), testicles (men)	• Regulates menstrual cycle • Sustains a pregnancy • Stimulates bone-building cells (osteoclasts) and increases the rate of new bone formation • Promotes energy production in the brain • Protects against nerve cell damage and brain aging

DHEA	Adrenal glands	• Precursor (building block) to sex hormones • Involved in sex drive • Maintains collagen levels in the skin for promoting smoother, younger-looking skin • Works as a natural antidote to negative effects of cortisol
Thyroid	Thyroid gland	• Affects all metabolic activity • Regulates temperature • Regulates heart rate • Increases fat breakdown • Controls metabolism of carbohydrate and fat • Lowers cholesterol • Keeps hair, skin, and nails healthy
Cortisol	Adrenal glands	• Keeps us awake and alert • Mobilizes sugar for energy
Adrenaline	Adrenal glands	• Mobilizes sugar for energy • Functions as a natural stimulant
Insulin	Pancreas	• Determines whether fat will be burned or stored • Involved in growth

Human Growth Hormone	Pituitary gland	• Controls chronic inflammation • Beneficial to organ systems, including the heart and brain • Protects immunity • Increases aerobic capacity • Protects bone • Regulates body composition by decreasing body fat and enhancing muscle tone • Provides energy and endurance • Lowers blood pressure • Improves memory • Improves vision • Enhances ability to deal with stress • Enhances sleep • Responsible for growth
Melatonin	Pineal gland in the brain; small amounts in retina and gastrointestinal tract	• Increases quality of sleep • Is a potent antioxidant and captures damaging free radicals • Activates thyroid hormones • Improves mood and relieves anxiety • Improves sleep disorders • Fights the growth of cancer cells • Improves immune system • Relaxes muscles and relieves tension

Estrogen

WHAT IT IS: Estrogen is one of the most powerful hormones in the human body; it is what makes a woman a woman. It is estrogen that gives women their softness, curves, and breasts and helps regulate a woman's passage through menstruation, fertility, and menopause. What many people don't know is that both men and women make estrogen. To be a woman, you need high levels of estrogen and low levels of testosterone. To be a man, you need high levels of testosterone and low levels of estrogen.

HOW IT WORKS: Estrogen is not a single hormone. It is a group of three different but related hormones (estrone, estradiol, and estriol) that perform functions we normally attribute to "estrogen." Approximately three hundred different tissues are equipped with estrogen receptors. This means that estrogen can affect a wide range of tissues and organs, including the brain, liver, bones, and skin. The uterus, urinary tract, breasts, and blood vessels also depend upon estrogen to stay toned and flexible. Many menopausal women have urinary "leakage problems" from losing estrogen, and many menopausal women have to urinate often; for some, it's constant throughout the day. This is remedied by bringing estrogen levels back to normal. The family of estrogens work in concert with progesterone to nourish and support the growth and regeneration of the female reproductive tissues as well as impart the characteristic female growth of body hair, breasts, and distribution of body fat.

Symptoms of an estrogen deficiency include

- unexplained weight gain
- apple- or pear-shaped body
- bloating
- itching
- sweating and hot flashes
- depression
- irritability
- weepiness
- trouble sleeping
- foggy thinking
- bladder infections
- incontinence
- watery eyes
- allergies
- low libido
- heart palpitations
- fatigue
- low bone density
- painful intercourse

HOW TO TEST: It is important to establish your estrogen levels with a blood or saliva test. Even if you are too young to experience estrogen loss, it is advised that you start getting a hormone panel done each year so that you can evaluate from year to year to see if there is an estrogen decline.

You also have to be able to evaluate the way you feel to understand when your hormones are declining or out of balance. The more you understand this, the more your doctor will be able to help you. One of my first symptoms of low estrogen is itchy arms. Normally, you wouldn't think to call your doctor about an itch on your arms, but when you are balancing hormones, a symptom such as this is information for the doctor. If you are in touch with your body and if you pay attention to the way you are feeling, your doctor will be able to help you balance your hormones and make you feel good again.

I suggest that you keep a journal for the first three months and mark down how you feel on each day of the month. If any of the symptoms listed are part of your day, mark it down and you will have an accurate record for your doctor to evaluate. Symptoms are signs of imbalance. This is not something to "tough out." Toughing it out only keeps you in an imbalanced state, and that is a dangerous and uncomfortable place to be.

USING BIOIDENTICALS: By replacing lost estrogen with bioidentical estrogen, a woman can restore her body to her healthy prime. Along with a good diet and exercise, a woman on BHRT can expect to feel good for the rest of her life.

Bioidentical estrogen has numerous benefits. First and foremost, your menopausal symptoms go away. Your sex drive comes back, and your memory and mood improve. Your fatigue dissipates, and your skin elasticity improves. You have a reduced risk of heart disease and bone loss. Your depression is relieved, and estrogen supports your immune function. No drug can do all this for you. Drugs only exacerbate these problems.

Bioidentical estrogen replacement is by doctor's prescription only and prepared for you by a compounding pharmacy. These pharmacies use only pure grades of estrogen. The strength and combinations of estrogens can be established by working closely with your doctor, but remember: You know your body better than anyone. Some women require large doses of estrogen to feel good. I am one of them. My body does not "sing" with low doses. Once you are on replacement, it is important to pay acute attention to your symptoms. If you are symptomatic, then you need to have your dosage evaluated. Talk to your doctor about it. A symptom might be as simple as "my leg itches," but even that can be a sign of low estrogen.

SAFETY AND SIDE EFFECTS: Many health care professionals, such as the doctors you will meet in this book, believe bioidentical hormones—including bioidentical estrogen—are safe. If you have any side effects such as weight gain, breast tenderness, bloating, or other symptoms, report these to your doctor. This usually means you are not completely balanced and your dosage needs adjusting. Generally, though, bioidenticals are well tolerated.

SYMPTOMS FOR WOMEN WITH EXCESS ESTROGEN (ESTROGEN DOMINANCE)

Often, too much estrogen supplementation can be at the root of your symptoms. Be sure to have your doctor do a blood or saliva test for levels and then have your hormones rebalanced. If you have gone through a period of high stress and now things have calmed down, the estrogen you needed during the stress is now more than you require.

Alternatively, estrogen dominance can be due to hormonal imbalance, and a complete evaluation of your levels must be done and a new prescription dispensed to fit your current needs. Some of the symptoms of estrogen dominance include

- bloating and puffiness
- heavy bleeding
- weight gain in hips
- fibrocystic breasts
- mood swings
- anxiety

- irritability
- depression
- frequent thrush
- yeast infections
- weepiness
- carbohydrate cravings
- no sex drive
- sore and swollen breasts
- scatterbrained (foggy thinking)
- fibroids
- headaches before periods
- migraine

EXCESS TESTOSTERONE FOR WOMEN

Women can suffer from too much testosterone. Often, this imbalance can be caused by consuming too much sugar and eating carbohydrates in excess. Having a blood test to evaluate your testosterone levels, then correcting any imbalances through bioidentical hormone replacement therapy, can also bring you back to balance. Some symptoms of testosterone excess in women include

- acne
- high blood pressure
- excessive hair on face and arms

- deepened voice
- polycystic ovary syndrome (PCOS)
- unstable blood sugar
- pain when ovulating
- infertility
- ovarian cysts

PROGESTERONE

WHAT IT IS: Progesterone and estrogen are two of the main hormones made in the ovaries. Progesterone is produced primarily in the second half of a woman's menstrual cycle and is the hormone responsible for the survival of the fetus in pregnancy. Men also produce tiny amounts from the testicles. Progesterone is further produced in small amounts in the adrenal glands in both men and women.

HOW IT WORKS: When women reach their thirties and forties, it is very common that the balance between estrogen and progesterone shifts heavily toward estrogen. This excess estrogen is commonly known as estrogen dominance and is often to blame for many symptoms experienced by women at this time, such as PMS, night sweats, and depression. Around this time, a small amount of bioidentical progesterone can help rebalance these hormones and relieve these symptoms.

Symptoms of a progesterone deficiency include

- painful, tender, swollen breasts
- anxiety and stress
- infertility
- painful abdomen
- aggression
- extremely heavy periods
- PMS
- night sweats
- early miscarriage
- weepiness
- trouble sleeping
- headaches associated with your period
- low bone density
- weight gain
- swollen extremities
- excessive water retention

HOW TO TEST: You can have your progesterone levels measured by a saliva or blood test. It is best to check hormone levels on days 12 and 21 of the month, if you are cycling rhythmically. If you are static dosing, check levels around days 18 to 21. If you are feeling that you can't ever achieve balance on your static doses, read about rhythmic cycling in chapter 5 and give it a try.

USING BIOIDENTICALS: Treatment with bioidentical progesterone may protect the breasts against cancer and benefit your bones, brain, and mood. It can help prevent excessive proliferation of both normal and abnormal cancerous breast cells. Trials conducted by Dr. Helene Leonetti at Bethlehem Obstetrics Clinic in Pennsylvania found that progesterone therapy reduced fibrous (benign) breast lumps.

Other benefits of bioidentical progesterone:

- Restores libido
- Protects against fibrocystic breasts
- Is a natural diuretic
- Protects against endometrial cancer
- Is a natural antidepressant
- Facilitates thyroid function
- Normalizes blood sugar levels
- Improves energy, stamina, and endurance

Please be warned: If you go to a health food store to get your progesterone, you are not getting progesterone. A wild yam cream **is not progesterone.** It contains phytoestrogens, which may increase the body's production, but it is not a hormone or a precursor to a hormone. In other words, you are not replacing progesterone by using a wild yam cream. True-grade therapeutic bioidentical progesterone can be supplied only by prescription through a compounding pharmacy.

Do not confuse natural bioidentical progesterone with Provera, and do not confuse natural progesterone with "progestins." These are synthetic chemical analogues similar to progesterone but different enough to have dramatic side effects. The progesterone molecule in progestins has been chemically altered in order to be patented and owned by the pharmaceutical company. Synthetic progesterone is foreign to the body and has actually been shown to inhibit the biosynthesis of progesterone.

According to Dr. David G. Williams, progestins can cause abnormal menstrual flow or cessation, fluid retention, nausea, insomnia, jaundice, depression, fever, weight fluctuations, allergic reactions, and the development of male characteristics.

Bioidentical progesterone, on the other hand, can relieve menopausal symptoms, reverse osteoporosis, enhance mood, and restore libido, provided you are working with a qualified doctor who understands how to achieve the correct ratio or balance between estrogen and progesterone.

The correct ratios between estrogen and progesterone are key. These two hormones are meant to work together to maintain hormone balance. Without balance comes mood swings and weight gain, among other symptoms. Even women who have had a hysterectomy need to balance their monthly cycle with progesterone ten days of each month. There has been controversy about this. Many doctors put women on continuous estrogen replacement (meaning estrogen every day of the month) and do not give them progesterone, figuring because they no longer have a uterus that progesterone is not needed. Here is where you need to really understand the template that the brain follows. If you are not ovulating (because without progesterone, ovulation is impossible), then the brain "knows" that you cannot reproduce; therefore, the internal shutdown begins. This woman begins to have all sorts of medical problems as a result. After a hysterectomy you must "trick" the brain into believing that "all is well, you are reproductive." This is why you continue to replace progesterone just as you did when you still had your uterus. Remember, this book is to empower you so that you can tell your doctor what you want and need. Natural progesterone is very useful to balance excess estrogen—a situation that happens to women in perimenopause (the stage prior to menopause)—and it is also useful to treat estrogen dominance.

SAFETY AND SIDE EFFECTS: Bioidentical progesterone has few side effects. It does not increase the risk of cancer or cause abnormal menstrual flow, fluid retention, nausea, or depression.

However, women need to be aware of the serious side effects when estrogen is administered alone and their progesterone levels are down: nausea, anorexia, vomiting, headaches, and water retention leading to weight gain. For some women with physical disorders, taking estrogen supplementation only can exacerbate high blood pressure, diabetes, migraines, and epilepsy.

DHEA

WHAT IT IS: DHEA is the most plentiful hormone in your body and can be converted into other hormones, including estrogen and testosterone.

HOW IT WORKS: Considered an antiaging hormone, DHEA has positive effects on the brain, immune system, reproductive organs, muscles, and other organs and tissues. DHEA also helps to maintain collagen levels in the skin, promoting smoother, younger-looking skin. French scientists studied the effects of DHEA replacement therapy in about three hundred men and women between the ages of sixty and eighty over the course of a year. One of the findings to come out of this well-known study (known as the DHEAge study) was that DHEA supplementation greatly improved the color, tone, thickness, and hydration of the subjects' skin.

DHEA begins to drop off after age thirty and can be almost negligible after the age of sixty. This drop-off parallels the general decline in our health and vitality as we age. Stress accelerates the natural decline of DHEA levels.

HOW TO TEST: To determine your DHEA levels, you can have your hormone levels checked by saliva or blood test. If you are a female of any age, you would want your levels to be at optimum, which would be between 150 and 350. If you are a male of any age, you would want your optimal levels to be between 250 and 450.

USING DHEA SUPPLEMENTS: DHEA is available over the counter as a nutritional supplement, but before you use it, make sure your levels have been tested and your doctor feels you would benefit from taking this supplement.

SAFETY AND SIDE EFFECTS: Too much DHEA in women can lead to some undesirable side effects (not serious ones) such as increased sweating, oilier skin, acne, or hair growth. These effects are generally not seen in dosages below 50 mg a day. If these side effects do occur, simply reduce your dosage.

With proper monitoring by your doctor, DHEA replacement therapy is a very safe and extraordinarily effective antiaging therapy for most people. However, those with certain types of cancer are an area of potential concern. This is why any hormones should be monitored by a qualified doctor.

THYROID

WHAT IT IS: The thyroid is a butterfly-shaped gland located in the lower part of the neck just below the Adam's apple. The thyroid secretes iodine-containing hormones, triiodothyronine (T3) and thyroxine (T4), which regulate body temperature, heart rate, and metabolism. Thyroid hormones have a profound impact on weight. They control how the body burns up carbohydrates and fats by increasing enzyme levels that produce energy. Thyroid function is very complex and exerts a profound effect on the function of nearly every other organ in the body. If your thyroid isn't functioning optimally, neither are you.

HOW IT WORKS: The thyroid takes its orders from the pituitary gland and the hypothalamus, which are constantly monitoring the amount of thyroxine circulating in the blood. When the level of thyroxine gets low, the pituitary gland releases thyroid-stimulating hormone (TSH), produced in the pituitary gland. As the name suggests, thyroid-stimulating hormone signals the thyroid to produce more thyroxine. As the amount of thyroxine in the blood increases, the production of TSH is suppressed. This in turn slows the production of thyroxine. This feedback loop between the pituitary and thyroid works to keep the level of thyroid hormone relatively constant in the body.

Once in the body, circulating T4 is converted to the active form of T3. As we age, the production of T4 diminishes. In addition, the conversion of T4 to T3 also diminishes, resulting in less stimulation of the cells.

When T4 is not converted to T3, hypothyroidism (low or underactive thyroid) occurs. The most common thyroid disorder, underactive thyroid, typically strikes after age forty but is underdiagnosed and undertreated. Untreated thyroid disease leads to elevated cholesterol levels, heart disease, infertility, fatigue, muscle weakness, poor mental function, depression, weight gain, and an increased risk of cancer. Endocrinologists estimate that one in five women and one in ten men over sixty suffer from underactive thyroid.

Dr. Philip Lee Miller says, "Astonishingly, one study found that 40 percent of patients who were already taking thyroid medication still had abnormally high levels of TSH, an indicator of low thyroid function." Because even "normal" TSH levels increase heart disease risk, Dr. Miller advises testing for TSH and other blood markers of thyroid function and working with an antiaging doctor to bring these values into the "optimal" range for peak thyroid function.

Some of the factors that cause a "sick" thyroid include:

• Selenium deficiency. Selenium is a mineral necessary for the conversion of T4 to T3. (Incomplete conversion results in high levels of reverse T3, an inactive hormone.)
• Estrogen dominance caused by stress and pollution. Estrogen suppresses thyroid function.
• Mercury, a toxic metal that can contaminate the thyroid gland.
• Stress, which causes decreased adrenal gland

function and prevents the thyroid gland from functioning optimally.

Hypothyroidism occurs when the thyroid gland does not produce enough "energy-generating" thyroid hormones. Weight gain is a classic symptom of this dysfunction. In such cases, levels of thyroid-stimulating hormone may rise in an attempt to spur more production and secretion of thyroid hormones from the thyroid gland.

Other symptoms include

- chronic constipation
- fatigue
- feeling cold, even when others are hot
- brittle hair, hair loss, or nails that break easily and split
- longer, heavier, and more frequent periods
- dry, scaly skin
- bruising easily
- depression
- mental confusion
- trouble sleeping
- low libido
- sensitivity to light
- recurrent infections
- headaches or migraines

HOW TO TEST: Thyroid function tests tell you whether your thyroid is working normally. When

TSH is measured, most doctors consider normal to be in the 0.2 to 5.5 range. However, the normal range is no longer considered optimal by antiaging doctors. Optimal is between 1.0 and 2.0. Higher than this, and you can experience premature aging and an increased risk of heart disease. Writing in his book **Life Extension Revolution,** Dr. Miller says, "If your thyroid levels are above 4.0 (still well within the considered 'normal' range), you are at increased risk of heart disease."

You may be going to your doctor with complaints that indicate your thyroid is too high or too low, but your blood work comes back in the normal range. Your doctor, therefore, may not treat your thyroid because you are "normal," and that could be one of the big reasons you are symptomatic and gaining weight. You need to know this. When you go to an antiaging doctor, bring these ranges with you so you can do your own evaluating. When the thyroid is not working at optimal range for you, you are not getting the full benefit of bioidentical hormone replacement therapy.

If you suspect that you have an underactive thyroid, blood tests should not be limited to the "faithful" TSH test. This method happens to be scientifically outdated, and not all doctors are up-to-date with this fact. To get an accurate picture of what your thyroid hormones are doing, you need to work with a physician who understands thyroid problems. Demand a full panel of tests, including TSH, free

T4, free T3, reverse T3, and possibly thyroid antibodies. Together, these are considered a complete battery of thyroid function tests.

Overweight women with a family history of obesity may have lower levels of T3 in their blood. Treatments to raise T3 levels may help reduce some metabolic risk factors associated with abdominal obesity in some overweight women. Also, it is not uncommon for women with thyroid problems to suffer from depression. One explanation for this is that T3 is actually a bona fide neurotransmitter that regulates the action of serotonin (the feel-good hormone) and norepinephrine and gamma-aminobutyric acid (GABA), two brain chemicals that are important for alleviating anxiety.

Whenever thyroid problems are suspected or treated, it is important to monitor adrenal function as well. Attempting to treat low thyroid levels without supporting the adrenals can deplete the adrenal glands. At the same time, if your adrenals are weak, symptoms of low thyroid may persist even after your thyroid levels have been restored. Recognizing and treating adrenal exhaustion in conjunction with thyroid treatment can bring the body relief from fatigue, anxiety, and depression. It can stabilize your mood and energy levels and could be a factor in losing the weight you have gained.

USING NATURAL THYROID HORMONE: There is such a thing as natural thyroid hormones, which can be helpful for a sick thyroid gland. Many antiaging doctors prefer to use Armour thyroid, a natural replacement for thyroid hormone obtained from porcine (pig) thyroid glands.

Low thyroid can also be easily corrected by augmenting the body's own production with bioidentical thyroid hormones. It's not just your individual hormone levels that matter, but the balance of all the hormones and a healthy lifestyle that helps you achieve optimal health and successful aging.

SAFETY AND SIDE EFFECTS: Natural thyroid hormone should be used with caution if you have cardiovascular disease. It may also increase the symptoms of diabetes. Always report any unusual side effects to your doctor.

CORTISOL

WHAT IT IS: Cortisol is your stress hormone. It is released by your adrenal glands and is one of the major hormones in the body.

HOW IT WORKS: Cortisol gives you energy, but more in response to stress. When you encounter a stressful situation, your adrenal glands release cortisol. If your child is trapped under a car, for example, your body will mobilize energy so you can lift the car and save your child. Or if you encounter a knife-wielding stranger, your body springs into action, thanks to cortisol, so that you can quickly run away. These are examples of cortisol in action. You cannot live very long without cortisol. It is that important.

However, the problem is that your body will secrete cortisol for whatever stress you encounter, including a bad day at work, stressing over the way your daughter is dressing these days, or a death in the family. Stress raises your blood pressure and uses up your energy reserves without much benefit to you. Using up your biochemicals is a waste because they are being used when there is no threat to your life. Our world is so full of stresses on a daily basis that most of us are running around with high cortisol all the time. It may give us a debilitating stroke, heart attack, or crippling diabetes—or worse, even kill us. Because stress is a wasted emotion that takes its toll on every part of your body, emotionally and physically, it is important to work at eliminating unnecessary stress and save your cortisol reserves for when you really need them, as in life-threatening situations.

There is a cortisol connection to getting fat. As I just explained, stress creates high levels of cortisol. High levels of cortisol, in turn, create insulin resistance, in which the cells of the body become resistant to the effects of insulin and higher levels of insulin are produced by the pancreas. When you are insulin-resistant, your body converts sugars and carbohydrates into fat rather than burning them as fuel.

When your cortisol is chronically elevated because of stress, it creates a devastating cycle of alternating high blood sugar and high insulin. This is why, after a while, your body loses its sensitivity to this cycle of alternating high blood sugar and high insulin. The dangerous progression from elevated cortisol to elevated blood sugar to insulin resistance is one of the major ways stress contributes to heart disease, obesity, diabetes, and even death.

Also, chronically elevated levels of high cortisol will eventually degrade your immune system. This is a dangerous place to be, since you will have difficulty fighting off infections, especially viral infections. Stressed-out people are more susceptible to colds and flu, as well as flare-ups of cold sores or shingles. Cancer patients with high cortisol have little ability to fight the cancer, which increases the chances that the cancer will metastasize throughout the body.

The stress connection goes on and on and is even harmful to your brain cells. It can impair "cognitive function," which means your memory, your reaction time, your problem-solving abilities, and your learning abilities. In short, high cortisol ages the brain.

HOW TO TEST: Cortisol levels can be determined by a saliva test, which you can obtain through any anti-aging doctor.

TREATMENT: The best treatment for high cortisol is stress reduction and stress management. Often, maintaining proper hormone levels and balance will resolve high cortisol, too.

ADRENALINE AND THE ADRENALS

WHAT IT IS: The adrenals are two triangular glands that sit on the top of each kidney. I like to think of hormones within the body as a concert. The adrenals are the orchestra leader. They communicate with all the other hormones, telling them what to do. Among other things, they produce stress hormones, including cortisol and adrenaline, which, once released, speed up heart rate, blood pressure, and other bodily functions to help you cope with stress.

HOW IT WORKS: Adrenaline is our engine. It pushes us forward. If we are leading a balanced life, our bodies release adrenaline when we need that surge of energy. Afterward, we return to a calmer baseline. But problems arise when we get addicted to adrenaline and put ourselves in situations that continually feed our bodies more and more. I describe a person in this state as being an "adrenaline junkie," meaning that he or she craves, and lives in, a high-energy state at all times. You know the type: Every minute of each day is filled with activities, responsibilities, and piles and piles of things on the to-do list, with lots of check marks ticking off completed tasks. It is often said, "If you want something done, ask the busiest person you know." There is truth in that statement, because the busy, busy people are running on adrenaline, and it's as though they have superhuman energy. It's akin to a caffeine high or even a drug high. And just like those stimulants, adrenaline can be addictive and dangerous to your health.

TESTING FOR ADRENAL FATIGUE: Saliva tests can measure cortisol and determine whether your adrenals are blown out. Also, some of the symptoms of shot adrenals ("adrenal exhaustion") include fatigue, heart palpitations, recurrent infections, achiness, and low blood sugar.

I know a little about adrenal exhaustion since I have been the worst offender. For thirty years I lived in an almost constant state of high adrenaline. I loved it, I craved it. I am a wife, a mother, and a grandmother first. Plus I work, travel, entertain, lecture, have seven businesses, remodel, decorate, write, perform—and oh, yes, I still cook and give perfect dinner parties for family and friends. Watching me go like the Energizer Bunny, my husband would tell me to slow down. But my body did not want to slow down! If I had some time left, it would be hard for me to relax. I would clean the house, organize a desk, or answer e-mail. Finally, my adrenals burned out.

I vowed never to do that to myself again. Though it was a big adjustment, I had to change my life. I reprioritized my daily schedule, made time for sleep, did yoga three or four times a week, and learned that relaxation time was as important as being so busy. I no longer stay up late at night, whereas I used to write until the wee hours of the morning. Now I try my best to be in bed by 9:00 p.m. and asleep by 10:00 p.m. It takes retraining. I have readjusted my social schedule so that I do not go out two nights in a row, and I try not to go out more than two nights a week. Had I not done this, I would have run into trouble down the road, since burned-out adrenals lead to chronic high cortisol and, ultimately, a heart attack or stroke.

My doctor told me this after I had experienced adrenal burnout for the third time. The body can't handle that kind of stress. It's not easy to make the choice to change your life for health's sake, but the way I look at it, what choice do you have? Look around you at the people who are on the adrenaline merry-go-round. Now that you know the facts, you can see where they are going. Is this where you want to go? If not, start making changes right now. This is your life.

When your adrenals are shot the way mine were, you have no energy, and you feel a "racing" inside that makes sleep impossible, further blowing out your adrenals. Why? Because burned-out adrenals put you in such a state of fatigue that sleep is impossible. This lack of rest exacerbates the situation; things get worse and worse. What do you do when you are exhausted? You drink coffee, a stimulant that gives a false sense of energy. Then, when you don't sleep soundly for days, weeks, even months, depression is the result. What do you do then? You go to your doctor, who prescribes an antidepressant like Prozac or Paxil.

Now you're in trouble. Antidepressants make you feel good at first, but after a while they produce lethargy, a false sense of well-being. Then you start to get fat. What would you expect? Antidepressants slow everything down, including your metabolism. No metabolism equals weight gain.

But you are already hooked. Once your body gets accustomed to antidepressants, it's hard to feel good without them. Thus, the addiction. Addictions develop because the antidepressants initially cause the release of a lot of serotonin into your brain, making you feel calm and happy. This is how we want to feel all the time. The irony is that these same toxic chemicals that give you an immediate release of serotonin also cause you to use up more serotonin. Then you start craving anything that will make serotonin levels rise, even if it is only temporary. Many people go to carbohydrates and refined sugars or self-medicate with caffeine, alcohol, or drugs to feel good. What they are really doing is trying to use these substances to raise their serotonin levels. Then they can't stop with the antidepressants because without them they feel depressed. Depression is an impossible state in which to live. It debilitates. It hurts. Any of us would do anything to get rid of depression when it arrives uninvited.

FACTORS THAT CAN BLOW
OUT YOUR ADRENALS

Almost everything and anything raises adrenaline levels in your body, because adrenaline is one of the hormones needed to access your biochemicals for use in the activities of daily living. Unfortunately, it is estimated that 85 percent of all Americans are walking around with burned-out adrenals. Here are some of the factors that can cause adrenal fatigue:

overwork

anemia

sleeplessness

high DHEA levels

high progesterone levels

high testosterone levels

high thyroid levels

high protein intake

low blood sugar levels

low estrogen levels

inflammation

infections

dietary imbalances

skipped meals

birth control pills

overexercising

pain

stimulants such as caffeine, nicotine, marijuana, ginseng, ephedra, Dexedrine, cocaine, and pure white sugar

So you see, it's not just junkies who get addicted. We are all driven by our deficiencies. Deficiencies cause cravings. We crave feeling good, and we will do anything to feel good, no matter what the consequences. It's not about willpower or intellect. Rather than cave in to cravings, it's better to make the decision to change your life. Start working on eating well, sleeping an adequate amount, managing stress, reprioritizing your schedule (yes, the world will keep on spinning without you running it!), and, of course, keeping your hormones balanced. Remember that all hormones talk to one another. If one is off, they are all off.

TREATING EXHAUSTED ADRENALS: No one of us can take on the whole world. All we can do is try to make the changes in our own lives. Part of this involves following a good diet of whole, unprocessed foods that avoids sugar and chemicals. These changes not only will affect our health positively, but will also have a positive impact on our immediate family.

INSULIN

WHAT IT IS: Insulin is a major hormone. It has many jobs in the body, one of which is determining whether fat will be burned off as energy or stored as fat. (This is why insulin is often called the "fat-storing hormone.") In my eating program, Somersizing,

I advise my readers that to lose weight, they must acquaint themselves not only with sugar, but also with foods the body converts to sugar, and then avoid those foods during the weight loss portion of the program. These foods promote insulin secretion and include white flour, white rice, high-starch vegetables, refined white sugar, and any food that contains sugar. By identifying and avoiding these foods, we can control our insulin levels and, therefore, our weight.

HOW IT WORKS: When we eat sugar or carbohydrates, our blood sugar is elevated. If our metabolism is working at optimum, our pancreas first secretes insulin. Along with sugar, the insulin travels to the liver, where the sugar will be converted to fat. The fat will be burned off immediately as fuel, or it will be stored as fat. Here's the hitch: If someone is "insulin-resistant," his or her cells will not accept any additional sugar. When the cells do not accept any more sugar or fats for energy, this initiates a further release of insulin from the pancreas, leading to even higher insulin levels. If blood sugar and fats are not burned as fuel, they will be stored for later use. Therefore, even fat-free carbohydrates like sugar and white flour can be converted to fat if we do not need the energy at the time we eat. With this information you can see how the elevation of blood sugar can lead to weight gain when we eat too many carbohydrates at one time.

With prolonged high insulin levels, you'll first notice fat deposits around the midsection. Men get that "beer belly" or "potbelly," and women get thick through the stomach, waist, and thighs. Think of your midsection as your "insulin meter." It doesn't matter if you are overweight or thin. When you are thick around the middle, your insulin levels are elevated.

Insulin resistance occurs naturally as we get older. Our metabolic processes slow down, and we do not need as many carbohydrates as we did before. But when we have too much insulin, we throw off our body's entire hormonal balance. Hormonal imbalance leads not only to weight gain but also to increased cholesterol and disease. Overproduction of insulin leads to plaquing of the arteries and accelerated growth and division of tumors. Breast, colon, and prostate cancers have been found to grow more rapidly under the stimulus of insulin. Anything that leads to chronic high insulin levels, including poor nutrition and lifestyle habits, can increase the risk of cancer.

High insulin also causes an abnormal increase of salt retention at the kidney level and is thus a factor in heart disease. Too much salt in the system increases water retention, and more overall fluid means higher blood pressure. Insulin also overstimulates the nervous system, and this increases blood pressure as well. With high blood pressure the amount of blood pumped out by each contraction of the heart is increased and the artery walls become stiffer—not good for heart health.

Women need to understand the estrogen connection to high insulin. When estrogen levels are low, we crave carbohydrates. This is why women are combing the cupboards for chocolate right before their periods, when their estrogen levels are at their lowest. A low estrogen state makes it impossible for a woman to avoid carbohydrate craving because estrogen is one of the hormones necessary for serotonin production. When she gives in and consumes the sugar, chocolates, or carbohydrates, her insulin levels shoot up. Now she craves more sugar and carbohydrates, and the merry-go-round begins.

If you continue your present high-insulin eating and lifestyle habits, both your immune and hormone systems will age faster, since prolonged insulin levels are one of the causes of accelerated metabolic aging. The best way to lower your insulin level is to keep yourself hormonally balanced, eat a well-balanced diet of real foods and real fats, and engage in some form of daily exercise. Remember this: **An important key to longevity is delaying insulin resistance for as long as possible.**

Here is a look at habits and factors that raise insulin levels:

- low-fat diet (yes, low-fat!)
- excess carbohydrates
- fake food, including saccharin, aspartame, mar-

garine-invented substances, refined and
processed foods
- consumption of soft drinks
- overconsumption of alcohol
- smoking
- recreational stimulants
- stress
- lack of exercise
- prescription drugs
- steroids
- diet pills

HUMAN GROWTH HORMONE

WHAT IT IS: Human growth hormone (HGH) is a
protein hormone released by the pituitary gland in
the brain. It is responsible for telling our bodies to
grow cells, bones, organs, and muscles and is beneficial to the brain, the cardiovascular system, the immune system, aerobic capacity, body composition,
and bone. HGH enters our bloodstream in bursts
during sleep, particularly after midnight. It heads to
the liver, where it is converted into insulin growth
factor 1 (IGF-1), a messenger molecule that travels
to all parts of the body and stimulates cell production and growth.

HOW IT WORKS: HGH promotes growth by helping transport amino acids (the building blocks of

protein) between cells and into cells. The body uses amino acids to create muscles and to build and restore organs, including the heart and skin.

Because this hormone is primarily responsible for the growth and regeneration of every cell in our bodies, low levels of HGH cause aging. HGH is in plentiful supply until about age twenty. Each decade thereafter, we lose approximately 20 percent of our HGH base level. So by the time you're sixty or seventy, your body has access to only 15 to 20 percent of the HGH you had in your youth.

Symptoms of a deficiency include

- thinning, sagging, wrinkling skin
- thinning bones
- loss of muscle strength
- accumulation of fat tissue
- decreased heart function
- lowered immunity
- thinning hair
- loss of libido
- decreased stamina and vigor
- depression
- anxiety
- fatigue

On July 5, 1990, the **New England Journal of Medicine** published a clinical study on HGH, hailing it as a fountain of youth. Injections of synthetic human growth hormone had turned twelve men, ages sixty-one to eighty-one, with flabby, frail, fat-bulging bodies into sleeker, stronger, younger selves. After just six months of treatment, the men gained an average of 8.8 percent in lean body mass and lost an average of 14.4 percent in fat mass. In addition, their skin thickened by 7.1 percent, the bone density of their lumbar spines increased by 1.6 percent, their livers grew by 19 percent, and their spleens grew by 17 percent. Finally, the subjects in this study showed a ten- to twenty-year reversal in the aging process.

According to Dr. Philip Lee Miller: "Perhaps more powerfully than any other hormone system, supplementing the body's waning production of growth hormone with bioidentical replacement hormones can reduce, and even reverse, the changes normally associated with the aging process. Growth hormone replacement therapy enhances the effects that we have already seen with testosterone and estrogen therapy: more youthful skin, increased lean muscle mass, and increased mental and physical vitality. But with the addition of growth hormone, the changes are even more dramatic and profound."

HGH is also great for weight control, doing something few other weight loss regimens do: It recontours the body, melting away fat and building muscle. In many cases, people who take HGH look as if they've shed not only years, but also lots of fat. Even better, the greatest loss occurs in deep belly fat, the area associated with increased risk of heart attack and diabetes. In a double-blind, placebo-controlled, crossover study on overweight women, HGH caused an average loss of more than 4.6 pounds of body fat, mostly in the abdomen. Most diets cause loss of muscle along with fat, but in this study the women's lean body mass increased by 6.6 pounds.

Loss of abdominal fat also has implications for type 2 diabetes, since there is a close association between central obesity and insulin resistance. According to Dr. David Clemmons, "While some early studies showed increased blood sugar and insulin resistance in GH-treated subjects, later studies showed that after six months of treatment, insulin sensitivity returned to baseline. While proof is still lacking, it is reasonable to assume that over the long run, stimulation of growth hormone could help to **prevent type 2 diabetes or even reverse the process.**"

HGH's disease-fighting and antiaging benefits are becoming more clear all the time. More than twenty-eight thousand different studies on HGH indicate that human growth hormone supplementation is indeed one secret to maintaining youth. (If you want to read some of these studies for yourself, go to www.pubmed.com.)

Dr. Julian Whitaker of the Whitaker Health Institute in California has been prescribing HGH to his patients with deficiency. In his view, HGH is most effective in combating the effects of chronic diseases that involve muscle wasting, stroke, chronic heart disease, and AIDS. He feels it can even be beneficial in treating burns and in helping patients recover from surgery.

For the record I, too, have become convinced and am enjoying the benefits of daily injections of HGH. My tests indicated I had a deficiency. In a few weeks of taking this hormone, my belly fat had all but disappeared. My skin appeared thicker and less wrinkled. My stamina, vigor, and vitality are now at optimum. Combined with a regimen of adequate sleep, good diet (most of the time), and exercise (but not fanatically), I find my hormone levels and all ratios are in line, and all my other tests are coming out in good to optimal ranges. These are very significant and encouraging results.

SUPPLEMENTING WITH HGH: The antiaging community has heralded HGH as the ultimate antiaging therapy. But it is prescribed **only** when there is a deficiency. For now, the conventional establishment continues to insist that growth hormone therapy is unproven and risky. Growth hormone is readily available as an FDA-approved drug and is the standard treatment for adults with a clinical diagnosis of growth hormone deficiency due to pituitary failure or disease.

As a cancer survivor, I have always been interested in understanding HGH, yet somehow I felt that a **growth hormone** certainly couldn't be a good thing for me. I mean, why would I want to encourage growth in a body that once housed the nastiest element of growth? But the more I discovered about this hormone, the more interested I became. According to Dr. Philip Lee Miller, "Perhaps more powerfully than with any other hormone system, supplementing the body's waning production of growth hormone with bioidentical replacement hormones can reduce and even reverse the changes normally associated with the aging process."

Virtually everyone over age forty has suboptimal growth hormone levels, and the earlier HGH is initiated, the greater the benefits. HGH is typically prescribed in small, regular doses to mimic the body's own natural secretions. Although supplementing with injectable HGH remains somewhat controversial, Dr. Miller argues strongly in favor of considering it as part of a comprehensive antiaging program. "Personally, I believe the antiaging effects of growth hormone are so profound and so beneficial to your long-term health that the benefits far outweigh the possible risks," he explains. "In addition, I firmly believe that when HGH is used properly, the risks are minimized. I not only offer growth hormone therapy to my patients as an option, but also personally use HGH injections as part of my own antiaging program."

At the moment, HGH injections are quite expensive. Most doctors I have spoken with say that the price will be going down drastically in the near future as this amazing hormone becomes better understood. If daily HGH injections are not a possibility due to cost, or if you find the idea of daily injections too difficult, you can try to jump-start your own body to make HGH on its own by supplementing with L-arginine, L-glutamine, L-ornithine, lysine, glycine, and niacin, all known to increase the body's internal release of growth hormone. Getting adequate sleep and exercising on a regular basis also stimulate the release of HGH.

SAFETY AND SIDE EFFECTS: I'm sure at this point you are asking whether growth hormone is safe. In my case, I first had blood work done to show that I had a growth hormone deficiency, probably due to the aging process and the natural occurrence of declining hormones. Then I wanted to know if using growth hormone could increase the risk of cancer, so I looked into this. The only evidence comes from children and young adults who were given growth hormone to treat growth disorders and later had a higher rate of certain cancers as adults. The dosages used in these cases were up to ten times those used today in antiaging therapies. The connection between cancer and growth hormone has also been observed only in patients who received therapy prior to 1985, when HGH was synthesized from cadavers. When synthetic forms of the hormone became available, the use of growth hormones from cadavers was halted.

To date, according to Dr. Miller, there is no conclusive data that connects the use of low-dose synthetic growth hormone with an increased risk of cancer. "The positive effect of growth hormone on overall health of the body, including the function of the immune system and other organs, is far more likely to decrease your chances of cancer and other diseases as you age," he emphasizes. "However, it remains an unanswered question that must be carefully considered by each potential user."

HGH can be prescribed only by a doctor under certain conditions—namely, that you are deficient. That stands to reason. Remember that with any hormone, you never replace a hormone that isn't low or missing, nor do you ever take more than your body needs.

Some of the negative side effects that have been reported from supplementing with HGH include carpal tunnel syndrome, arthritis, water retention, and the growth of precancerous cells. Some men whose hormonal activity has been reawakened by HGH supplements find themselves growing small breasts. Finally, long-term HGH use in higher than physiological amounts has been known to cause enlargement of the bones of the hands and feet, particularly in bodybuilders who overdose. Recent studies have indicated that most, if not all, of the undesirable side effects are reversed when the patient stops taking HGH or the doses are reduced.

For antiaging purposes, however, HGH is prescribed in small, regular doses to mimic the body's natural secretions. Doctors have discovered that this protocol cuts out most of the risks associated with taking excessive amounts.

Normally healthy young people under thirty should not receive HGH injections. However, they can ensure maximum production levels through diet, exercise, vitamins, minerals, and natural hormone supplements.

For more information on HGH, read Dr. Ron Rothenberg's interview in chapter 28.

MELATONIN

WHAT IT IS: I first learned of melatonin when friends of mine started flying back and forth to Europe and were using it to help them with jet lag and to get them back on regular sleep cycles. It was then hailed as the wonder drug for sleep, although it was actually a hormone available as an over-the-counter sleep aid, but without the side effects of sleeping pills. At the time, it seemed to me that a glass of wine might be a better solution. How wrong I was!

Melatonin is the hormone of sleep. It is secreted from the pineal gland located in the brain. (Very small amounts of melatonin are also produced in the retina and gastrointestinal tract.) The main function of the pineal gland is to help govern those of our biological rhythms that take place over the day, such as the sleep-wake cycle. Researchers see this gland as important in coordinating and controlling our other hormone-release and immune responses. The pineal gland communicates with these other systems through its messenger, melatonin. The pineal gland knows "how old we are" and when we are past our prime. It responds by producing lower levels of melatonin, signaling our other systems to break down, and causes us to age. If we can keep melatonin raised to optimal levels as they begin to fall, we would once again be tricking our bodies into believing that we are still young. With optimal levels of melatonin, we can continue to produce high levels of sex hormones and keep our bodies operating with a well-functioning immune system to fight off disease. Chronologically we would be older, but biologically we would be younger.

Melatonin is synthesized from an amino acid called tryptophan, which in turn is converted into the brain chemical serotonin. Ultimately, serotonin is turned into melatonin. See how all hormones speak to one another? With adequate amounts of melatonin, you sleep soundly and deeply, and you dream and wake up rested in the morning. Melatonin is also responsible for making you yawn. As night falls, melatonin release induces sleep; dawn shuts it off, waking you up in the morning.

HOW IT WORKS: It is important to understand that melatonin is produced naturally in the body. Aging, work, travel, and stress can cause changes in sleep patterns and are likely to have adverse effects on melatonin secretion. However, you can achieve optimum release of melatonin by going to bed three hours before midnight and coupling this practice with BHRT if you are in hormonal decline. These three hours of melatonin production reset prolactin production. Three hours of melatonin production is always followed by six hours of prolactin production at night to rev up the defensive arm of your immune system. If you do not go to bed three hours before midnight, you only provoke one and a half hours of prolactin production, possibly suppressing your immune system.

Changes in melatonin set off a range of responses, such as puberty, menstruation, and sleep. Melatonin also alerts our bodies to produce antibodies to combat disease. So you can see how important the presence and maintenance of the correct level of this hormone are for the optimal functioning of our bodies throughout our lives.

Melatonin is known as a wonder drug because of all its other incredible effects. In fact, melatonin may extend our life span by 25 percent or more, possibly because it acts as a powerful antioxidant, keeping the body young by doing battle with free radicals—those toxic agents that pummel and mutilate DNA. It is the only antioxidant capable of penetrating every cell of the body and is the most active and effective of all naturally occurring compounds. For example, in certain tests melatonin proved to be five times more powerful than glutathione and at least twice as effective as vitamin E, another potent antioxidant.

In 1995, an Italian researcher demonstrated that melatonin boosted the immune system of people under extreme stress. Not only that, melatonin helps prevent cancer and improves sexual functioning. Additionally, it helps prevent heart disease by lowering blood cholesterol. It also combats AIDS, Alzheimer's disease, Parkinson's disease, asthma, diabetes, and cataracts. Melatonin can also extend your youth, enabling you to enjoy work, sex, and social activities with the same zest and vigor that marked your life in your twenties. Author T. S. Wiley says that with less melatonin in your system, you accelerate aging by four years for every one you live.

SUPPLEMENTING WITH MELATONIN: There are plenty of reasons to supplement your hormonal system with melatonin. Because melatonin production drops off sharply around age forty-five, supplementation should begin then and not before. The idea is to start taking melatonin when your levels drop.

To find out how much you need, have your melatonin levels checked with a saliva test. Melatonin in the range of 0.5 mg to 12 mg is usually effective. It's best to start on low doses such as 0.5 mg to 2 mg; increase this dosage if you find it does not help. With melatonin, less is more. Although melatonin plays an extremely important role in our bodies, it is present in only tiny amounts, even at our youthful peak. Larger doses of melatonin won't help. You can find melatonin in your local health food store, or your doctor can recommend or prescribe the type he or she feels best.

Take melatonin supplements only at night, since the production of this hormone is initiated by darkness. If you take them during the day, you confuse your brain. You don't want to do that, since there is more to this hormone than sleep regulation. Melatonin also governs which other hormones are released and when. Additionally, taking melatonin generally makes you sleepy, so you definitely want to take it prior to bedtime.

SAFETY AND SIDE EFFECTS: There are no harmful side effects with melatonin and no long-term dangers because it is not a drug, but a substance that occurs naturally in your body. Even so, people with autoimmune diseases, leukemia, or lymphoma should consult a doctor before use. Melatonin can also interfere with fertility and should not be taken by those who are pregnant or nursing. On the other hand, women on BHRT can take melatonin without fear of any ill effects.

CHAPTER 3

TRANSITIONS

Three old guys are out walking.
First one says, "Windy, isn't it?"
Second one says, "No, it's Thursday!"
Third one says, "So am I. Let's go get a
beer."

We women go through a lot. Our bodies are constantly changing and in transition owing to the hormone balance that shifts with age and with the environment to which we are exposed. We are chemical beings, and we live in a world that is environmentally hazardous. We have chemicals in our water. Our food supply is damaged from the soil in which it grows and from the acid rain that falls from the sky. Our food is loaded with preservatives and chemicals that our bodies were never meant to assimilate. When you factor in the daily stress we are all coping with—noise pollution, traffic, airplanes, angry drivers—along with major stresses like a death in the family, serious illness, and accidents, it's no wonder we have so many problems associated with our changing bodies, from PMS to perimenopause to menopause and beyond.

They say in today's world we experience more stress in a single day than a person in Elizabethan times experienced in their entire lives. Think about that . . . this is why these transitions have become so difficult. Transitions are a part of aging, and each passage that occurs involves changing hormone levels. How you get through these transitions, or passages—successfully, with your health intact—has to do primarily with balancing your hormones. That's what we'll look at in this chapter.

PREMENSTRUAL SYNDROME

PMS is real. The dictionary description is as follows: "a disorder causing a range of symptoms such as nervousness, irritability, bloating, depression, headache, fatigue, tenderness of the breasts and acne, that occur each month following ovulation and leading up to menstruation: usually five to fourteen days before." The very existence of this definition in the dictionary proves PMS is a real syndrome!

We are not given sympathy for this syndrome, either, because we are so difficult to be around while experiencing its symptoms. We know inside that we can't help it when we fly off the handle, but it takes so much effort and maturity to try to cope with it.

If you suffer from PMS, there are two things you can do: The first is to find a doctor who understands bioidentical hormone replacement therapy. So often a blood test will reveal that your "chemical imbalance" is hormonal in origin. This finding makes the syndrome easily rectified.

You have to understand that hormone replacement is not the sole domain of older women. Teenagers with "raging hormones" can feel and act crazy from hormonal imbalances. Additionally, in teenagers with PMS, painful periods and cramps are often a result of a progesterone deficiency. Add to that scenario that they do not yet possess all of their "common sense," and parents have a recipe for disaster. Getting a blood test to determine the existence of an imbalance and then a prescription for real progesterone, short-term, until the girl is balanced, can save a lot of heartache. If she needs it for a deficiency, then it cannot be harmful, only helpful.

Perimenopausal women experiencing PMS may be suffering from an estrogen deficiency that makes them feel crazy and irritable. This can start in the early thirties and continue for years. Again, a blood test to identify the imbalance and then replacement with real hormones for what is needed can change a person's life and outlook.

PMS can be so serious that it can ruin relationships and marriages. No one understands it, least of all the woman herself. This brings me to the second thing you can do about PMS: You have to get a handle on yourself. Understand that your hormones are acting up and that the feelings you are experiencing are magnified by the chemical imbalance. Right before your period is usually the worst and most dangerous time. You can experience true rage; then two days later when your chemicals have calmed down, you feel so bad for all the terrible things you have said and done.

I remember being terribly PMS-y in my early thirties. When I think about it now, I was definitely hormonally imbalanced. Remember, I was also on those original birth control pills, and they could make you feel crazy. I wonder how much of my craziness was chemically induced by those harmful pills I was taking. I would do terrible things: throw a beautiful vase across the room, try to jump out of a moving car, cry, or scream, all of which was truly embarrassing behavior. My anger at my husband and kids felt real.

I was extremely stressed dealing with my newfound and tremendous fame and blending our two families. My schedule was crazy. My eating habits had not been formed. I drank a lot of champagne and ate too much sugar. I went out too much, didn't sleep enough, and prided myself on the tiny amount of sleep I got each night, as though outworking everyone were something to be proud of. In other words, I had zero understanding of my body as a temple to be revered and taken care of. I abused my body and mind during those years, and the craziness the week before my period was always inevitable. I am extremely lucky that my husband tried his best to understand what I was going through. But the truth is, I did not understand it myself, and as a result, I could have lost everything.

Yes, PMS **is** real, but you have to accept that your lifestyle and diet choices can affect it, good or bad. Poor sleeping habits, poor diet, consumption of chemicals and preservatives, and other bad choices will have a negative effect on your quality of life. Have your doctor order a hormone panel to see if it is imbalance that is making you this way. See a therapist to try to unravel the confusion of your life. I did this because I was in anguish from leftover childhood issues and new issues relative to putting a family together that didn't want to be together. My therapist helped me change my life and attitudes. I also changed my diet and reprioritized my life.

Hormone replacement has let my true nature emerge. I no longer get PMS. When I do feel irritable or bitchy, I ask myself, What is going on in my life? Is it real stress, can I handle this stress better, or is this chemical? I go over my eating patterns for the prior couple of days to see if too much sugar had been in my diet in any of its forms, such as processed carbohydrates, bread, desserts, or wine. These foods can cause PMS even in menopause, even if you are on bioidenticals. Diet affects your hormones and, thus, your moods. If I find my diet was not good, I will give myself a talking-to and remember that the irritable feelings are from my choices. Then I get a grip. It's not fun to be around a PMS-y woman, and it's not right to take things out on others. In the end, the one who loses out the most is you.

PERIMENOPAUSE

Perimenopause, which is the transitional stage from normal menstrual periods to no periods at all, is not given a lot of attention because it's seen as a precursor to menopause and not the real deal. Perimenopausal women are emotional; yet because they are still getting a period, most doctors toss it off as "nothing serious." But here is why you should be concerned about perimenopause: You are in a severe state of hormonal imbalance that has potentially dangerous consequences. One day your estrogen goes sky-high, one day it's low, one day your progesterone levels are off the charts, and the next day they are nonexistent. Perimenopause is about hormonal surges. It's these surges that are causing new, unexplained weight gain. It's these surges that are causing mood swings. It's these surges that can set the stage for cancer, as you'll learn later in this chapter.

Perimenopause marks the beginning of hormonal decline, and with hormonal decline comes withdrawal symptoms. These symptoms vary in severity from woman to woman, but unexplained feelings, emotions, hot flashes, sleeplessness, lack of sex drive, weight gain, and irritability are all part of the pro-

cess. The falling hormones you experience in perimenopause are the opposite of what you experienced
as you entered puberty, yet there are parallels. Back
then, your hormones were building up to get you
ready to be a reproductive person. Remember all the
crazy feelings you had inside you? Remember that
lack of understanding you had when you would
suddenly break into tears or that teenage rage that
seemed so inappropriate? Except now, in perimenopause, the situation is reversing, so on the way down
you are going to experience the same emotional and
physical havoc that you experienced when your hormones first started building up. It's no fun.

You must understand that in perimenopause you're
running nearly on empty. That's why you don't feel
"right." As author T. S. Wiley explains, "You still
have just enough estrogen to make a thin lining in
your uterus and cause unopposed hormonal growth
elsewhere in your breasts and body, but not enough
to cause an estrogen peak. That's why your periods
are getting shorter and shorter, your breasts lumpier
and lumpier, and your mind far less agile. The fact
that you don't peak estrogen with any regularity anymore, and you haven't since your late twenties, is the
hallmark of perimenopause."

As fully reproductive women, we make enough estrogen each month so that it reaches its peak on the
twelfth day, stops the growth of cells, and makes
progesterone receptors. Without an estrogen peak,
your brain can't send the signal to release any of the

eggs you have left. T. S. Wiley further says, "With no peak of estrogen, there's no feedback information to shut off follicle-stimulating hormone, so FSH pours constantly, overstimulating your ovaries and ripening all at once most of the eggs you have left. The loss of this rhythm in perimenopause actually triggers the destruction of the rest of your eggs through the action of excessive FSH, using up the remainder of your eggs. At about this time, you begin to feel the heat of hot flashes. That's how the system effectively shuts itself down for good. This process can take a decade."

You can find out whether you've gone from perimenopause to actual menopause by having your FSH blood tested. An FSH score higher than 5 is the clinical diagnosis of menopause. So have your blood work done and ask your doctor what your FSH score is. You can stop the destruction, essentially achieve feedback, and shut off FSH with estrogen replacement.

Having no more eggs means having no more estrogen, a situation that, of course, leads to no more progesterone either. Since you've stopped regularly producing the small amount of progesterone that you would from a normal menstrual cycle, and there's no steady increase of it either (that is, you're not pregnant), nature "thinks" that you're back in "adrenarche," the increase in activity of the adrenal glands just before puberty. Because your estrogen is so low and you're producing even more testosterone than before, thanks to your sleeplessness, the pubertal picture is complete.

Wiley goes on to say, "After we reach thirty, nature identifies falling (low) estrogen and higher than normal (rising) testosterone as the beginning . . . again. This is a perfectly reasonable conclusion on the part of nature. You must be in adrenarche, because nature knows no other template for not ovulating except pregnancy and lactation . . . unless, of course, you're a man. Now nature tries to send you on your way to puberty. Only it can't. The whole point of puberty is to get you to the next level of existence . . . ovulation. There's the hitch. That developmental milestone takes eggs, and we don't have any. It's too late to start puberty again, but the outcome of puberty, a normal rhythm of estrogen and progesterone in youthful quantities, is something you can achieve with natural hormone replacement. You can try to fool nature by covering the fact that you're missing eggs if you replace the hormones that they would generate in exactly the amounts and rhythm in which they would occur."

The important thing to remember is that when you are in perimenopause, you have almost no eggs left, which means you no longer have much estrogen left, either. This is an uncomfortable place to be. Without estrogen, we can't think, we can't control our body temperature, we can't sleep well, we have no protection for our heart, and among many other things, we lose our sex drive. There is simply no sexual feeling. It's as though the motor has died. Most women are mortified to admit this. And really, no one has to know, right? We can still "do it," but there is no sensation and no pleasure. Any participation on our part is a loving gesture. We can enjoy the closeness; but without any feeling, it is actually more pleasurable to read a magazine.

This is the unfair part. At this point in life, our men (if they are around the same age) are at their virile peak. They would like to have sex every day and more than once if they can. How can we keep up with them? How long can we go on participating in this intimate activity without getting any pleasure? Add the lack of pleasurable feelings to the fact that without estrogen there is no lubrication, so sex can be uncomfortable, or it can hurt. Additionally, yeast infections and other conditions take hold because of the imbalance that is going on in our bodies.

Testosterone levels fall significantly throughout perimenopause and menopause and will affect desire from an early age. Circulating levels of testosterone play an important role in the psychological and sexual changes that occur in menopause. That's why women respond positively when testosterone is added to their hormone replacement program. Testosterone helps with problems such as fatigue, poor concentration, depression, inability to have an orgasm, and lack of sex drive.

You have to understand that hormonal imbalance is a dangerous place to be. It is in hormonal imbalance that disease can proliferate. Here is a scenario that I am going to be explaining over and over in this book, because it is very important for you to understand the "nature" in you: The brain considers a fully reproductive woman to be a valuable member of the species. Remember, there really is one reason we are all here (biologically speaking), and that is to reproduce, to keep the species going. When we are reproductive, we make a full complement of hormones. There are no surges and no imbalances. Everything is working perfectly. Each month, we are capable of making a baby; whether we choose to do so or not is up to us and nature. But when we are in hormonal **imbalance,** the brain thinks "aha, this person is amiss. The hormones are leaving her body, meaning she is no longer making a full complement of hormones. Therefore, this woman is no longer capable of making a baby due to loss of eggs." The brain now wants to eliminate you because you are no longer a productive member of the species, since we are here only to reproduce so that the species can perpetuate itself, according to biology.

Now, of course, with today's advancements in medicine and technology, we know this is not the end but the beginning of the second half. But the brain doesn't know this. The brain knows only that this body is no longer working properly. The hormones that nourish and regenerate the organs and all parts of the body are missing. Here is where it gets dangerous: Cancer, viruses that live in all of us, and other diseases are allowed to proliferate. This is why when a woman hits age fifty, she has a one in seven chance of contracting cancer. She didn't wake up one morning and find cancer in her breast. It started years ago in **perimenopause,** during the first throes of hormonal imbalance, when the disease that was hanging around inside her body had an opportunity to grow.

Disease doesn't develop when hormones are in perfect balance. It doesn't need to. There is no reason to grow a new "self" (cancer) when everything is in balance. For this reason, you need to take perimenopause seriously. Don't count on your doctor, either. You have to remember that until the medical establishment catches up, we of this generation are on our own. Unless he or she is one of the cutting-edge doctors, your doctor most likely knows nothing about hormones, perimenopause, or menopause. Your emotional complaints will probably be met with pats on the back, antidepressants, and sleeping aids. At the moment, that is all most of our doctors know how to do. As I have said many times before, it's not their fault; they were not taught in medical school. But I have to say, I am losing a little patience and am getting tired of defending their ignorance in this area. Let me ask you this: If you were an MD, an OB/GYN, or an endocrinologist, and there was so much chatter about bioidentical hormone replacement therapy, wouldn't you by now have made it your business to find out about it, read up, and take courses to keep up with the times? With all the negative information out there on synthetic hormones, with the alarming reports from the Women's Health Initiative relative to synthetic hormones, with all the complaints from female patients, I have to say I find it shocking that most doctors in this country are still prescribing synthetic hormones and telling women to use them only as long as it is necessary and then get off them.

Now that you know how important it is to replace hormones with bioidentical hormones, not for a short while but for the rest of your life, you can see how uninformed a doctor has to be relative to the importance of hormone replacement to put you on synthetics and then say get off them as soon as these nasty symptoms subside. This means that this doctor doesn't have a clue as to the importance of hormones. Hormones are what make us run; without them we die. In fact, if you look up **death,** it will say "loss of hormones."

Without hormones, there is no quality of life. Try not sleeping for days or months on end (remember, sleep deprivation has been used as a form of torture in times of war), and see how you feel. Try having no working internal thermostat so that your body is in a constant state of "high" all the time, and see how you like sweating. It's both embarrassing and uncomfortable. This is just the tip of the iceberg. Any doctor who tells you to "tough it out" is doing you a disservice. It means he or she doesn't get what's happening to you while in perimenopause. Run, don't walk, from this doctor. You can continue to go to him or her for your other needs, but when it comes to hormones, you want someone who is knowledgeable and sympathetic.

Here's something else about what happens hormonally in perimenopause: When estrogen rises without progesterone (in other words, your estrogen is surging higher and higher but with no progesterone to create the right rhythm), this elevation turns off a powerful cellular growth controller called epidermal growth factor (EGF-1 and EGF-2). This particular growth factor is the major player in HER2-neu breast cancer. You need the estrogen rising to high enough levels (in other words, to reach an estrogen peak and then cascade down as it does in nature) to turn off the EGF-1 and EGF-2, or you may end up with cancer. A simpler way to explain this is to understand that imbalanced hormones are at the root of cancer. When you are in perimenopause, your natural rhythm is off; that is why perimenopause is a dangerous time for women.

By the time a woman is in her late forties, she has spent anywhere from ten to twenty years in this hormonal confusion. Most women go from doctor to doctor during perimenopause with myriad complaints. Everything gets treated—from her allergies, to backaches, to depression, to weight gain, to headaches and migraines, to sleeplessness and a hundred other maladies—with some form of drug treatment.

The drugs are Band-Aids, taking away the symptoms but never addressing the underlying causes. Rarely does a woman find a doctor who actually realizes what is really happening.

The real problem is hormonal loss. The sooner you start putting back what you've lost hormonally, the better you will feel. It's never too early. If you are low, you're low. But you will have to drive this train. No one is going to do this for you. This is your life. Start now. Perimenopause is a call to action. Your body is starting to shout at you. It wants help. Please listen, hear the call, and save yourself.

When I discussed this potentially dangerous stage of life with T. S. Wiley, she told me perimenopause is problematic because as far as the brain is concerned, women are hormonally in first-trimester pregnancy range. The specific hormone ratios of early pregnancy are insulin (high) and estrogen (low) and thyroid (functioning). These levels are mimicked in perimenopause. This hormonal environment triggers fetal oncogenes to start flipping on, and oncogenes contribute to the production of a cancer. However, perimenopausal women are stranded with no source of progesterone to give the growth or death command (of the cells) to turn those same genes off, because they don't have enough estrogen to peak in order to ovulate anymore with any regularity, and there's no placenta on board. Without the progesterone from the remains of an empty egg sac, their low chronic estrogen is never turned off, either. The state they are in is now life-threatening. This is the backdrop for cancer.

Take perimenopause seriously!

The good news is that bioidentical hormone replacement therapy can rectify the entire scenario of perimenopause. It's a little tricky and will need constant tweaking from your doctor because of your surging hormones. But a good, qualified doctor will know how to handle this. Stress will change your hormone levels, and the fact that the surges come and go will change your hormone levels. This is the exciting part of this new medicine, however. When you are working with your doctor to balance your hormones during this tricky phase, you should call when you have even the smallest symptom, because every symptom is an indicator that things are not in balance . . . and balance is the goal.

MENOPAUSE

Actually, menopause should be called egglessness! You're out of eggs! Once you hit menopause, you're in serious hormone decline. Hormone decline is exactly that: a decline **in you.** You cease to be the vital, vibrant person you have been. It's as though your soul gets sucked out. Women start to experience a variety of symptoms—if you have read **The Sexy Years,** then you know I call them "the seven dwarfs of menopause": Itchy, Bitchy, Sweaty, Sleepy, Bloated, Forgetful, and All-Dried-Up.

When all seven dwarfs (or even a few of them) come knocking on your door, it takes away your quality of life. But that's not all. Have you ever wondered what is going on inside you as your hormones are draining out? That's the scary part. Symptoms are only one part of this scenario—the big problem is that you don't feel the effects of internal hormone loss and the havoc it is beginning to wreak on your heart and other bodily systems until much later. There is no way to know if a cancer is forming in your breast, or lung, or brain, or ovaries.

Every woman experiences this passage differently. Some have an easier time than others, but I have noticed—and this is my own unscientific observation—that high-powered successful women often have a harder time of it than others, although there are always exceptions. I know of one woman, for example, who was a major player in the fashion world. Internationally known and respected, she was at the top of her game, with her designs in all the major fashion magazines. Then menopause hit. This woman "took to her bed," as they say in the South— and I mean **literally.** She doesn't come out of her bedroom. She doesn't bathe. She doesn't fix her hair or put on makeup, whereas she used to wear the most beautiful fashion makeup. She has gained a tremendous amount of weight. She is depressed and angry. She yells at her husband as though he's the cause of all her problems. This behavior has gone on for a number of years, and now her husband is leaving her for a younger woman. I don't believe they would have ever broken up had this not happened. I used to see them all the time, and they were in sync, happy, and creative together.

I feel so bad for her because it was all caused by a lack of understanding of the hormonal system, ignorance on the part of her doctor, and her inability to talk about her problems with someone who could have steered her to the proper doctor. Unfortunately, after a while a woman like this who doesn't get a handle on her hormone problems becomes too difficult for others to be around. That's the lonely part.

When I was a girl, women were routinely sent away to sanitariums "for their own good" when these violent reactions to hormonal loss occurred. Just think of all the poor women who were "put away" because of menopause and the lack of understanding. They were drugged, and most of them never came out. This is a big part of why our mothers never spoke to us about this passage. They didn't want to draw attention to the fact that they could no longer sleep, that they were depressed, and that their insides were screaming to be heard. They remained silent, because to be vocal could mean you'd end up in the loony bin; so they "toughed it out." Women of my mother's era got fat and lost their shape, they accepted their sexless lives, and they all lived in a place of silent desperation . . . just getting through each day the best they could.

A woman who is having a violent reaction to loss of hormones can become truly suicidal, or worse— she can even kill another human being. It happens. Look at Andrea Yates. She killed her five children. Perhaps it was schizophrenia, or another mental illness, or the tremendous hormonal drain of progesterone after five babies that created her delusions. If her doctors had been more in tune and understood hormones and their effects, they might have blood tested her; and if, in fact, it was low progesterone, they might have been able to save the lives of those children by putting this woman on hormone replacement until she normalized. I know this is an extreme example, but our bodies do respond in dramatic ways to hormonal change during and after pregnacy, perimenopause, and menopause. This is a tough passage, and women need help, but so far it hasn't been there for them. The times, they are a-changin', though. We are mad as hell, and we are not going to take it anymore!

Yes, I realize there will always be the woman who sails through menopause and hardly notices it. I have a hard time believing that, but let's say that woman exists here and there. They are the exceptions, and most likely these are women who have high human growth hormone levels for longer. You learned all about this remarkable hormone in the previous chapter. The rest of us have to white-knuckle this passage without assistance. Bioidentical hormone replacement therapy can make menopause the best time of your life. I know because I am living it.

In my search to get to the bottom of this very difficult passage called menopause, bioidentical hormone replace therapy came like a godsend to me. For the first time in my adult life, I was truly balanced. When your body is working at optimum, the internal concert sings in tune. You can feel it, and once you have felt this way, nothing else will do. We have come to accept the aches and pains and illnesses and stiffness as part and parcel of aging. But we don't have to.

Once you understand the benefits of restoring your body to its healthiest prime through balance, I can't imagine you won't want to go the bioidentical way. While you get to feel good again, BHRT also heads off disease at the pass. It's such a blessing. So many women have accepted the decline in quality of life as unchangeable, and that is extremely sad. Their emotions and bodies are out of control, and they learn to white-knuckle each day. Life is not meant to be endured; it is to be enjoyed. But how can you enjoy it when you feel awful all the time?

Hormone replacement is really pretty simple; unfortunately, the medical community is still having trouble grasping it. The good news is that, as outlined in this book, many, many doctors are now beginning to get an understanding, and some of them are in full grasp of the necessity to replace what has been lost in the aging process. What a difference this will make in your life! All the feelings of loss of control over your body will dissipate when you are back in balance. As Dr. C. W. Randolph Jr. points out in his book **Hormone Hell, Hormone Well**: "If you replace what is missing, your body will work better." It's that simple.

As time goes by, you will be able to understand your own hormonal needs, and your doctor will encourage you to dose up your estrogen a little or lower your progesterone or other variants. You will figure out what your body needs through trial and error. I know that I need massive amounts of estrogen to feel good and be in a happy mood. My body doesn't like a lot of progesterone. It has taken me quite a while to figure out my "needs," but now that I have, I am not so reliant on my doctor. This is a good thing.

The more self-reliant you become, the easier it is to take care of yourself. Once I found the right balance for me, it was bliss. It still needs adjusting from time to time, depending upon my stress levels. That's just the way it is. Hormones fluctuate all the time. That is why the "one pill fits all" theory of synthetic hormones was such a joke. No woman's needs are the same as another's, and no woman takes the same amount all the time. Even when you find your blissful dosage, a world event like 9/11 will upset your balance, and you will have to be readjusted. A near

miss in a car will change your needs, as will an argument with your partner. Usually in a daily routine,
when one of these crises dissipates, your hormones
will settle down; but something like the death of a
loved one will change your needs significantly.

No matter what is going on in their day-to-day
lives, women are desperate for answers and solutions.
For the first time, their doctors have lost a little of
their luster. Whereas we used to listen to and respect
everything told us by our family physician, now we
stand back and question, or at least we should. Too
many of us have been patted on the back and told to
be good girls and take our pharmaceuticals. When
we complain of depression and weepiness, we are
given a prescription for an antidepressant. It shuts us
up and gives our doctors a solution. They are, after
all, very good people who want to help us. But antidepressants are not the answer for menopause. Once
doctors understand this, we will all be better off. The
answer is hormone balance, and it is worth it for you,
the patient, to be patient and do the work to get the
balance just right for your needs. Once you are in
balance, you won't be depressed.

Those doctors who "get it" know that the answer
lies in bioidentical hormones. Yet despite the fact
that there is sound scientific research and clinical
data to support the safety and efficacy of bioidenticals, this option for hormone replacement is still not
widely acknowledged as a safe and effective alterna-

tive treatment. Fortunately, there are several studies ongoing at the moment.

The Women's Health Initiative cost the medical community the faith of many women. Gone is the absolute trust we once had in our doctors. As with all negatives, maybe this ultimately will be a good thing. By losing faith in our doctors, women have been forced to be proactive about their health. We have been forced to find new cutting-edge doctors. We have been forced to understand that different doctors have different areas of specialization, and just as the "one pill fits all" therapy no longer flies, the one-stop doctor is no longer viable. For hormones, you want a doctor who has chosen to specialize in bio-identical hormone replacement therapy. Ask the doctor whether he or she prescribes BHRT; if the answer is no, move on. This is your life. This is your quality of life. The longer you wait, the more trouble you will be in. It's not a game; these are not passages to "tough out." By not replacing the lost hormones, you are signaling your body to wind down and age faster. Even if that doesn't bother you, understand that the "winding down" is going to be uncomfortable, painful, and lonely, and ultimately you will probably be very sick. But if you choose bioidentical hormones, plus a healthy lifestyle to support your quality of life, you'll be bursting with youthful energy and a great quality of life.

COMPOUNDING PHARMACIES

Compounding pharmacies are the best source for finding a doctor who specializes in bioidentical hormones. So many women write to me that there is not a doctor in their area who understands this way of treating BHRT. Your compounding pharmacy is where a doctor in your area will call to fill prescriptions. Usually your local pharmacist will be able to assist you in finding a doctor who understands real bioidentical hormone replacement.

As with so many things in life, it is important to understand that there are "cooks" and then there are "chefs." Likewise, some compounding pharmacists are better than others. To find a certified pharmacist near your home, access the following website: www.iacprx.org. Or contact the Menopause Institute at (877) 5menopause or www.menopauseinstitute.com.

CHAPTER 4

EFFECTS OF AGING

The nice thing about being senile is that you can hide your own Easter eggs.

We weren't expected to live this long. Seventy-five years ago, we did not have access to the technology we have today. Seventy-five years ago, sewage was a problem and antibiotics were not available. Surgery had not advanced to the point it has today. Seventy-five years ago, women routinely died at age forty and forty-five. Why? Because our purpose (biologically) as part of the human species is to reproduce.

Up until recently, women lived through their reproductive years and bore their children; then, as the internal hormonal faucets turned off after their childbearing years, so too did the internal protection that the hormones provided. That factor alone began to allow the diseases to take hold that are now taken for granted as diseases of aging: high blood pressure, angina, diabetes, heart problems and heart disease, arthritis, allergies, joint pain, senility that was a precursor to Alzheimer's disease, and, of course, cancer. Senility in particular was always seen as a part of aging. We all had our senile old aunts and uncles, and we accepted it, because we never realized that replacing estrogen and human growth hormone just might be the answer to keep our memories intact—and perhaps, as some researchers now suspect, the best way to ward off Alzheimer's disease. The bottom line is that all these diseases were simply not as prevalent then as they are today for the simple reason that we are living longer.

From the age of twenty-five, we all begin to experience gradual declines in our hormone production, causing a slowing down or decline in many of our normal bodily functions. If your hormones are not functioning properly, are unbalanced, or have been affected in any way, you may suffer some form of illness associated with aging. In fact, one of the diseases that can come from hormonal imbalance is breast cancer, which is now considered an epidemic. Many doctors and researchers feel that it has much to do with the chemicalization of women of our generation. We are the sickest women on the planet in this country, probably because of the amount of chemicals we knowingly and unknowingly ingest and the poor diets consumed by most Americans.

By contrast, French women are among the healthiest on the planet. They are not as plagued with cancer and menopausal symptoms as we are here in

America. They take fewer pharmaceutical drugs than we do, probably because they shop daily for fresh food and eat quality food. In Europe (France included) doctors first try to heal homeopathically and then prescribe pharmaceuticals as a last resort, plus they have been using bioidentical hormones for fifty years. In America we immediately go to pharmaceutical drugs for the slightest problem. We can now see that all these chemicals and drugs that we have taken and exposed ourselves to without thinking have been a prescription for disease. We are sick as a result, and getting sicker all the time. We have to stop this insanity now.

As men lose their hormones, they get grumpy and big bellies. They don't want to go out so much anymore. They start to check out. They lose vitality. Their muscles start to shrink. Along comes the risk for prostate cancer, which is the male equivalent to breast cancer. As their hormone levels decline, men begin to see a rise in their prostate-specific antigen (PSA) tests. A new theory, though one not shared by all doctors, is that putting back a man's lost hormones will quash prostate problems. It's worth looking into instead of the male nullification that the main prostate drug, Lupron, has to offer. In its life-debilitating effects, Lupron for men is similar to tamoxifen for women. Both mess with your hormones.

The change we notice in a man's energy is so normal as they age that we have come to accept this as the way it is, but the entire scenario can be rectified and reversed for men who choose hormone replacement. Men get to feel better, look better, have more energy, and build muscle. The benefits of BHRT to their hearts, brain, and ability to prevent cancer are astounding.

Lifestyle habits such as bad diet, lack of exercise, overuse of stimulants, stress, and smoking all elevate levels of insulin and will lead to increased risk of heart disease and cancer. The reason excessive body fat is linked to cancer is that elevated insulin levels cause excessive body fat, rapid cell growth, and an imbalance in every other hormone system of the body. When hormones are imbalanced, the possibility of abnormal cell division (cancer) increases.

For years, the medical profession advised people to eat a low-fat, high-carbohydrate diet. This advice has been problematic, however. You need fats in your diet. Real fats—butter, cream, sour cream, full-fat cream cheese, and olive oil—are essential building blocks for your cells. They are essential for the production of hormones, and hormones regulate normal cell division and keep your immune system functioning. Every cell in your body requires protein, fat, and carbohydrate to reproduce itself. Think about it: As human beings, we are a bundle of **cells reproducing.** That is how we stay alive. So does it make any sense to avoid one of the essential elements of the makeup of a cell? By avoiding fats, people were left defenseless against cancer-cell growth. Remember, abnormal division of cells is the definition of cancer.

So if you are avoiding one of the building blocks (fats) of the makings of a cell, there is no way a cell can reproduce properly. The low-fat movement was a big mistake, and it partly caused the alarming rise of cancers for those who adopted this way of eating. Yet today patients are still being advised to go off fats.

I see similar bad advice all the time in the treatment of diabetes as well. The standard advice to the diabetic is to avoid sugar, which is good advice, and to also avoid fat, which is incorrect advice. The correct advice for a diabetic (or anyone, for that matter) should be to avoid sugar and to avoid **fake** fats: trans fats, hydrogenated oils, and anything that comes in a bag or a box. These packaged foods are what I call "cancer in a box."

The body can't handle any more chemicals. This point is essential to understand for survival; it's that serious. Besides, what is better than butter, cream, or cheese? I think of all the years I ate margarine because I was trying to do something good for myself—what a waste! I always tell my readers to shop the periphery of the supermarket. That's where they keep the real food—meat, chicken, fish, dairy, fruits, and vegetables.

Although no one really knows where cancer comes from, whether it's diet or something else, the best prevention is to keep your hormones balanced. In fact, the doctors I have interviewed for this book all concur that the best prevention for the diseases of aging is balanced bioidentical hormone replacement. Think about it: Young people, with their full complement of hormones, rarely get cancer, heart disease, or Alzheimer's disease.

In this chapter, I don't want to delve into those diseases specifically, because you'll "hear" the doctors in this book talk about them and how they're related to hormonal loss. Mainly I want to talk about some of the effects of aging that you may be experiencing (and that I experienced): age-related conditions and illnesses like gastrointestinal (GI) problems, osteoporosis, and hysterectomy.

GI TRACT: WHY AM I BLOATED?

Bloating, bloating, bloating! Do you know one woman who doesn't complain about bloating? It starts around age forty. Your once flat stomach now looks like the Pillsbury Doughboy's. You feel that if someone stuck a pin in your stomach, all the air would come out. It is uncomfortable. Not only that, nothing fits when you are bloated, and bloating makes you look ten pounds heavier.

It is extremely important to understand that the GI tract can be healed, and eating well is the largest component of fixing the problem. With the help of a qualified doctor who specializes in the GI tract, you must identify the foods that you are allergic to. All of us have foods that we are unable to process. When you know what they are and avoid them, the problem begins to dissipate. There is a test you can take to help identify foods that offend you. If your doctor is not aware of this test, you can find information about it by going to Dr. Diana Schwarzbein's website at www.schwarzbeinprinciple.com.

Another major factor in GI problems is stress, which can partly be resolved through adequate sleep. Thus, if you can get eight to nine hours of sleep each night, you can go a long way toward ridding yourself of uncomfortable bloating. When you get a full night's sleep, the release of melatonin lowers your body temperature, and this, in turn, kills off the bad bacteria in your gut. Exercise (with the right type of exercise for your current metabolism) is also vital for relieving stress.

There are other measures you can take: Avoiding chemicals to self-medicate is helpful. It is also necessary to recolonize your intestines regularly and daily with acidophilus. The culture in acidophilus puts back the friendly flora and helps to restore balance. As you will read in Dr. Prudence Hall's chapter, she first gets the "bugs" out of the intestinal tract before she recolonizes. Recently I had to take antibiotics, which in the past have always given me a yeast infection. This time I took acidophilus like candy, two and three times a day, and I never got a yeast infection.

If you are taking bioidentical hormones, it is important to take them correctly. (See chapter 5 for guidelines.) They should mimic your normal physiology, meaning that you are trying to replicate the hormones you made naturally in your younger years when you were completely balanced. If you remember, when you were young and balanced hormonally, bloating was not even an issue. It is not until we start losing our hormones in the aging process, coupled with a lifetime of antibiotics (unnecessary in so many cases), that the bacteria in the gut finally go on overload.

BONES AND OSTEOPOROSIS

It's pretty crazy that we don't realize that osteoporosis, a bone-thinning disease, is rectifiable and in some cases reversible with bioidentical hormone replacement. Think about it: Did you have weak and fragile bones when you were young? No! The reason you didn't is that your hormones were perfectly balanced. But hear this: Bone loss is not a condition that has to accompany middle to old age.

At menopause, we begin to worry about and even expect bone loss. Since most of us have already started to experience some bone loss at this point, our doctors order bone density tests. Osteoporosis is insidious because you can't see or feel what is happening. Most people who have the disease don't know it. And then a bone breaks.

Each year, half a million Americans wind up in the

hospital because of fractures related to osteoporosis.
Hip fractures, which represent about three hundred
thousand of that total, are devastating. One victim in
five dies within a year, and half are never able to live
independently again. Most of us know someone who
has suffered a hip fracture, but you may be surprised
to learn that complications of this injury kill even
more women every year than breast cancer. Preventing osteoporosis is really a life-and-death matter, like
preventing cancer and heart disease.

Hip fractures are just the most obvious part of
the problem. Millions of women suffer distressing
symptoms that they don't connect to fragile bones. A
woman may not realize that her chronic back pain
comes from little crush fractures in her spine. Ever
felt a shooting pain in your back as you bent to pick
up something? If you are experiencing bone loss,
each one of those sharp pains could be fractures happening in your spine. Fragile vertebrae can gradually
crumble under the ordinary stresses of everyday life.
Osteoporosis can make a woman look old before her
time. She may have no idea that her slumped posture
and protruding stomach are caused by fractures in
her spine. As a woman, your odds are one in three of
suffering from osteoporosis in your lifetime. You can
beat those odds through bioidentical hormone replacement given in the correct ratio and balance.

Osteoporosis affects women eight times more than
men. One in two women over age fifty will suffer at
least one lifetime fracture from osteoporosis. When

we run out of estrogen and progesterone, our bones start to die very quickly. Bones have their own life cycle or metabolism. According to author T. S. Wiley, "A rhythm of growth and death governed by estrogen and progesterone is the falloff of estrogen in perimenopause, which means there is no peak of estrogen activity to make progesterone receptors that would build bone. This is the beginning of osteoporosis."

She goes on to say: "Estrogen controls osteoclast activity. Osteoclasts are bone cells that eat up old bone for disposal. Progesterone controls osteoblastic activity. Osteoblasts are bone cells that build fresh new bone. Progesterone, in this case, grows bone, and estrogen takes it away so that new bone can grow again next month. Without this balanced interplay, one of two things can happen: Without estrogen, bone would overgrow into a cancerlike state, or without progesterone, unopposed estrogen [taking estrogen only every day] would make bones thin, fragile, and porous . . . in other words, osteoporotic."

This process gets confusing. Estrogen is prescribed for menopausal women, and it does help with osteoporosis for a little while because it prevents apoptosis—that is, the birth, death, and rebirth of cells. (A good way to understand apoptosis is through our monthly periods: We build a lining, slough off a lining [bleed], and then rebuild a lining again for next month, in hopes of making a baby. Every cell in our body goes through this apoptosis every month.) However, estrogen prevents apoptosis in the bone-building cells, the osteoblasts. Unless progesterone comes in to **stimulate** osteoblasts, not much bone grows from estrogen replacement alone.

Basically, it is the decline in three hormones—estrogen, progesterone, and testosterone—and not just estrogen, that causes bones to become thinner and more brittle. Evidence suggests that bioidentical hormone replacement therapy can help slow down osteoporosis, and in some cases, it will reverse bone loss in women. Ten years ago, I was experiencing bone loss. Today, after a decade of replacement, I have reversed the loss. With a full BHRT regimen, including HGH, bone loss reversal is possible for most women.

Unfortunately, though, there are two synthetic drugs given to women with osteoporosis: Fosamax and raloxifene. Fosamax prevents the osteoclasts from doing their job of breaking down bone. There are no long-term studies on Fosamax, but a drug that interferes with the cycle of bone growth can't be good. It is not natural. It is a drug.

Raloxifene blocks estrogen in an attempt to slow down bone degradation. Its side effects are similar to those of tamoxifen, including menopausal hot flashes and vision changes.

Bioidentical hormone replacement can do what none of the drugs can do: revive your bones. In other words, taking bioidentical hormones in the correct ratio and rhythm prevents osteoporosis. That's all we want. Other crucial ways to keep strong, healthy bones include exercising, light weight lifting, and following a healthy diet. Calcium helps some, but taking vitamin D with your calcium can affect you dramatically. Vitamin D is needed to absorb calcium and turn it into bone.

Men are also prone to osteoporosis, and an estimated 2 million men already have this disease. In fact, a man is more likely to suffer an osteoporosis-related fracture during his lifetime than he is to get prostate cancer. Most men, and even their doctors in some cases, are unaware of this problem.

Low testosterone levels are responsible for about half the cases of osteoporosis in men. When a man shows symptoms of low testosterone—low libido, decreased facial and body hair, enlarged breasts—it's time to get his bones checked. There are many men who have low testosterone with no symptoms at all, however. But the point is that hormonal stimulation and balance are just as important for men's bones as it is for women's.

Men with a light frame and low body weight, as well as men with eating disorders, are particularly at risk for osteoporosis. So are competitive athletes in sports with weight classifications. Anyone who has been a yo-yo dieter or had anorexia or bulimia is at a higher risk for osteoporosis. Other risk factors for men and women are inactivity, high alcohol consumption, and smoking (current or past).

But the big answer to osteoporosis is bioidentical

hormone replacement therapy. There is nothing that can build and revive bones like real hormones.

HYSTERECTOMY

Do you realize that more than 1 million hysterectomies are performed each year? Now that I am among these statistics—my uterus was removed in February 2005—it makes me wonder how many of these operations are really necessary. Do 1 million women really **need** to have a body part or parts removed? Is that what nature intended?

A hysterectomy is the option that most physicians commonly recommend for women who have fibroid tumors, severe endometriosis, cancer, or constant heavy bleeding. A complete hysterectomy involves surgical removal of the entire reproductive tract, including the uterus, tubes, ovaries, and cervix. According to Dr. Randy Randolph, "Unfortunately, up to 90 percent of the time a woman's pelvic organs will be removed for benign disease that could have been treated by nonsurgical approaches." Ninety percent!

It's unbelievably sad that so many women of any age have complete hysterectomies without being told that their bodies will immediately enter menopause as a result. If hysterectomy is necessary (and there are circumstances when hysterectomy is definitely necessary), a woman needs to be informed as to all the ramifications of removing a body part. So many women are led down this path, trusting their doctors. Worse, they're often told, "As long as we're in there, we might as well remove your ovaries and cervix; that way you'll never have to worry about ovarian or cervical cancer." What a crock!

Here is where you have got to do your homework, ladies. Unless you find a doctor who really understands bioidentical hormone replacement and puts back the hormones in a template the brain understands, you can be a serious candidate for these cancers that the removal was supposed to correct. Here's why: No ovaries, no cervix, no uterus, and you are no longer a reproductive woman. I'm sure by now that in reading this book, you know the serious consequences when the brain no longer recognizes you as reproductive.

The job of the brain is to send signals to the rest of the entire system (the body) that all is well. When a full complement of hormones is running through our systems and all the hormones are talking to one another in their unique and brilliant language, the brain recognizes this person as reproductive. The moment the hormones start to decline, it is a signal to the brain that things are amiss and that this person does not have the capacity to reproduce. Then gradual shutdown happens.

Because estrogen and progesterone have bottomed out, the immune system revs up so high that it starts attacking the cartilage and other tissues. This can result in stiff joints, weakened bones, arthritis, and even cancer of the bones. The immune system also attacks the mucous membranes, leading to runny, watery eyes, allergies, sinus problems, and infections, among other symptoms. Without estrogen and progesterone (made in the ovaries, which you no longer have), a host of other symptoms begins to occur. One of these is high blood pressure, though it is just the beginning. Other symptoms can include anxiety, sleeplessness, unbelievable itching, skin rashes, fungus infections, hot flashes, night sweats, depression, weepiness, irritability, foggy thinking, bloating, weight gain, no—and I mean **no**—sex drive, and obvious physical aging: wrinkling, shrinking, and a tired-looking body. As a result of this radical removal of a woman's organs, the body goes into a kind of shock.

The problem is that most women do not have it spelled out to them like this. If it were, believe me, 1 million women wouldn't volunteer to walk into that operating room every year.

I'm sorry, but the lack of knowledge and insensitivity of doctors who think that by removing organs unnecessarily, they are protecting women from cancer is truly disturbing! I will not even venture to think that somewhere in this scenario is a financial gain. Let's hope that has not been a factor.

By having their organs removed unnecessarily, women are not only not protected but they are also left wide open for other cancers, heart disease, and

Alzheimer's. I choose to truly believe that doctors are doing the best they can with the information they have on hand. Unfortunately, many of them don't know enough anymore about our changing bodies in a changing world. You must know this and get more than one opinion when you are dealing with something as serious as your own body.

When a woman has a complete hysterectomy, so many doctors make the mistake of prescribing only estrogen. This is a recipe for disaster. If the hormones prescribed are also synthetic and not bioidentical, then forget it. Trouble lies ahead.

Estrogen alone can foster estrogen dominance. When this occurs, it can be very dangerous for the body. After a complete hysterectomy, a woman's body will need a new and balanced supply of **all** her sex hormones: estrogen, progesterone, and testosterone. Remember, they took out your ovaries and cervix. The sex hormones are made in the ovaries. If you don't replace these hormones, what do you think is going to happen to your body? Many doctors feel that without a uterus, you no longer need progesterone because you are never going to have a period again. But the **brain** needs the progesterone. Don't forget: You now have to "trick" your brain into believing you still have your body parts. Without progesterone, reproduction is impossible, and you know what that means. Besides, it's about the correct ratio. Estrogen needs to be balanced by progesterone. That is how your body did it when you were young and still making a full complement. Without a uterus, without ovaries, without tubes, and without a cervix, you need to refill the tank daily with the hormones that were all a part of your female process. Although you have now been "castrated," you can still fool the brain into believing you are intact.

Do not let them take body parts unless there is no other recourse. Do read up and learn how your body works so you can ask the right questions. If you must have part of you removed, do not let them take your ovaries or cervix unless there is cancer. This is important. Most often, the only reason to remove your ovaries and cervix is to remove cancer.

I believe my condition required removal of my uterus. I have no regrets over it. My doctor and I felt we had no other recourse. I certainly didn't want cancer again. But be cautious. Question and read. Go forward only if you feel sure. It costs a lot more to do a hysterectomy than to replenish lost hormones with bioidentical ones. Hysterectomy is big business. Imagine: 1 million hysterectomies a year! Imagine the profits!

Hysterectomy is life-saving when cancer is present. You have no choice. But do know that you can put yourself back together again after removal with hormones in the right template. Loss of your female organs does not have to be the end of your life as you know it. You can be put back together again, but make sure you are with a knowledgeable doctor.

According to Dr. Randy Randolph, "I believe that

every gynecologist should make it standard protocol to attempt to intervene medically before reaching for a knife. I first try treating my patients with non-invasive measures, including bioidentical hormone therapy. Often, I find that these nonsurgical interventions prove successful in shrinking fibroid tumors, reducing uterine bleeding, and improving pelvic pain. Surgical intervention is always my last resort."

That's the kind of doctor to look for: forward-thinking doctors who are trying to save your body parts.

Incidentally, "hysterectomy" comes from the word **hysterical.** Unfortunately, when hormones are not put back correctly after a hysterectomy, a woman often becomes hysterical. Life quality goes downhill, and it is not gradual. It happens immediately.

Now here's another thing: Artificial menopause can also occur as a result of radiation or chemotherapy or by the administration of certain drugs that catalyze menopause (such as to shrink fibroid tumors). Dr. Randolph points out, "Because there is no opportunity for gradual adjustment to the hormonal drop-off, the symptoms of artificial menopause can be sudden, severe, and debilitating, requiring an immediate intervention of supplemental hormone therapy."

There is no expendable body part or "accidental" organ. We were given all of them for a reason. A woman's female organs serve many purposes beyond reproduction. Remember that the ovaries play a crucial role in producing the sex hormones long after your reproductive years. Estrogen, progesterone, and testosterone are produced in the ovaries and play a huge role in maintaining your health, vitality, and sex drive.

Removal of the uterus is downplayed, as though "you're not going to miss it," but the uterus and cervix (the tip of the uterus) serve a purpose beyond housing a fetus in pregnancy. They also provide an ongoing blood supply to the ovaries through the uterine artery. When this artery is cut, blood flow to the ovaries reduces the production of hormones.

The uterus has another role within the body that shouldn't be overlooked: It contributes and intensifies a woman's sexual pleasure. Dr. Randolph says, "During sexual intercourse, penetration can stimulate uterine contractions. The consequent rhythmic response has been found to contribute to an enhanced feeling of sexual pleasure. Many women report that after removal of their uterus, they experience less satisfying orgasms."

Dr. Randolph's point is serious, and any woman facing hysterectomy should give it a lot of thought. As I said, if it's cancer, then you have no choice. But if you can try to correct the problem with hormone replacement, that is always the best way to go at first.

Fibroids, heavy and endless bleeding, endometriosis, and unrelenting pelvic pain are symptoms that can change the quality of your life. These are the other reasons for hysterectomy, but first try to treat the problem noninvasively. If you do not respond to natural treatments, at least weigh your options and know the consequences and ramifications of hysterectomy. You don't want to be sorry later on.

Keep in mind that we live in a society where Western medicine is disease-oriented, meaning that we wait for the disease to take hold and then treat the disease. Fortunately, cutting-edge medical thinking urges us to start living a healthy life as early as we become informed and to focus concentration on staying well so that we live in an optimal "well state" and disease and other effects of aging do not have to be a part of our future.

CHAPTER 5

BIOIDENTICAL HORMONES AND AGING

Getting old is when getting a little action
means you don't need fiber today.

Aging can be difficult. But it doesn't have to be. Bioidentical hormone replacement makes aging and its stages simply "passages," and enjoyable ones at that. When your hormones are replaced in perfect balance, you look, feel, and act younger, plus you are protected against some of the worst diseases and effects of old age.

"Bioidentical" means biologically identical to human hormones—exact replicas of what we make in our own bodies. Made from soy, wild yam, and other plant extracts, bioidentical hormones are synthesized in a lab to exactly replicate human hormones. Bioidentical hormones are not drugs, however. They are completely different from synthetic hormones, which are made from the urine of pregnant mares and have nothing to do with what we make in our own bodies. In times past, your doctor would simply give you a prescription for Premarin or Prempro—a one-pill-fits-all type of regimen—and tell you to have a nice life. On these synthetic hormones, you would get fat and/or have brittle bones, lose your sex life, and get depressed and bloated, among other symptoms. Great, huh?

These synthetic hormones are not hormones; they are drugs that have been proven to be harmful to our health by creating hormonal imbalances. Synthetic hormones do not replace lost hormones. Instead, they simply cover up some of the nastier symptoms of menopause and other issues related to aging. Remember, hormonal imbalance is an opportunity for disease to proliferate, especially cancer. This is why synthetic hormones are dangerous to our health. It's not just me saying this; read for yourself the Women's Health Initiative 2002 and get backup for this statement.

Again I say this: I am not against pharmaceuticals. I willingly take drugs as a last resort when necessary, and any of us who have gone through a major illness know the blessings of pharmaceuticals. But when it comes to hormones, I believe (and many doctors concur) that the pharmaceutical companies are working against us. According to Dr. C. W. Randolph Jr., "The big drug companies have twisted and manipulated the idea of hormone replacement to capitalize on a business opportunity."

For background, synthetic hormone replacement started fifty years ago, even though bioidentical hormones existed. This was the first tragedy for women. By 1970, HRT was a common term. We didn't know about bioidentical hormones because no drug company was interested in them: They were not patentable (because they were natural). Without a patent, there was no profit. As women started to live longer, the drug companies knew they would have female customers waiting in the wings. And were we ever . . . we would take anything so the hot flashes would stop, so sleep would come back as a nightly event, so the depression and weepiness from lack of sleep would subside. "Oh yes," we said. "Give them to us." So we started downing these synthetic hormones and exclaimed for all to hear that we felt great again. (Well, relatively.) At least the hot flashes calmed down. At least we were sleeping pretty well. But why were we getting fat? Must be part of aging, we surmised. We accepted high blood pressure as part of aging; we accepted breast and ovarian cancer as simply the unlucky lottery. We all prayed we wouldn't end up a statistic of those dreaded diseases.

The drug companies were ecstatic. Oh boy, these were expensive prescriptions that a woman would take for **life!** Yippee! What a financial bonanza! Then came the baby boomers . . . they were really going to need hormones, because this group had decided to outwork their parents. Yep, this was a stressed-out group. Hooray . . . another bonanza for the drug companies. After all, stress blunts hormone production, and we were not going to change our stressful lifestyles. It got even better for the drug companies. Younger and younger women were running out of hormones because of their stressed-out lifestyles. "Superwomen" we called them. This meant more revenue for the pharmaceutical companies. We baby boomers decided early on that we wanted more: a better life, so our children could have all the things that we never had—TVs in their rooms, all the toys you could dream of, swimming pools, and private schools.

As we baby boomers entered this passage, we willingly downed our synthetics. We didn't even give it a thought. After all, we were well introduced into the world of chemicals. Chemicals were in our food. We had already embraced fake food and fast food filled with chemicals. We thought nothing of taking our synthetic birth control pills. They told us the pills were safe, and we believed them (by the way, who are "they"?). We decided to not breast-feed our babies. What were we thinking? Breast-feeding is nature's antidote to immunizing our babies and ourselves from the destiny we are now experiencing. Lactation and the production of prolactin are natural wonders, but we decided it would be better to have careers. Gloria Steinem (well-meaning though she was) told us so. We burned our bras, and we had fewer children. Some of us waited so long that we destroyed all chances of conceiving. But we had big careers and big houses, and our children had everything they ever dreamed of.

Over the decades, the pharmaceutical industry touted the praises of synthetic HRT as the female fountain of youth. From a business perspective, the drug companies were winning, but we were losing big-time. But then the double nature of synthetic HRT started to be exposed. What was happening to us? By 2002, breast cancer was an epidemic. Statistics changed dramatically. At the turn of the century, the statistics indicated that one in ninety-one women would get breast cancer. In 2002, the stats were one in eight. One in eight! Did you hear me? Why? What had changed?

Then came the really bad news. Mounting clinical evidence began to emerge that taking HRT long-term was dangerous because it manifested more chronic health problems. No one mentioned that these so-called hormones they were reporting as dangerous were **not** bioidentical, "real," natural hormones, but the deadly synthetic hormones being pushed on us by our doctors because of the influence of the pharmaceutical companies. In her book **The Hormone Solution,** Dr. Erika Schwartz says, "You must understand that it has been proven that once broken down in our bodies, conjugated equine (Premarin) becomes toxic to the very DNA that keeps us healthy or makes us sick."

So we women started getting sick . . . in greater and greater numbers, everything from breast cancer to autoimmune diseases, and we also started gaining weight. The new statistic on overweight adults in America is now 65 percent and rising.

Yet as I write today, doctors all over the country are still prescribing synthetic hormones. Why? Because most of the information the doctors receive is fed to them by the pharmaceutical companies. Very little instruction on hormone replacement and prescribing hormones is given to our physicians in medical school. There is no way for doctors to learn about another method unless they look outside the "standard of care" to find a better method, as the doctors interviewed in this book have done. No drug company is going to say about synthetic hormones, "Hey, this is dangerous stuff." No way. So for the last fifty years, the drug companies have been "pushing" the one-pill-fits-all regimen of HRT. They have ignored the fact that each woman's body has a genetically predetermined hormone balance that directs the interaction of all her sex hormones (estrogen, progesterone, testosterone, DHEA, and others) uniquely for her.

So here we are today, with recent clinical studies showing that synthetic HRT can be more harmful than helpful and can foster many long-term, and potentially terminal, health concerns. According to Dr. Randolph, "The pharmaceutical industry had misinformed physicians. If drug companies were truly patient advocates, they would educate the medical community about hormone testing and natural bioidentical hormone therapies."

But this is about business. I don't like it, but the pharmaceutical companies have a bottom line—a big bottom line, I might add. How can you blame them? Business does not have a conscience when so much money is at stake. A patented "one pill fits all" is a lot easier to distribute, and it is certainly much easier for the doctors.

By 2002, Wyeth-Ayerst's top-selling synthetic HRT drugs accounted for approximately 70 million prescriptions and $1 billion in yearly sales revenue. Even though it's such big business, women are suffering and dying from synthetic HRT. Instead of proving to be a safe and effective solution for women suffering from symptoms of hormone imbalance, synthetic hormones actually unlocked doors leading to health dangers. The problem with synthetic HRT is that it is not an exact fit for the human body's hormone receptor sites. It doesn't fit. Just like the glass slipper didn't fit Cinderella's evil sisters' feet, the "glass slipper" of synthetic hormones doesn't fit!

No wonder that in all the alarming reports on HRT, it is never mentioned in the media or in the actual studies themselves that they are talking only about synthetic hormones. These reports never strive to clarify the difference between synthetic and bioidentical hormones. They don't want us to know that something else exists; they don't want us to know about nonpatentable bioidentical hormones. But **you** must know the difference if you are to make an educated choice, and you must know the difference if you are to stay in the game and remain vital and healthy. This is your life we are talking about.

THE NATURAL SOLUTION

As consumers, our health is at stake. We must look outside the pharmaceutical protocols at safe, real hormone replacement. I cannot say enough about bioidentical hormones. They have changed my life and given it back to me. These hormones have allowed me to enjoy this passage better than any of the previous ones. Yes, I have some wrinkles, and I'm not twenty anymore, but I really don't care. I'm frisky and vital and energized. My brain is working perfectly, my health is great, my cholesterol is perfect, and my insulin levels are at optimum. I'm "the elder of my tribe," and I'm digging it. I have never had so much fun.

Thus, the beauty of bioidentical hormones is that they are natural hormones. You see, bioidentical hormones have a molecular structure that exactly matches the molecular structure of the hormones produced by the female body. According to Dr. C. W. Randolph:

Bioidentical hormones enter the bloodstream and look and perform just like the original hormones they were designed to replicate. Bioidentical hormones are molecular keys that the body can automatically recognize and utilize. In other words, bioidentical hormones are the perfect fit for a woman's genetic hormone receptor lock. When used for hormone replacement, bioidentical hormones enter the bloodstream, attach to their appropriate receptor locks, and safely and effectively reestablish optimum hormonal equilibrium. Bioidentical hormones replace what is missing so that the female body has what it needs to feel and perform the way it was originally designed.

I ask you, when the fit is this perfect, why would you take a drug when there is a nondrug exact-replica hormone exactly as your body once made?

WORKING WITH THE RIGHT DOCTOR

Replacing lost hormones is an art form and must be embraced not only by the patient, but by the doctor as well. You have to find the right doctor, and you have to find a doctor who is willing to put in the time it takes to achieve balance. Each person (women and men) has different needs.

As I explained in my book **The Sexy Years,** I started on my bioidentical hormone replacement therapy with my dear friend Dr. Diana Schwarzbein, a Western-trained endocrinologist who has dedicated herself to helping her patients achieve hormonal balance. I will always owe her a deep debt of gratitude for helping me turn my life around. She got me off sugar, and she taught me about the importance of keeping my adrenals intact. She taught me about the insulin connection and the effects of high cortisol. She taught me the importance of healing my metabolism. After the merry-go-round of going from doctor to doctor, I felt that I had finally found "home" when I sat in her office for the first time. Finally, here was a doctor who "gets it."

Through Dr. Schwarzbein, I discovered that the miserable existence I was experiencing was physical, not emotional, and that putting back the hormones I had lost in the aging process could alleviate my uncomfortable symptoms. Sure enough, within a short period of time I began to feel good again, and by the end of the year I felt wonderful—maybe better than I had ever felt in my adult life. (Incidentally, Dr. Schwarzbein is no longer taking patients but has decided to devote her time and energy to teaching other physicians the correct way to prescribe hormone replacement therapy.)

With bioidentical hormone replacement, your doctor may or may not take a blood test at first. If you are complaining about symptoms, it will be pretty evident to your doctor that by your age, you are in hormonal decline. After about three months, your doctor will take a blood test, approximate your hormone levels, and prescribe the same amount of estradiol every day of the month (this is referred to as "static dosing") and, on days 18 to 28, a static dose of progesterone to approximate what your body once made when you were making a full complement of hormones. At the end of each cycle will come a period. I discuss different forms of bioidentical hormone replacement in detail at the end of this chapter. The Menopause Institute is a good place to get set up with bioidentical hormonal replacement (see Resources, page 611).

Now, you've got to know that there's no free lunch. It's not as simple as taking your hormones every day; you must be attuned to your symptoms and your stresses. Exercise is a major component, the quality of the food you eat is important, the amount of food is crucial, plenty of sleep, fighting the environmental effects, and a happy life are all part of reversing the aging process.

So if you are considering bioidenticals or just starting to use them, remember that they require patience. You may make many phone calls to your doctor to complain of various symptoms, so he or she can tweak your dosage or the delivery system you use to take the hormones.

Here is a pretty serious example of what I am talking about: A woman I know is experiencing **severe** hormone loss. She calls me crying on a regular basis. She goes into a dark place, and the only way out for her is to contemplate suicide. I encouraged her to get to one of my doctors, in this case a gynecologist in L.A. who treats with BHRT. Some cases are tricky. This woman is now on bioidenticals, but in the beginning stages. She feels great for three weeks of the month, but when the week of her period comes around, she goes to that dark place where she wants to kill herself. She has no recollection of how good she has been feeling during the other three weeks. This darkness takes over, and the woman runs away—literally. Last month, she was found in a small town two hundred miles outside of Los Angeles but does not remember how she got there. Her husband then has to calm her **down** enough to get her to her doctor's office. While the answer to this instability is achieving the correct ratio between estrogen and progesterone, this patient is very "tricky" chemically, so it takes some time to get that ratio. Getting this woman regulated is possible, but her symptoms at present are so severe that there is worry she might not survive these dark phases. Her doctor hopes she will stay with it until she is regulated. Otherwise, she possibly faces a life of emotional pain and most likely antidepressants.

This case illustrates patience, especially when symptoms are this severe. But when you can't sleep night after night after night, you're sweating and hot flashing constantly, the result is depression and weepiness. How could you be anything else without sleep? And because you are not getting the proper sleep, your cortisol levels are sky-high, which in turn raises your insulin levels to the moon, and now you get fatter and fatter. That causes more depression, more weepiness.

The lack of sleep causes high insulin, which makes you crave processed carbs—cakes, pies, bread, cookies, chocolate—the only pleasures of the day. Eating carbs like this all the time can lead to diabetes. Incidentally, I've heard many doctors say that they would rather have cancer than diabetes; that statement should give you some insight into the dangers of high insulin and high cortisol.

Now are you getting the picture about the importance of replacing lost hormones?

Without patience you will get frustrated and probably walk away from all of it, but I am telling you the only loser in this will be you. I can't say it enough or in too many different ways: Without hormones your body begins to disintegrate. Without hormones the diseases of aging begin to take hold. It isn't normal to have high blood pressure. It isn't normal to have aching bones. It isn't normal to lose your sex drive. It isn't normal to have memory loss. It's normal only if you are no longer a reproductive person.

Once again: The idea of HRT is to "trick" the brain into believing that we are still functioning, reproductive beings. What? you say. That doesn't sound right—why trick our brains into anything?

Well, what do you think you are doing when you have heart bypass surgery or a hip replacement? You are "tricking" your body into believing that you still have a perfect heart or that your bones are still young and strong and not falling apart because of lack of hormones. If we weren't going to live so long, then let the chips fall; however, technology will keep us alive until we are ninety or a hundred years old. Don't you want quality of life for those years? Or do you want to be the one who is gradually disintegrating in front of everyone's eyes?

Bioidentical hormone replacement therapy offers extraordinary benefits for men and women, but the public remains shockingly ignorant about the readily correctable effects of diminishing hormones. The doctors in this book clearly distinguish between desirable bioidentical hormones and the thoroughly discredited side effect–prone synthetic versions. Working with a Western-trained antiaging doctor is the new way to develop and periodically reevaluate your hormonal needs. A doctor who understands can individually customize the dosages that are perfect for you in order to ensure optimal balance among all the various hormones.

That is the goal. When you find hormonal balance individualized just for you, your body sings. You will feel the best you have ever felt. That has been my experience and the experience of millions of my readers.

This balance doesn't come easily. If there were a

way to give you a sneak peek so you could feel what it is like at optimum, you would be more than willing to do the work to get there. A lot of people get impatient and give up too soon. It takes time to lose hormones, so it's going to take a little while to "tweak" until balance is reached. Your doctor can only approximate the dosage for you the first time based upon talking to you, then after a couple of months having your labwork done. Sometimes doctors get lucky, and the song begins immediately. Sometimes the song is off-key. Even though you are feeling better, you know it's not exactly right. That's when you want to start talking to your doctor about how you feel. It is important to be in tune with your symptoms. Remember those seven dwarfs: Itchy, Bitchy, Sweaty, Sleepy, Bloated, Forgetful, and All-Dried-Up.

Having symptoms like the seven dwarfs is an indicator that your system still needs tuning. But oh my, when all these symptoms go away, the result is heavenly. Here's a list of what to expect: energy, vitality, creativity, brainpower, strong heart, loss of wrinkles (yes, adequate amounts of estrogen plumps up the skin), perky breasts, a vagina that's moist and ready, renewed sexual desire, and sleeping through the night. Plus, you don't itch, and you aren't bitchy. You don't have hot flashes, so Sweaty says good-bye; and best of all, if you are eating correctly, your excess weight starts to melt away.

For men, your grumpiness dissipates. You get your

energy back. Your libido wakes up. You want to go out, have fun, and continue working. That fat around your belly now has a chance of going away, provided you are eating correctly and exercising in moderation. I will go into detail about men's hormonal needs in chapter 12.

Teenagers can also get relief from the mood swings and horrible cramping that accompany weight gain. Of course, they have to watch their carb intake, but many doctors I have talked to, like Dr. Erika Schwartz, believe in bioidentical hormones for teenagers who are heavy bleeders and victims of raging hormones.

Bioidentical hormone replacement therapy is a huge antiaging opportunity—the true fountain of youth that can keep your insides young. What a concept!

OPTIMAL REPLACEMENT

Once you are in the care of a good doctor who has chosen to specialize in bioidentical hormone replacement or a good antiaging doctor (there are referrals at the back of this book), you can get to work optimizing your entire hormonal system. First, your doctor will get rid of the uncomfortable symptoms from major and minor hormone loss. This is no small task. Again, it takes time and patience. The good news is that you will start feeling better almost immediately, but just know that the best is yet to come. Once you get there, you will want to continue with this type of medicine because you will realize just how joyous and vibrant life can be. You will never look longingly at the young people. In fact, my husband and I are often amused at the fact that most people are probably not making love on Saturday afternoons as we often do. Alan and I have completed our child rearing, and as hormonally balanced people, we are "in the mood" more often than not. It's a beautiful thing, and believe me, with what I know is going on in our home, I don't ever worry about younger beautiful women. In fact, I love being around them myself! They are having a great time, and so am I. They may have better skin, but I have wisdom. I prefer the trade-off.

When it comes to replacement, **optimal** is the operative word. So often a patient goes to his or her doctor and asks for a hormone panel (through blood work) to be done. When the results come back, he or she is told that everything is normal and there is nothing to worry about. "Normal" for what? "Normal" for a fifty- or sixty- or seventy-year-old person? You don't want normal for your age. A fifty- or sixty-year-old is in hormonal decline. Yet that is how most doctors treat their patients in this country. They figure if you are "normal" for your age, everything is okay.

Optimal, on the other hand, describes hormonal balance for a person who is much younger and at his or her healthiest prime. That's what you want—not hormones that are declining. The goal of bioidentical hormone replacement therapy is for you to enjoy vibrant good health throughout a long lifetime. This means that most of the standard reference ranges must be discarded in favor of optimal ranges. Working with a qualified physician to measure, assess, and correct your medical tests is strongly recommended. Obtaining the best results means working with a doctor who understands the difference between **normal** and **optimal** and is willing to take preemptive action against aging. If your doctor doesn't understand this, you need to find another doctor for your hormonal needs.

METHODS

If what I have said so far has convinced you that bioidentical hormone replacement therapy is the way to go, if you are convinced that BHRT is the true fountain of youth, then let's look at your options. You have two choices: static dosing or rhythmic cycling.

STATIC DOSING

With static dosing, your doctor will most likely start you on low-dose bioidenticals according to your symptoms. After a couple of months he or she will order a blood test, approximate your hormone levels, and prescribe a static dose of estradiol every day of the month. On days 18 to 28, your doctor adds in a static dose of progesterone, based upon your lab-work. This regimen is designed to match what our bodies once did when we were making a full complement of hormones. It brings about a period at the end of each cycle (at the end of the month). This approach is how it happens in nature and is used by some of the cutting-edge Western doctors (but not all of them) to replicate nature. Based upon the research I have done and information from the dozens of doctors I have interviewed, I will go on record and say that I believe cycling in this fashion is not an option but a necessity if we are trying to mimic normal physiology.

So far, static dosing sounds simple, but here is the complex part. As you will read in chapter 16, stress affects and blunts hormone production. So if you are going through a stressful period in your life (and all of us are stressed regularly in this country), it changes your needs. To compensate, you may need to dose up a drop or a fraction of a milligram or dose down. If the stress is severe, you may need to have another blood test to determine where your levels are. This is what I mean by the "art form" I mentioned earlier. It is important that you work closely with your doctor and communicate your symptoms so he or she will adjust your dosages until you get it just right.

RHYTHMIC CYCLING

Rhythmic cycling is a new concept in bioidentical hormone replacement, but one that is based upon the ancient cycles of nature. In fact, it goes all the way back to early man, who was attuned to the planet in a way that is completely inaccessible to us in the modern world.

There were no executives or career women at that time—just people living in tune with the cycles of the moon and the tides, reproducing as often as was possible, and then seeing that each baby occupied a year of a woman's life, followed by breast-feeding for another couple of years.

It was all so perfect back then. In summertime, early humans ate all the abundant carbohydrates that were available, danced, and made love by the light of the moon. Women menstruated to the cycles of the moon, and we fattened up in the summer with all of the abundant food. Then winter arrived, and darkness came earlier. We had no more carbohydrates, we ate meat, we went to sleep earlier because there was no light, and we could stay warm with one another. As women, our bellies grew with the baby we had made during the summer months. We lived off the fat supplies that we had accumulated by eating all the carbohydrates in the summer, and we slept more. With spring, we gave birth. The sun began to shine, and the process started all over again. Simple.

This was nature working at optimum before **we**

got involved and messed with it. When electricity came, it was declared a miracle, but it also changed our rhythms. Now we could stay up as late as we wanted. Without the proper amount of sleep, the work of all the healing hormones—which normally happened from getting enough sleep each night— was disrupted, so we slept less. Stress became a part of our lives and blunted our hormone production. We stopped cycling to the lunar calendar, we had fewer children, we breast-fed less, and in general we became weaker as a species.

In ancient times, women cycled to the rhythms of the moon. Our bodies would produce estrogen in increments: The first three days was one amount; the next three days another amount (each woman required or made the amount perfect for her); and by the twelfth day, our estrogen would peak, which happened to coincide with the full moon. Then the receptor sites opened to receive progesterone, and the lining would shed. As the estrogen fell, the progesterone would rise until it reached its incremental peak, only to rebuild the lining of the uterus to be ready next month to start this process all over again. According to T. S. Wiley, "That is the beginning of life. Anything else is death."

Rhythmic cycling exactly mimics our healthiest prime, which would be us when we were our reproductive selves, when our hormones would rise and fall in peaks . . . a rhythm. Without a rhythm, the body perceives things as "not exactly right for reproduction," and it is in this imbalanced state that disease cells can begin to go wonky. Bioidentical hormone replacement therapy given rhythmically appears to be an important way to avoid cell proliferation and thus keep organs intact. Rhythmic cycling is using the model of early man when our bodies were operating at their prime and we were our healthiest.

Rhythmic cycling is worth looking into. It resonates. It makes sense. We do ebb and flow as human beings with the moon and the tides. It would make sense that our cycles would do the same. As a young woman, when I was cycling naturally, there were days I felt light and free, and there were days I felt heavy and intense. Some days I would be in a perfect mood; other days I was not. These were my rhythms, or cycles. A few days before my period, I would feel bloated or cranky—signs of chemicals moving around in my body.

To cycle rhythmically, you need to work with a doctor who understands how to do it. (See Resources, page 410, for the names of doctors who prescribe rhythmic cycling. You can also check out the Wiley Protocol or ask your compounding pharmacist. The Wiley Protocol website and the number for the Professional Compounding Center of America are also in the Resources.)

This protocol must be prescribed by your doctor. It sounds complicated, but really it is as simple as looking at the calendar that accompanies your prescription. You look at the date of the month, and it shows you what amount to take that day. That's all it is. The thinking has been done for you.

As I said earlier, I felt that it was important to try this protocol on myself so I could report to you my findings. I have been cycling rhythmically for almost two years as of this writing, and I have to say I feel great. I have no bloating, nor have I gained weight. In fact, I am experiencing weight loss, but I am also injecting HGH, which promotes weight loss. My weight is exactly where I want it to be at this age: 127 pounds at five feet five. For the last few years, my weight had been around 137, even 140 at times, although I have always eaten correctly and exercised. A lot of that weight gain I attribute to my radiation treatments for breast cancer. I know that it takes seven years for complete cell turnover, so that weight was most likely induced by hormonal imbalance created by the radiation treatments, even though I have been on bioidenticals.

I am enjoying quality of life cycling rhythmically. Both ways have given me back quality of life. Because I was on birth control pills for twenty years, I can honestly say that the way I feel on bioidentical hormone replacement therapy is the best I have ever felt in my life. This is all such a personal choice, and just being on bioidenticals is a step in the right direction.

T. S. Wiley is knowledgeable yet somewhat controversial. Some doctors will react with horror at such amounts. But according to Ms. Wiley, it's not the amounts, it's the correct ratio that makes you feel good, and the ratio between progesterone and estrogen must be correct.

I have spoken to a lot of women and doctors about this protocol. Some women cannot stop rhapsodizing about how they feel on this protocol. They love it, they love life, and they have their sex drives big-time.

Other women feel it is too much work and stop the protocol. There is such rampant fear of hormone replacement because of the alarming reports that have come out on synthetic hormones that these amounts seem to be crazy. Yes, the Wiley Protocol advocates large dosing, but we are talking about **bioidentical,** not synthetic HRT. That is a big difference. We are talking about real hormones. We are talking about regular blood tests and striving for perfect balance. If this protocol interests you, look into it. Do your homework, and then you can make an informed decision. The problem with these passages and transitions is that our doctors are so poorly informed that you are really on your own.

In the interviews with doctors that follow this chapter, it is important that you read carefully and absorb what each of them is saying. Every one of these doctors is on to something. What you can learn about aging well, antiaging, detoxification from the environmental pollutants, and bioidentical hormone replacement therapy will set you on a path of joy and good health.

But I'll say it again: No one will ever care about your health the way you do. No doctor can understand your body as you do. No one will lose out as much as you do if you don't make the right choices for yourself. This book is meant to empower you with knowledge. We have to question our doctors. No longer do we have to take their word as gospel. In this era of specialization, you, the patient, now need to understand how **your** body works, what is happening to it internally as the years pass, and what you can do to reverse the destructive process brought about by the environment, bad diet, and poor lifestyle habits and choices.

Think of your body as a finely tuned machine. You have to feed it the right fuel, the best fuel, and you have to take care of the engine and give it regular fine-tunings. This is just common sense. You will be the recipient of negative consequences if you put into your body chemicals and bad oils (that is, trans fats, hydrogenated oils, artificial food, and poison), if you don't sleep properly and long enough, or if you load up with pharmaceuticals without thought about the effect they are having. If you don't think good thoughts, if you wallow in negatives, what do you think will manifest?

We are what we eat, think, and drink. We need sleep to give us the fuel to have the energy to live and love. It's really all up to you, and what you put into yourself from this point on will have a direct effect on who you will be and the state of your health down the road. There are no "lucky ones." There are only people who understand that we can live a long time and be productive in society and within the family structure while they are alive. This isn't rocket science . . . just good common sense.

Hormones are the "juice of youth." This is what we have all been looking for, and they are real and natural and available. We are lucky to be alive at this time. Our daughters will certainly have an easier time of it, because by then bioidentical hormone replacement will be the accepted way of dealing with aging. We are the pioneers, and we are blazing the way for the next generation . . . once again.

CHAPTER 6

GLORIA: A FIFTY-TWO-YEAR-OLD SUCCESS

I first met Gloria several years ago. She is a fantastic aesthetician. My regular treat to myself is to have her work her magic on my face. I have been a client of Gloria's for a couple of years. You can't help but be struck by her beauty: long sun-streaked natural wavy hair, beautiful olive skin, and green eyes, a combination of Italian and Swedish heritage. The combo is striking.

The day I first met her was not our best day together. I could tell she was agitated. I had no idea why, but it was not exactly the vibe you want when you are getting a facial. As she began "slapping" my face around, it was clear that she was not in a good mood. She was full of complaints and bitchiness. It was when she said to me, "No man will ever take me out more than once because I am such a bitch. Plus, I haven't slept in four years," that I knew I was dealing with a severely hormonally imbalanced woman. It was stealing her life from her.

I said to her rather tentatively, "You don't know me, but I think I could help you." I sent her to Dr. Prudence Hall, a gynecologist in Santa Monica, California. (Read her interview on page 204.)

Wait until you read Gloria's story. If this doesn't convince you to embrace bioidentical hormone replacement, then I will be at a loss.

SS: Yours is such a success story that I can't wait for my readers to hear it. One of the things I feel is so remarkable about your story is your family history.

Gloria: Well, my grandmother was the first one that I knew of in the family to have severe menopause symptoms. My mother didn't have them as bad, because, as I am educating myself, I realize that when you have eight children like my mother, and you are pregnant and nursing that long, your menopause is not as severe. So that's what saved my mother. She did go through symptomatic menopause, however, because I remember her sweating all the time. She had other symptoms, but they weren't life stopping like they were for me. Also, my mother stayed home to raise her children. Even though she was very busy, she was still within her safe environment while going through the "change," whereas I was a businesswoman. I had my business to run, and I had to work with people every day. I was expected to be at my optimum every day. Giving facials, I can't afford to have daily mood swings. My customers come here to relax and get beautiful, and they expect me to be up and in a good mood and creative. All of a sudden, feeling happy was almost impossible, and I didn't understand why.

SS: Is this what happened to your grandmother?

Gloria: My grandmother's curse was that she and my grandfather were one of the wealthier couples in her community. They survived the Depression. My grandfather was a hardworking immigrant who was able to be successful a few times in his life. That he could provide my grandmother with whatever she needed became her curse.

SS: Why?

Gloria: Because he had the money to send her to whatever doctor she wanted to go to, and the more they did for her, the crazier she got.

SS: What were they doing to her?

Gloria: They gave her different drugs. I don't know which ones, though, because no one wrote anything down in those days. She was on drug after drug to try to suppress her menopause symptoms, and this triggered her pituitary gland to grow. Her body became bloated. Her features became abnormal as a result of the medications that she was on. Her nose got huge, her hands swelled, and her legs and feet couldn't fit into any shoes. No shoes were big enough for her. She used to be tiny. If you could see her wedding picture, she was a very small woman—maybe ninety-three pounds.

SS: What was her mood like?

Gloria: Just angry all the time. I was the only one

who had the patience to even want to know her. Otherwise she was secluded and reclusive and lived behind huge walls with a big dog.

SS: Would people talk about the fact that she hadn't been like that prior to menopause?

Gloria: Yes. My grandfather adored her. When they were young, they were so happy. Extremely talented. She was an artist and one of those people who could make anything. She had gardens that the whole neighborhood envied. When menopause hit, her whole life fell apart.

She gave up her zest for life. She could no longer paint because her hands were too swollen. She couldn't get out into the garden and work because she was physically in pain, sore, and swollen, and not feeling well. She could barely walk. She still did a little cooking, but no more sewing, whereas before, she used to crochet beautiful doilies.

SS: Would it be fair to say that menopause sucked the soul out of her?

Gloria: It stole her life. Then the doctors got to her and made things worse, much worse. My poor grandmother went into menopause, and then to top it off, my grandfather died. She was only forty-three at the time.

SS: So let's go to you.

Gloria: I don't know why, but I always had a feeling that I was going to take after my grandmother genetically because I am physically most like her. I'm the only one out of five sisters who was small and blond like my grandmother. All my sisters are five feet seven inches, with dark hair and features.

SS: What was your first symptom?

Gloria: My moods. I started noticing that people were telling me that I was a bit touchy at times. Touchy, and maybe a lack of patience, nervous, tense. People would say to me, "You don't have to be so uptight; it's not a big deal." But I wasn't able to let things bounce off me the way I normally would. I was starting to become a sponge, absorbing everything: Everything went in, everything was personal. That was probably the beginning. Then one day I was sitting in a restaurant, and all of a sudden, I stopped talking and said, "Oh my God. I think I just had a hot flash."

Next, I started gaining weight. I used to be kind of a babe, but I had gone from a size two to a size ten just in a matter of a year. Before, I was the kind of person who never had to watch her weight. I once had a doctor put me on a diet of three malted milkshakes a day just to keep my weight on. I was so thin that if I turned sideways, you wouldn't be able to find me.

SS: Must have been a shock to change that quickly.

Gloria: Right. All of a sudden, I had to start watching my weight. I had always been into exercise, but now exercise became this difficult chore.

SS: Had your vitality been drained out of you?

Gloria: Yes, just everything. No matter what I did, I didn't know myself anymore. I would eat less and gain weight. It was all screwy. Everything I knew about myself was no longer valid. If I exercised for two hours a day, it didn't do a thing. Before if I had done that, I would have been in Olympic shape. I was ready to just throw in the towel. I felt like I was ready to go over the edge. I was almost there when I met you. I was feeling despondent.

When I met you, I was already on antidepressants—a very high dose of Effexor. I was given the prescription because a friend of mine who was a therapist said to me one day, "You're not going to make it. You need to be on something." So she took me to a doctor who gave me the prescription.

SS: Were you still having your periods?

Gloria: I was pretty much done. It had been almost two years since I had had a period.

SS: And if you don't mind my asking, what happened to your sex drive?

Gloria: What sex drive? I think this is also what started to cause the depression. It started happening to me at age forty-three. I felt like somebody struck me down in the prime of my life. I was a single mother, and I was just getting to the point when my daughter was old enough that I could start to have some sort of life of my own again. I had made my daughter a priority while she was young. I didn't want to have a revolving door with men with a little daughter at home. So I waited until she was in high school, and I thought, Okay, now I can start dating again. That's when it hit. The idea of someone coming near me was repulsive. And then you walked into my day spa.

SS: I guess there are no accidents in life.

Gloria: You called Dr. Schwarzbein for me, and even though she was no longer taking patients, you talked her into treating me, along with Dr. Prudence Hall.

SS: Yes, because Dr. Schwarzbein is now only teaching, but she has passed on to Dr. Hall all she knows. Dr. Hall has access to Dr. Schwarzbein whenever she wants information.

Gloria: When I started feeling good again, I was like a kid in a candy store. I was in love all over the place. I wanted to love everybody. I was just so happy to have my mojo back.

Dr. Hall got me started on bioidentical cyclical static dosing of hormones. So I was taking the same thing every day and adding in progesterone on days 18 to 28. At first, it was helping, but not much, not enough. I remember you saying to me that I was getting there, but I had to be patient. I had been at absolute zero on everything. At first I wasn't on testosterone, so I still didn't have any sexual feelings. My mood was improving. I had a boyfriend at the time, so that should tell you something, but it was strange to have no feeling.

Then I found out that the compounding pharmacist had given me the wrong dosage. I thought I would kill him. I had lost time. I wanted to feel good, and this held me up. We got the dosage right, and then things started changing rapidly. The effects were almost immediate. In twenty-four hours, I started to notice the difference.

SS: What was different?

Gloria: The first thing you notice is that you can actually sleep at night. And the hot flashes aren't there anymore. You wake up in the morning, and your first thought is a good thought. And you know, life is so wonderful that I just want everyone to know that it's not your environment so much as it is your physiological state. You can have a good time doing almost anything if you are healthy and well. We don't even know what that is anymore because we're moving so far away from it in this drug-riddled world that we live in. We are getting so far away from nature that our bodies are almost in a constant state of immune defense response. You couple that with hormone imbalance, and I don't know how anyone can live a good life.

Then I read about the Wiley Protocol, and I thought it made total sense to cycle with the rhythms of the lunar calendar. So that's what I am doing now, and I feel unbelievable. I hang a calendar on the wall and I write what dosage I am supposed to take every day and each morning I look at it. What's so hard about that? You don't have to be a rocket scientist to figure this out.

SS: Yes, I have written about the Wiley Protocol in

this book and explained for my readers the essence of rhythmic cycling.

Gloria: I've also had Dr. Hall add in a little testosterone, and I was just so "Oh my God!" I just have to thank God for my three dogs and all the time it takes to care for them, or else I would have been out there preying on young men all day. (That's a joke!)

SS: Like T. S. Wiley says, "It's nice to be alive while you're alive."

Gloria: You can say that again. My alertness is so much better. My body is even getting better. I'm losing that tire around my middle. I'm actually feeling my hip bones again. I feel so lucky. It got so bad for me that I now have seen both sides. And I don't ever want to go back over to that other side again. Now I'm coming back. I get to reverse all the stuff that was going on. I'm never depressed anymore. Never! And when I think back on it, I was depressed a lot when I was young, so I'm beginning to realize that I was probably never completely hormonally balanced.

SS: Well, it sounds like in your family history there may be something that is hormonally off.

Gloria: I think so, but the only thing to cure it is to have fifteen children, which we are not going to do these days.

SS: But I don't think women understand the value of pregnancy and nursing and what the birth control pill did to us.

Gloria: I agree, but also what society did to us. Women are moving further and further away from what our bodies were really designed to do. As we have fewer and fewer children, become more career-oriented, run businesses, and go against the nature in our bodies, there has got to be some payback for this.

SS: How do you feel now about having a period again?

Gloria: Oh, it's like my best friend. Every month I get my period, and I know my body is working right. I don't ever want it to go away again. I never thought I'd love having my period so much.

SS: Now that you are feeling so well, how is your teenage daughter doing? I remember your telling me that she had to miss a week of school every month because her periods were so severe and that it made her moods very difficult.

Gloria: It could be genetic, but I think it's because of our diets. We're eating food that has been altered, and it's throwing off the delicate balance that these girls have in their bodies. So many girls are starting their cycles earlier and earlier. I have a niece who started her cycle at age six!

I took my daughter to Dr. Hall around age sixteen (she's eighteen now). Dr. Hall prescribed a little bit of natural progesterone after looking at her blood test to be sure that was the problem. I was so glad she wasn't going to give her birth control pills like other doctors are giving to young girls. This just causes them to act more crazy and gain weight. Now my daughter has no more mood swings, and her periods are regular. Things in our house just couldn't be better. I'm fifty-two years old, and I have never felt better or happier.

It wasn't too long ago that my daughter wanted to put me in a cage and only let me out at certain times of the month. I feel better than I did at thirty or forty years old. I think it's because I've gone one step further. I am cycling rhythmically, in which I am taking different levels every day, reaching an estrogen peak. Then later in the month, I reach a progesterone peak. That's how my body did it when I was younger.

SS: I know. I was speaking with Dr. Hall, and she said, "You should see Gloria. She looks so beautiful. She's in love, she's thin, and she's happy." I was so happy for you that I almost started to cry.

Gloria: I feel beautiful. I have a boyfriend now, and it's a wonderful feeling to be in love. I will be the first one to testify that I've seen life on both sides of the fence. I really have, and it wasn't worth living the other way. It really wasn't.

SS: I understand.

Gloria: That's what I appreciate about you. You were the first person who was out there informing everybody about hormones. I was always trying to seek information. I needed to know as much as I could because that's how I was going to survive. I'm even making a dress from scratch. That's something I used to do, and now I'm doing it again because I'm back to the old me. See, this is a great thing for me. I wanted the life I once had, and now I have it again because of bioidenticals. I'm calm enough again to put in a zipper without losing control. I'm also gardening again. I'm getting my life back. And it's the life we all should have. Because I feel so good on these hormones, I finally have the courage to go back and fix the stuff that caused me to be dysfunctional in other areas. I never would have been able to do that.

I've changed everything about my life. We now eat only organic food. It's amazing how much better an organic pear tastes than one that has been tampered with. I bring them into the spa, and clients say, "That's a pear!" I don't buy junk food. I cook at home. I don't like eating out very much because I don't trust the food. I won't even put an aspirin into my house anymore. The only thing that even resembles a drug are my hormones.

ss: And you know enough, because of the work you have done to learn about your body and how it works, to know that this hormone you are taking is not a drug.

Gloria: The first thing women say to me is, "Gloria, what about breast cancer?" Know what I say to them? "Read Suzanne's book, then come back to me, and we'll talk about it." It really pays to inform yourself, because no doctor in the world is going to have the time to sit down, educate you, and figure out exactly what you need. If you don't educate yourself, you're going to end up the loser. This is your life.

ss: Amen. What a great thing that you work in a

day spa. Think of all the women coming in that you are going to educate. Good luck to you, Gloria, and thank you.

Postscript: Gloria is getting married. Look what bioidenticals did for her!

CHAPTER 7

DR. JULIE TAGUCHI: BREAST CANCER

Dr. Taguchi is my personal cancer doctor, and it gives me great relief to work with a doctor who will support the use of bioidentical hormones as my choice for preventing a recurrence of my breast cancer. She is a medical oncologist at the Sansum Medical Clinic in Santa Barbara, California, and currently the principal investigator for the Sansum Clinic conducting cutting-edge cancer research. Her interest in hormones led her to coauthor the book Sex, Lies, and Menopause. **She is also conducting clinical trials on the use of BHRT.**

SS: Thank you for your time, Dr. Taguchi. I know how busy you are. So let's begin. When I was diagnosed with breast cancer, the first thing I was told was that I had to discontinue taking my bioidentical hormones.

JT: I know, but it's unlikely that is what caused your cancer. It is my conclusion that balanced real hormones (also known as bioidentical hormones) are important to keep aging women healthy. If you're going to replace hormones, they should be rhythmic because it makes the most sense. The hormones that medicine in general had been prescribing for the past forty years has been with Premarin alone and Prempro, daily. Prempro is not good for women because it is associated with a higher incidence of breast cancer as discovered by the Women's Health Initiative 2002. Now I see that there are commercials for low-dose Prempro, which makes no sense at all.

SS: That seemed crazy to me also. When it comes to hormones, too much is too much and too little is too little. It's about perfect balance. So women who gave up their synthetic hormones when this report came out were left adrift. They threw away their synthetic hormones but then didn't know what to do. Menopausal symptoms are so devastating, and if these women didn't know about bioidenticals, then the idea of "low-dose Prempro" would probably make them feel that these are better for them.

JT: Yes. I don't blame women for being terrified. The party line in medicine is that hormones can cause cancer. That's the dogmatic thought, and physicians have been ingrained with this information or this limp belief based upon weak information that's been around for years. The thinking originated when they would have postmenopausal women with breast cancer give up and/or block their hormones, that breast cancer sites would shrink or disappear.

The standard in traditional medicine is to take away hormones so as not to "feed the tumor." But we have several single-institution studies on women who have been treated for breast cancer who are on bioidentical hormones, and even Premarin and Prempro, who actually do better in several different parameters.

SS: Even with synthetic hormones? Why is that, because even small amounts of horse estrogen are beneficial? If that is so, imagine the benefits of real bioidentical hormones.

JT: We don't know. Maybe because the small amount of cognition is better; maybe because they feel better because the hormones make them feel better and they have more will to fight. On hormones the quality of life is better. And who knows? Maybe the hormones may even be protective in ways we have not discovered yet. There are several studies that are being done, but mostly with synthetic hormones, that show improvement. I'm sure bioidenticals have been thrown into the mix, but bioidenticals are rarely looked at . . . that's why we are running a clinical testing with ten doctors at the moment to see the effects of bioidenticals in perimenopausal women without breast cancer first. From my experience, I think the results will be impressive.

SS: Normally, a cancer doctor would be oblivious to bioidentical hormones. What made you interested?

JT: Observing an elderly physician with recurrent

metastatic bladder cancer go into remission by taking and applying natural progesterone, suggested by T. S. Wiley. This got my attention. I then became a partner working on the book **Sex, Lies, and Menopause** with T. S. Wiley. It was the theory of replacing hormones based upon the original hormones and cycles of women. We studied the physiological levels, the physiological highs and lows, and we found that there were important biological reasons for those highs and lows of both hormones during a woman's menstrual cycle.

SS: You're talking about the rhythm of women's cycles, estrogen peaks and progesterone peaks . . . the highs and lows, the ebb and flow of our cycles?

JT: Yes, I'm talking about estradiol and progesterone levels. You're right, there are low levels of both hormones on days 1, 2, and 3. What happens at that point is your pituitary is pouring a message to your ovaries to make more estrogen. By day 12 you have your highest level of estrogen in your system as a reproductive woman to cause an egg to pop at ovulation. Then, throughout the cycle in the rest of the month, there are different estrogen levels that lower just before your period. After ovulation, progesterone is produced starting with a low level and slowly rising until a peak is reached on day 21, and then it falls again. Once the progesterone falls, it signals your body to have a period. This style and type of hormone replacement has not yet been studied. That's why we are conducting a second clinical trial using bioidentical hormone replacement in this fashion. I have several women who have had breast cancer who choose to use this particular program, and they are doing very well. The problem is because there is no data using this type of treatment, I can't recommend it . . . **even though I believe in it.** I must first recommend "standard of care." But when I get a patient such as yourself, who wants other options rather than the "standard of care," it's very gratifying because I feel we can really achieve good health and quality of life together.

SS: Give me your thoughts. I took birth control pills for twenty years, had the dry-up shot to prevent lactation as a teenager; throw in the environmental mess and the stresses that accompany everyday life in America, and you have a pretty good picture of myself and a lot of other crazed women in America. By switching to rhythmic cycling with bioidentical hormones, even though I am nearing age sixty, should I expect to be in pretty good shape for the rest of my life?

JT: I would hope so, and that's what I am hoping for with other women. I'm not trying to be negative, but there's a combination of things. I had a ninety-one-year-old patient who had a mastectomy when she was sixty because she had breast cancer. She did not have chemotherapy, radiation, or tamoxifen. I saw her thirty-one years later, and she had tiny nodules on the skin over her mastectomy site. This was her recurrence thirty-one years later. What it taught me was that if she had died a year before the recurrence, everyone would have considered her cured from breast cancer.

SS: But it was never really cured?

JT: It was never really cured.

SS: What you are saying is that the mastectomy didn't really do anything for her?

JT: Well, the mastectomy probably gave her peace of mind for thirty-one years. I quote this for my patients . . . If you have a mastectomy, there's a 9 percent chance that the tumor will come back to the chest wall. The reason we began to do lumpectomies and radiation is that the number of local or breast recurrence is also about 10 percent, so we consider the outcome the same. But even with lumpectomy, radiation, or even a mastectomy, there's still a chance that certain breast tumors can come back to the skin area.

SS: What do you think about radiation? Because isn't it radiation that can **give** you cancer?

JT: It's an odd paradox . . . I tell my patients that if you have a lumpectomy and you do not have radiation, your chances of the tumor coming back to the chest or skin are one in three. However, if you have radiation added to your lumpectomy, it reduces the risk of it coming back to one in ten. So that's worth it.

SS: Add chemotherapy to that equation.

JT: Depends upon the patient and the tumor. When I evaluate a woman with breast cancer, I take many things into consideration, such as the age of the patient. Is she menstruating? Is she hormonal? You look at the tumor characteristics such as size, histology estrogen receptor status, and HER2-neu expression. How many nodes were positive, if any? With this information or staging, we try to predict the treatment benefit for women with these different profiles and deliver our best shot.

But this is changing now, because of molecular biology and genomics. Soon we'll be able to take a tumor, plug it into a machine, and it's going to tell us the genetic mutations and where the problems are located. This will allow us to be able to fine-tune and target therapy much better, instead of giving a hundred women toxic chemotherapy and having a mere 20 percent of them getting a benefit.

Women who have positive estrogen receptor breast cancer tend to have a better long-term prognosis than women with estrogen receptor negativity disease. But this latter subset is doing better with newer therapies.

SS: How would that work, like a laser?

JT: It will most likely be either oral or infusion. Tamoxifen is a form of targeted therapy and blocks the estrogen receptor of the cancer cell, causing it to become dormant. However, tamoxifen also targets your uterus, your brain, and activates your clotting system.

SS: I find tamoxifen a troubling drug. I refused to take it when it was recommended to me. The side effects didn't warrant the so-called benefits as far as I was concerned. Is tamoxifen the female version of Lupron for men with cancer of the prostate?

JT: No, Lupron basically shuts off hormones at the brain. It shuts off the ability to give the signal to make hormones. Tamoxifen is a receptor blocker, so it actually works on the cell itself. It has a dual action. If it sits on an estrogen receptor, it can either stimulate or block. That's why you can block the receptor cells to the breast, yet the uterus is stimulated and you can get cancer.

SS: Sounds like trading a stomachache for a headache. The side effects of tamoxifen take away quality of life. Weight gain is a supposedly small side effect, but excess weight is undesirable and makes women unhappy. Then there's the possibility of depression because this woman is without hormones, plus a 40 percent increased risk of heart attack, stroke, or pulmonary embolism. Doesn't sound like the benefits are worth it.

JT: You are correct about the side effects of tamoxifen, but it doesn't interfere with the ability to make hormones . . . it interferes with the ability to read the hormones in some parts of the body. Remember, tamoxifen can block or it can stimulate. It depends upon what organ we are talking about. But you're right, tamoxifen can cause horrible effects in women; yet some women can take this drug and feel fine.

SS: What's that about?

JT: In my practice it seems that the older women, the longer they've been menopausal, the more likely they may tolerate the drug better than the younger women.

SS: Maybe it's because they've been in hormonal imbalance longer and have gotten used to feeling lousy. Why do you think we get breast cancer?

JT: First of all, I can tell you age is the biggest risk for any cancer.

SS: So that means loss of hormones equals increased risk?

JT: Yes, or lack thereof of hormones, if you're looking at breast cancer specifically. Seventy-five percent of the breast cancer diagnoses are made after the age of fifty, which is after the time of menopause, when women are hormoneless. What's also interesting is that the largest group of women to get cancer at any one time are ages forty-five to fifty.

SS: Think about it, at forty-five they are in perimenopause.

JT: Exactly, because there is the hormonal change from balanced, rhythmic hormone levels to which a woman then experiences hormonal falloff to menopause. You can't ignore the fact that lower and erratic hormone levels have an influence on some kinds of breast cancer.

SS: Then perimenopause should be taken very seriously as a condition and hormones should be followed very closely at this age as a preventive measure against cancer. Yet I must say, having been diagnosed at age fifty with breast cancer, not one, **not one**

of my doctors ever mentioned perimenopause as a serious condition. In fact, it was treated kind of as a joke.

JT: It's a good idea for doctors to take perimenopause seriously. But there are many people who are not happy that "perimenopause" has been made into a disease, since most women go through it and survive "the change." Perimenopause is a transitional state for aging women, and the frequency, type, and intensity of symptoms vary; 10 to 15 percent have no symptoms when they stop having periods, and you've got 20 percent of women with symptoms so severe that they cannot function. And then you have this in-between range.

SS: What is the difference? Is it the difference between women who have had children and have breast-fed and those who have not?

JT: Yes, breast-feeding is very important for women, but that is just part of the whole picture. Breast cancer is one disease, but I've seen so many variations in the women who get cancer.

SS: Add to that scenario the women who have been on birth control pills.

JT: I think the birth control pills and certainly the older birth control pills of the sixties and seventies have been associated with an increased risk of breast cancer. The current third generation of birth control pills does seem to have a slight increased association with breast cancer. They are interfering with a natural hormonal process, and we don't know the ultimate outcome of the big picture due to this altered state. Birth control pills (which are more like having a controlled menopause) delay pregnancy in young women. This has risk associated with it. The other factor is that women who tend to be highly educated and in business or whatever are the same women who are delaying pregnancy until their late twenties and into their forties. We know that a pregnancy after age thirty can increase the risk of breast cancer. Early pregnancies and breast-feeding for years are things we don't do very well in this country, and they are the two things that strongly reduce the risk of breast cancer.

SS: I have read that the best age to have your children is no older than twenty-eight, but most women don't do that anymore.

JT: Yes, twenty-eight is considered to be a "geriatric pregnancy," according to OB/GYN textbooks. If you look at the biology of women, it's kind of like "use it or lose it." You've got this reproductive system. You see, years ago women would marry at eighteen and have their baby at nineteen and breast-feed. When you do that, there's a protective mechanism. Protective changes happen to the breast tissue at a younger age when you have first-term pregnancy. That protective effect does not happen after the age of twenty-eight or thirty.

SS: But take a woman who has breast-fed, and let's

say she started having her children at thirty, thirty-two. She's still in better shape than the woman who hasn't yet done it at all, right?

JT: Can't tell you. But long-term breast-feeding is beneficial for both the mother and baby, no matter what.

SS: So if it's really about early pregnancy and early breast-feeding, then no wonder there's a cancer epidemic in women of my generation. We burned our bras and wanted equality in the workplace. Plus, we could have all the sex we wanted because of the pill. We wanted to get paid like men and work like men. . . .

JT: And end up like a man. I'm forty-seven, and I grew up in the 1970s when we thought we could have it all, and I feel like I have been sold a bill of goods. I had children at age thirty-one and thirty-four, but I was working literally a hundred hours a week. Total craziness. Somebody else was bringing up my children during the day, and I didn't snag very much sleep. There is a price to pay.

SS: The bill of goods was that baby formula was better than breast milk.

JT: Yes, and in the 1970s, which was the peak, 85 percent of all babies in this country were fed formula. You start putting all these things together and you see a pattern forming, as T. S. Wiley did.

SS: What's the future for breast cancer?

JT: Targeted therapy . . . better targeted therapy

and prevention and patient education. More and more, I am finding that some of my patients who have been through the "standard of care" now want to be treated with bioidentical hormones. Some are like you, have evaluated the research and information and choose not to undergo the standard of care.

What's important for me as an oncologist is the issue of choice. I offer all women the "standard of care," which is surgery, lumpectomy or mastectomy, radiation, chemotherapy, and possibly hormone blockade (like the aromatase inhibitors, tamoxifen, or raloxifene). With a lumpectomy plus or minus you might need radiation therapy to the chest; or if you have a lot of lymph nodes at the time of the section, we would also suggest radiation. Then it depends upon the tumor types and characteristics and how old the patient is. If she is premenopausal, the data shows us that chemotherapy is beneficial. If the tumor is estrogen receptor positive, then it's tamoxifen or raloxifene for five years.

But we really don't know much about it just yet. These drugs and this treatment could be curing breast cancer or just delaying it from coming back sooner.

SS: What about someone like me who says no to most of the options of standard of care?

JT: Well, these patients still need to be followed, but I offer it and say what is recommended. But if someone comes to me and says, "I don't want to do that, I want to do something else," or, "I want my hormones back," I review the pros and cons of not having standard treatment as well as the risks and benefits of hormone replacement or the unknown risk of complementary options. Once a woman understands her informed choice, I do offer rhythmic hormonal cycling using mostly compounded bioidentical estradiol and progesterone. There are always some women who don't want to do that much work to get it right. For doctors it's really more work.

SS: Yes, because prescribing hormones bioidentically is an art form, wouldn't you agree?

JT: Yes, because you are tailoring it to that particular woman. The physician has to be tuned in to . . . what this woman is going through every day. How is she sleeping? How is her libido? Her vaginal dryness? How many hot flashes? Is she having normal periods? It's an art form trying to get this right. It also depends upon the pharmacy that makes the hormonal preparation, which can vary widely.

SS: What's your hunch? There's standard of care. Then there's the bioidentical approach.

JT: Good question. I'm in this interesting position because I certainly have been trained to be a mainstream oncologist. And certainly I read all the data, and there's tons of data that say that women given tamoxifen after breast cancer have fewer breast cancer relapses. We consider them curable. I rarely use the word **cured** when it comes to breast cancer. The point I am trying to make is that there's European data right now that followed premenopausal women who had breast cancer, and at twenty years they continue to relapse.

SS: What do you think about Iscador as a cancer treatment? Iscador is an anthroposophic medicine. Not FDA approved, but legal in this country with a doctor's prescription. I have been injecting Iscador for five years, and I'm still alive and well.

JT: I have prescribed it to a few women because of you. There are some studies that show there is no major effect or harm. Yet there are a few promising published studies that also show an improvement in other areas such as relapse. It would be wonderful to have clinical trials studying Iscador. There is no real financial incentive to do studies on a natural substance or treatment that is not patentable. Western medicine has not looked at options like Iscador yet, but I bet it is coming.

Eli Lilly makes a chemotherapy used for several cancers called Gemzar, and I read that Gemzar has similar properties as those found in mistletoe, which of course is what Iscador is made from. So I found that interesting. But Gemzar does not work as an immune booster as Iscador apparently does. Gemzar becomes part of the cell's DNA. So when the cells are going to replicate, they can't.

I get frustrated because doctors don't want to look anywhere else. My gynecologist found fibroids on my exam. She gave me the party line as the reason for them: "Because you take hormones," she said. She informed me that it isn't a matter of how much you take, it's that uterine fibroids are stimulated by estrogen. I asked, "How could that be?" Young women in their twenties and thirties are flooded with estrogen, and they don't get fibroids. Fibroids happen when you're in your forties and perimenopausal, when your hormone levels are starting to fall. And, of course, we know that fibroids shrink after menopause.

SS: I believe the problem is lawsuits. Doctors are afraid to prescribe outside the standard of care.

JT: Yes, doctors are not encouraged to think anymore, and they are too busy trying to make a living because of the way insurance works and reimbursements are handled. Quite a lot of the information we are fed comes from drug company–sponsored studies. There's no time to sit there and do research on your own and come to your own conclusion if there are no studies available that address your questions. Also, I realize there's a huge world of information we doctors don't know about and for the most part are too busy to find out about.

SS: Like Iscador.

JT: Yes, and they don't want to tear it down with poisonous chemicals that are supposed to help. We know that chemotherapy does this. As I told you, I can give a hundred women chemotherapy, and 20 percent at most are going to get the benefit. So as oncologists we know that eighty women out of a hundred get this toxic drug exposure for nothing.

If there was a guarantee . . . but there isn't, so as an

oncologist it's heartbreaking. That's why I'm more open to women making other informed choices.

SS: As an oncologist . . . what do you dream about?

JT: I hope in the future I will no longer have to poison people to treat cancer. My major job as an oncologist is giving and managing the effects of toxic drugs. We honestly believe we are helping people, and we do see results with these drugs, but in the future I hope there's another way.

SS: Thank you for your time . . . I hope your dreams come true.

DR. TAGUCHI'S TOP FIVE ANTIAGING RECOMMENDATIONS

1. Pay attention to perimenopause; a long symptomatic perimenopause might be a risk factor for breast cancer.

2. Work with a doctor who not only will advise you on the standard of care, but is also open to exploring other options.

3. Replace your hormones using bioidentical hormones given rhythmically because it makes the most biological sense.

4. Know your odds if faced with breast cancer. With a mastectomy or with lumpectomy and radiation, there is a 9 to 10 percent chance the tumor will return to the chest wall.

5. Treatment for breast cancer is based upon the tumor type and characteristic and the age of the patient. Be informed on these issues as you consider your treatment options.

CHAPTER 8

DR. MARC DARROW:
BONE HEALTH

Dr. Marc Darrow, a professor of medicine at the UCLA School of Medicine, has an established practice in Los Angeles, where he specializes in sports rehabilitation. As my personal sports doctor, he has never given me a drug for any of my injuries. He is of the thinking that unless a drug is necessary, it is better to allow inflammation to do nature's work. However, as a Western-trained doctor, when drugs are needed for pain, he will prescribe them.

SS: Tell me about bone health.

MD: Bones are a living part of our body just like the heart, the brain, or the muscles. As pieces of hard material, they are built with calcium in a crystal-like structure permeated with blood vessels, nerves, and specialized cells. For example, bones have active, live cells called osteoclasts that actually chew little canals through the bone to create an opening so that other cells called osteoblasts can bring in new bone. In a process called remodeling, osteoclasts remove old bone tissue, while osteoblasts build new bone.

SS: So our bones are constantly regenerating?

MD: Yes. A healthy body is constantly regenerating bones. However, if you don't keep them regenerating, you are at greater risk for fracture. As we get past age thirty, all the hormones in our body start diminishing, and these hormones include pregnenolone, thyroid, melatonin, and testosterone, among others. For healthy, strong bones, both men and women need testosterone. Testosterone builds bone.

SS: What can interfere with the process of regenerating our bones?

MD: Diet, for one. Eating too many processed carbohydrates has a very bad influence. As a kid, I would drink a six-pack of cola a day. I'd beg my mom for money to buy it. This habit led to osteopenia, or bone thinning, in my hips, because soda leaches minerals from the bones. Osteopenia means there is some demineralization of the bone, whereas osteoporosis is severe demineralization.

Excessive exercise is another problem. All day long, I deal with athletes in my medical practice. Athletes have a lot of stress—the stress to succeed—and as a result, they work out too much, which is not good. The body is not meant to take this kind of treatment; the body will use up whatever resources it has inside—hormones, neurotransmitters, or proteins—to compensate. This situation blows out the adrenal system, along with cortisol and testosterone. Add to this the stress of trying keep up the appearance of looking successful, and then at the end of an athlete's stressful day, he or she goes to the gym and uses up more biochemicals. The energy that is spent is not replenished with deeper levels of sleep, which is required to regenerate growth hormone.

SS: What kind of nutrition is best for bone protection?

MD: I believe in a diet called the Paleolithic diet, in which you eat only foods that you run after, catch, grow, or milk. In other words, real foods. Back in the days of early humans, there were no grains. Yet today, carbohydrates are the "drug of choice," especially processed carbohydrates such as sweets, candies, snacks, and commercially baked goods. We grab processed carbs because we know they will give us a rush.

SS: Talk to me about balanced hormones relative to our bones.

MD: The best bone-management program involves hormone replacement with bioidentical hormones. I like to get people on these hormones as early as possible, and I mean early, like in their thirties. That is because we now know that women start losing bone in their twenties. Our healthiest prime for bones is when we are eighteen or nineteen years old, when our hormones are the highest.

SS: Where does a drug like Fosamax fit in?

MD: This is a drug known as a bisphosphonate, and I don't like bisphosphonates. They block osteoclasts from breaking down the bone, thereby interfering with the remodeling and construction of new bone.

SS: What about calcium?

MD: Calcium does only a little good, because the body doesn't absorb it very well, particularly as we age.

SS: What about women with those tiny spine fractures along with those large stomachs?

MD: Multiple small fractures brought on by osteoporosis can cause the spine to form a dowager's hump, medically known as kyphosis. This condition occurs when the vertebrae actually get squished down, and it can be very, very, painful. Although surgery is sometimes indicated, this area can be pumped up with a new type of glue or cement (for lack of a better description) that will alleviate the person's pain within minutes after the procedure.

SS: What is your approach to treating a disabling condition such as arthritis?

MD: People diagnosed with arthritis have been on painkillers, generally anti-inflammatory drugs supposedly designed to reduce inflammation in the body. The problem with these drugs is that they allow pain to go deeper and deeper into the body. Here's why: Inflammation is the body's way of healing itself and rejuvenating itself to its preinjury state. When you constantly take away the inflammation through the use of anti-inflammatories, you drive the pain further into the tissue. These drugs, in effect, block the inflammatory cycle, which in turn blocks the deposition of collagen, the main structural protein of the body. Without collagen holding us together, we would be a bag of nerves just sitting there unable to move. In short, blocking the pain is blocking the healing. We are left with an incomplete healing.

SS: But isn't it a part of our culture that we would rather have a painkiller?

MD: Absolutely. So often, when I get a referral from a pain medicine doctor, all the patients look like zombies. They have been on anti-inflammatories and antiseizure medication, not to stop seizures but to stop neuropathic pain. They are taking opiates such as Vicodin and Percocet, as well as antidepressants. When I ask them how they are feeling, their response is usually, "Uh, I feel pretty good today." When I ask them why they are not working, they say they can't because they are disabled. But the real answer is that they are drugged. What I do is try to get them to think more positively, encourage them to exercise moderately, and put them on a healthy diet of protein, vegetables, water, and some fruit. I try to get them off caffeine and nicotine, both of which weaken bones. And I use prolotherapy to heal the areas that hurt.

SS: Prolotherapy goes right to the pain. How does it work?

MD: Prolotherapy is a very simple process of naturally stimulating the body to produce healing by bringing and rejuvenating more tissue to the area of an injury. Prolotherapy uses a glucose (sugar water) solution, injected into the ligament or tendon where it attaches to the bone. This causes a localized inflammation in these weak areas, which then increases the blood supply and flow of nutrients and stimulates the tissue to repair itself.

I use the thinnest needle I can find in the form of a Dermojet, with an anesthetic beforehand. It blows lidocaine (an anesthetic) onto the tissue, under the skin. The injection stimulates collagen growth and cartilage growth. The results are amazing. A person can walk in with intense pain and walk out the door after an injection and play sports.

Prolotherapy is useful for many different types of musculoskeletal pain, including arthritis, back pain, neck pain, fibromyalgia, sports injuries, unresolved whiplash injuries, carpal tunnel syndrome, chronic tendonitis, partially torn tendons, ligaments and cartilage, degenerated or herniated disks, and sciatica.

Surgery is the very last resort for anything, as far as I'm concerned. Surgery seems to lead to more surgery down the line. If you come to my clinic, my hallways are littered with people who have had surgery that failed. Prolotherapy may not work on 100 percent of the people because they feel so good on it that they overexercise or they sneak anti-inflammatory drugs.

SS: Give me your top five strategies for optimum health.

MD: Number one: sleep. Number two: adequate

nutrition. By that, I am talking about low-glycemic-index foods that do not cause blood sugar to rise too quickly. Number three: moderate exercise. For some people, this may be a good walk every day for twenty to thirty minutes to oxygenate and get the blood going and raise feel-good endorphins in the body. Number four: hormone replacement using bioidentical hormones. Number five is a philosophy of life: Don't hurt yourself, and don't hurt other people. If you can manage to do just these things, you really don't have to do anything else.

SS: That's a great place to finish. Thank you.

DR. DARROW'S TOP FIVE ANTIAGING RECOMMENDATIONS

1. Change your lifestyle: Get enough sleep, adequate nutrition (avoid processed carbohydrates in particular), and moderate, not excessive, exercise. Get off nicotine and caffeine; both can weaken bones.

2. Watch overuse of anti-inflammatory drugs. They block the inflammatory cycle, drive pain farther into tissue, and interfere with the deposition of collagen, the main protein that holds us together. Inflammation is a necessary process that helps the body heal itself.

3. Pursue bioidentical hormone replacement therapy, including testosterone replacement, if necessary, since testosterone is required for strong bones in men and women.

4. Consider prolotherapy as a way of stimulating tissue repair for orthopedic-type injuries, arthritis, sports injuries, or fibromyalgia.

5. Develop a positive philosophy of life: Don't hurt yourself, and don't hurt other people.

CHAPTER 9

DR. PRUDENCE HALL: DISEASES OF AGING AND NATURAL HORMONE BALANCE

Dr. Prudence Hall is a practicing OB/GYN in Santa Monica, California. Along with her husband, Dr. Howard Liebowitz, she runs the Hall Center for Rejuvenation and Vitality, specializing in bioidentical hormone replacement for men and women coupled with antiaging medicine. Dr. Hall is dedicated and passionate about helping men and women through the often difficult and tricky passage of hormonal decline. She has much to say on the subject, and her passion will win you over instantly. She is also an expert at getting to the root of problems involving the GI tract. Women sing her praises. Her approach is unique and thorough, and she doesn't need to fill you with drugs to do it.

SS: There is a lot of talk about the relationship between our GI tract and disease. What is your take on this association?

PH: One of my big concerns in dealing with patients for the last three years has been toxicity coming from their GI tracts. European medical practitioners who believe in gastrointestinal health are exactly right, because health begins in the GI tract. That's where 70 percent of our immunity is coming from, yet every day our gastrointestinal tract is constantly exposed to offending agents that are very bad for it.

SS: Is this because of what we eat or our lifestyles?

PH: It has to do with food intolerances, such as gluten, wheat, eggs, soy, and so forth—foods that many people simply cannot handle. In addition, GI health is adversely affected by taking antibiotics that kill off the good bacteria in the gut, leading to intestinal yeast and overgrowth of bad bacteria.

SS: A lot of women are prone to yeast infections, so taking antibiotics twice a year or more often can upset the balance. Should these women be recolonizing with acidophilus?

PH: Acidophilus is a wonderful way to recolonize the GI tract and restore healthy bacteria. That approach, however, is not the first action I take when trying to restore health to the GI tract. First, I want to start healing the GI tract for about six to eight weeks in order to kill off the bad "bugs." Once those bugs are killed, then you recolonize the tract.

SS: Do you think the primary complaint behind the bloating problem for women is GI tract problems? Or is it intolerance to progesterone?

PH: That is a very interesting question. The way I got interested in functional medicine (which is getting to the root of the illness) is through the GI tract. What I started to notice was that my menopausal patients had stomach problems and digestive problems, and they would come in complaining of bloating, gas, and a variety of irritable bowel symptoms. As I became more curious about this, I began to realize that as we age, we lose acid in the GI tract, so some of this bloating is that we're not digesting our food very well. Partly digested food results in a reflux of acid up the esophagus and also causes bloating and gas. In the aging process, our hair loses its luster, our skin loses its elasticity, and our GI tract loses its acid, with bloating and indigestion as the result. Gastric acid is important because it helps protect the gastrointestinal tract from harmful bacteria.

SS: How do you put acid back and balance it?

PH: We give a supplement called betaine HCL, which is not a drug. My patients simply take 2 to 4 capsules with meals, and lo and behold, they get tremendous relief from bloating and gas.

SS: How does betaine work?

PH: Betaine is a source of hydrochloric acid, a naturally occurring stomach acid. It puts the acid back. So in the GI tract, where people have acid reflux and too much acidity, ironically it really is a result of not having enough acid in the stomach and partially digested food refluxing up into the esophagus, resulting in a heartburn type of phenomenon.

SS: It seems like everyone should be on betaine, because acid reflux is an epidemic. Just look at the amount of space devoted to heartburn in the drugstore.

PH: Yes, it's an epidemic, but the problem is that patients are usually put on precisely the wrong medication for them. They are put on Pepcid or acid blockers. But what these patients really need is acid. When they block the acid, the patient feels better temporarily. But in the long run, it's not good for their health—they are not extracting the food and the nutrients they really need from their food because they lack the acid to do so.

SS: This may be somewhat confusing, because the goal is to have more of an alkaline body, correct?

PH: You want an alkaline body, but a very acid GI tract for digesting food. Without an acid environment in the GI tract, some of your food goes partially undigested. You can develop what is called a "leaky gut," in which large spaces develop between the cells of the gut wall, and bacteria, toxins, and food can leak in.

SS: I was diagnosed with that before I became hormonally balanced. It was no fun. I was out of energy. It developed when my mother died, and the stress involved with her death seemed to manifest in my gut.

PH: Having a leaky gut wreaks havoc on your immune system. A lot of my patients come into my office with the same symptoms you mention—exhaustion and fatigue. I look to the GI tract as a possible cause, and I look into the burden of toxicity they may be carrying around. I also look at hormonal balance, making sure their thyroid is healthy and their sex hormones are where they should be.

SS: Do you recommend detoxification to your patients?

PH: Yes. Patients with PMS in particular can be greatly helped by detoxifying the body, for example. I often put my PMS patients on a low-toxicity diet, taking them off wheat, dairy, and alcohol. If you eat correctly—and that means real food—your health keeps getting better and better. This passage is a great time to clean up your life, to get healthy, and to start instituting a healthy lifestyle pattern for the next fifty years. Taking care of yourself now will carry you through to a radiant age.

I also put my patients on vitamins and supplements. In addition, I work on cleansing the liver so we can move those hormones through faster. I get their GI tract going so they are properly eliminating waste and do not become constipated. These patients end up feeling great.

Next, I go to work on their adrenals by encouraging them to start resting and sleeping. Sleep is such an important component in healing the hormonal system. Both perimenopause and menopause require a multipronged approach, and this is one of the reasons I enjoy this work so much. There are steps to wellness, and when I get a patient who is committed, we can absolutely turn their health and quality of life around.

SS: How important is the mind/body connection in all of this?

PH: Thoughts are important because the body follows the mind. Understanding the power of our minds and the way we can use our minds can enhance our bodies and frankly elevate the consciousness of the whole human race.

SS: And changing thoughts if you tend to think negatively?

PH: Yes. It is not only a toxic GI tract or a toxic liver. It's also toxic thoughts. Those must be detoxified as well.

SS: Tell me about your approach to bioidentical hormone replacement.

PH: Understanding the benefits of bioidentical hormone replacement must become mainstream medicine. I trained at USC and took my residency there. We were taught to administer daily synthetic hormones with Premarin and Provera (nasty synthetics, in my opinion). What I discovered is that when you give continuous combined hormones like this, this protocol increases insulin resistance and diabetes.

SS: But how did those conditions manifest themselves? Did your patients get fat?

PH: Yes. They gained weight, and they became

bloated. Many women are allergic to Premarin, which is synthesized from horse urine. These women also became depressed due to so much progesterone in their bodies, because this form of HRT puts the body into a hormonal state similar to a permanent pregnancy. Pregnancy can actually cause diabetes because it keeps insulin so high. Physicians always screen pregnant women for diabetes. What's more, abnormally elevated blood sugars increase your cancer risk by elevating insulin, a hormone that can increase the risk of cancer. So if you were to ask me what causes cancer, I would say increased insulin. Fifty percent of people with diabetes develop cancer. Add to that situation toxicity and an abnormal GI tract. When you take estrogen and progesterone continuously, cortisol levels soar in the body, and that creates numerous problems that could also lead to heart attacks.

SS: How do you feel about periods? Many of the doctors I've interviewed for this book feel, "If a woman doesn't want to have a period, how can I insist?" But when I speak with T. S. Wiley, Dr. Diana Schwarzbein, or Dr. Julie Taguchi, they say there isn't a choice. There's a right way and a wrong way, and having a period is the right way.

PH: What I do is explain to my patients the benefits of having hormones in their bodies—for example, a lower risk of diabetes, heart disease, osteoporosis, Alzheimer's disease, stroke, and hopefully breast cancer. I tell them that in order to get these benefits, one of the side effects is that they will have a period. Surprisingly, most women are open to the idea; it reminds them of being young. Estrogen builds up uterine lining, and then progesterone sloughs it off, hence a period. It's not that having a period is the goal; balanced hormones are the goal. To balance them correctly, the woman will have a period.

SS: Amen. Now let's talk about perimenopause. Most women do not realize when they are in peri-menopause, nor do they think that they need HRT because they feel they are too young.

PH: Perimenopausal patients are a little tricky because it's a time of fluctuating hormones. One minute, we'll measure estradiol levels that are 400 or 500, and the next time the levels are 30. I measure on day 21 of their cycle, which is the progesterone peak. If they are experiencing PMS, I know that often it is due to the presence of progesterone because women never have PMS in the first two weeks of their cycle when progesterone is absent. Progesterone blunts your estradiol, so the last two weeks of your menstrual cycle or two weeks before your period, we see fairly high levels of progesterone and declining levels of estrogen in perimenopause.

SS: How do you figure out how to dose them when their numbers are all over the place?

PH: I say, "Let's try plan A for one month and see

how you feel." I give them .05 mg of estradiol. That's a very low dose, and it's one or two drops in the second half of their cycles. But other women have low progesterone, so I'll measure their levels. If they are at, say, 6 and it should be around 15 to 25, I can clearly see this patient needs progesterone. So that's how you individualize this therapy.

I realize that every woman is different, and what works for one might not work for the next. I've been using bioidentical hormones for twenty years, with every possible permutation, from progesterone drops to capsules to rings to patches. While there are many different forms of transport you can access, the ultimate goal is to mimic a natural menstrual cycle. Every woman is different, and every woman absorbs differently.

SS: So where do you start?

PH: I have a standard dosage that I begin with. If a patient is older and hasn't had a period for four or five years, I'll start her on .05 mg of estradiol twice a day. I tell her to take this dose every twelve hours to spread it out. With some women this works better if I divide it into three times a day to keep a steady stream coursing throughout her body—just as when she was young and in her prime.

Then on days 1 through 14 or days 15 to 30 (fourteen days out of the month), I start with a relatively low level of progesterone, usually sublingual progesterone drops. Then as I cycle up with estradiol (for those who need it), I also increase the dosage of progesterone accordingly. If you give patients progesterone who have no estradiol, they will not feel well. They will experience PMS, among other symptoms.

SS: Once you get them on progesterone, what is the ratio of estradiol to progesterone?

PH: It's usually .1 mg of estradiol to 4 to 6 drops of progesterone. I never give estradiol orally in capsules. I just don't like it, but progesterone is tolerated quite well in capsule form. Sometimes I have women insert their morning dose vaginally. Some women have less breast tenderness when I do that.

SS: I've read about that, to give the progesterone vaginally on days 19, 20, and 21 of the cycle to open up their receptor sites.

PH: This is important. High levels of progesterone are good because progesterone actually decreases cancers through apoptosis.

SS: What is apoptosis?

PH: Apoptosis is the death of unneeded cells—in other words, the menstrual cycle, which is the sloughing off of the lining of the uterus each month to make new lining for the next month. It's all about the brain preparing the body to make a baby, each month. Even though at menopause we no longer have any eggs left, it is still important that the brain perceives us as reproductive.

It takes time and patience in the beginning, but the good news is that even when we haven't attained perfect balance, my patients usually feel so much better than they did when they first came in that they are willing to ride it out with me. In time we find balance, and that is a joyous experience for both my patients and me. That is why I became a doctor: to make people well. It's what keeps me going.

When you have patients who feel dramatically better, they have their sex drive back, they are no longer diabetic or have high blood pressure, this is a patient who is sold. So it's not about me trying to convince them. It's about them seeing the results for themselves and the benefits they now have as a result. When you add to this the spiritual dimensions and understanding the power of our mind and the way we can use our mind to enhance our body, and to know by doing this you can help elevate the consciousness of the whole human race, it truly is the best work I can think of to do. This is not just medicine; this is helping our patients to love themselves enough to pursue this kind of care. It requires self-respect, and self-love. These go hand in hand with good health.

SS: You helped me work out the problem I was having with severe hyperplasia (precancer) in my uterus. Through your wisdom and advice, you guided me through my hysterectomy. I was at the time very concerned about losing my sex drive, which I have worked so hard (through hormone replacement) to restore. Because you are my doctor, and because I was informed about hormones, we both knew that we were going to remove only my uterus. I say this because one of the tragedies that befall women with bleeding problems and hyperplasia are those doctors who tell women, "As long as we're in there, let's also remove your ovaries and cervix so you never have to worry about getting cancer." Excuse my French, but what a crock! How many women have lost their ovaries and cervix (which is the equivalent of female castration) for no reason?

PH: It is so unnecessary. There are a number of reasons women get hysterectomies; one of the major reasons is fibroid tumors. These are abnormal growths on the uterus that can be very painful and can result in a lot of abnormal bleeding and pain.

SS: Where do these fibroids come from?

PH: There are a number of causes, but one of the causes is inflammation. You can measure inflammation with a simple blood test, the C-reactive protein (CRP) test.

SS: The CRP test is one of the most important tests to prevent heart attacks.

PH: I agree. Inflammation stems from, number one, imbalanced hormones; and number two, food intolerances and allergies to foods such as wheat, dairy, soy, citrus, and so forth. Where food intolerances exist, I put patients on an oligo-antigenic diet, which means a nonallergic type of diet. Then we again deal with the GI tract. An unhealthy GI tract fuels inflammation in our body, and nutrients cannot be adequately absorbed, setting you up for vitamin and mineral deficiencies, even chronic fatigue. But back to fibroids: Most are caused by a hormonal imbalance. This imbalance causes bleeding and pain.

SS: It truly is a tragedy that doctors have been so eager to remove the entire reproductive system of women when it is not necessary. This old thinking of proactive removal is truly debilitating. Most women are not informed of the consequences physically and emotionally from having this radical surgery. At this point, a woman is left an emotional mess. Now there are no hormones left to keep her healthy and happy, and no sex drive at all.

PH: The irony is that **without** balanced hormones, she has a much greater chance of contracting cancer. No body part should ever be removed unless it is absolutely essential to a person's survival. Removing parts "proactively" makes no sense at all.

SS: For all those women reading at this moment and saying, "My God, that's me," let's try to sort this out for them. In my opinion, one of the biggest mistakes doctors make after a woman has a hysterectomy is to tell her that she no longer needs progesterone. Most women are put on that fake synthetic Premarin continuously, creating a template that the brain cannot understand. The brain perceives her body as part of the human species that needs to be eliminated because she can no longer reproduce.

PH: You are absolutely correct. One of the goals of BHRT is to "trick" the brain into believing all is well. Without progesterone, all is not well. Progesterone helps the body to balance itself, and progesterone is very important for the brain in terms of calming the body. The balance of cycling (even without a uterus) makes our bodies feel fertile; in doing so, women are protected against unhealthy aging. Also, this balance protects our bones and prevents cancer. Think about this: Breast cancer reaches its peak the further we get away from estrogen and progesterone production. For example, a ninety-year-old-woman will have a very high chance of developing breast cancer. She has no estrogen and progesterone left. By this time her bones are brittle, and her brain is no longer functioning well. If we keep cycling going (even though this woman cannot have a period), we offer the best protection for women against dreaded diseases. I realize this is a controversial statement, but I'm going to stand by it.

The whole idea of bioidentical hormones is to mimic the way our bodies once worked when we were in our healthiest prime. The way it happened in nature is that we made estrogen every day of the month in its dosages, and it made progesterone fourteen days of the month. Why would we change that?

SS: So for a woman who has had to have a hysterectomy, you still need to create a template hormonally that replicates nature. To only give a woman estrogen once she no longer has a uterus is not anything that ever happened in nature. In doing this, a woman will potentially have problems, ranging from emotional problems to cancer.

PH: Exactly. I'll say it again. Why would we try to reinvent women? This brings up another discussion I often have with my patients, who say: "Well, Doctor, maybe I should just do the natural thing and let my hormones decline." Now, I am a very natural person, and I am opposed to patients taking lots of medication, but what I tell them is this: "When you lose hormones, your body starts to age internally, and that's when the problems start. If you develop heart disease, you'll get a bypass. If you develop hypertension, you'll take medication. If you lose your bones, you'll be on Fosamax. If you get depressed, you might take antidepressants," and on and on. People consider all of this "natural," even though they are now on six or seven medications by the time they are age sixty-five, all of which is most unnatural. I offer them a way to reinstate their hormones that truly **is** natural and usually obviates taking any of the above measures or drugs.

SS: You walk the fence between static dosing for some woman and rhythmic cycling for others.

PH: What I do with a lot of my patients is start with one dose of estradiol, and when they're on progesterone days 18 to 28, I up their dose of estradiol during this phase, because progesterone blocks estradiol slightly during the second half of the cycle. If I don't do this for some of my patients, they can get

PMS symptoms on a static dose of estradiol. I find that upping the estrogen to balance the progesterone helps tremendously.

SS: Do you think we have to get sick just because we are getting old?

PH: No, no, no. Being sick as we get old is the result of unsuccessful aging, and under no circumstances do I feel we need to age with disease. My goal for my patients—and for everyone, for that matter—is to age with vitality, with their minds intact, and with their organs intact as much as possible, and be able to pedal a bicycle at age 110.

SS: What a lovely thought. Thank you.

DR. HALL'S TOP FIVE ANTIAGING RECOMMENDATIONS

1. Supplement with acidophilus to recolonize your GI tract with healthy, friendly bacteria. With a healthy GI tract, your body can better extract the nutrients it needs from food and reduce chronic inflammation.

2. If you have acid reflux disease, get to the real cause of the problem rather than taking the over-the-counter acid blockers. Real causes are low stomach acid, bad bacteria, and food allergies.

3. Detoxify your system with a diet that removes wheat, dairy, and alcohol. Eat natural, unprocessed food instead.

4. Work with your doctor to tailor a vitamin and mineral supplementation program that addresses your specific needs.

5. Take bioidentical hormones to help reduce your risk of diabetes, heart disease, osteoporosis, Alzheimer's disease, stroke, and breast cancer.

CHAPTER 10

DR. DANIELA PAUNESKY:
BIOIDENTICAL HORMONE
REPLACEMENT

Dr. Daniela Paunesky is board certified in internal medicine. She spent two years at the Cleveland Clinic and then moved to Atlanta, Georgia, and started specializing in antiaging medicine. She likes to refer to it as "age-management medicine." She has been prescribing bioidentical hormone replacement for five years. I was very impressed with her compassion, dedication, and understanding of the importance of restoring the hormonal system: how it works and the vital necessity of replacement. She understands that hormonal decline is difficult and requires patience on the part of the doctor. She is willing to give that time to her patients, and as a result, people are flocking to her.

SS: You are very passionate about your work. This spirit alone will affect the quality of many people's lives.

DP: Thank you. I do care a lot. My aunt, who lived in Yugoslavia, had breast cancer, and we brought her to the United States. My mother didn't trust the doctors in Europe. She wanted her to be treated by American doctors. The money it cost to take care of her devastated our family. She didn't have insurance, and her treatment cost around a hundred thousand dollars, but we would have done anything for her.

I felt that her doctors completely missed the boat on so many levels. She had several cysts, yet they never did an ultrasound. They stuck a needle in one cyst (she had four) and said there was no cancer. I told my mother that we didn't know whether there was cancer or not because they did not do a needle biopsy of the other cysts. Not wanting to hear this, my mother felt these doctors knew what they were doing. In less than two years, my aunt was diagnosed with metastatic breast cancer. We were all devastated because the doctors had told us not to worry, that it was not cancer, and that she didn't have to come back for three years. It was too late.

They could have found it in time, and I knew it. That's when I dedicated myself to becoming a better doctor. I decided that I would spend as much time with a patient as was necessary to really know what was going on and that I would have a different kind of practice.

This is a long answer as to why I am so passionate about my work and my patients. Also, this is why I do not give oral synthetic estrogen, because it sets up so many adverse conditions in the body. It increases inflammation, and it increases clotting factors. What's more, it increases 16 alpha-hydroxyestrone. I wouldn't take the chance for these things to happen.

SS: Let's talk about hysterectomy and bioidentical hormone replacement.

DP: There is a big difference between women who have had hysterectomies and women who have had bilateral oophorectomies [surgical removal of one or both ovaries]. Women who have had ovaries removed with their uterus need all their hormones replaced, and the sooner the better.

I had a very powerful, very intelligent woman come into my office last week. She was in tears. She had had a hysterectomy to remove fibroids. Her doctors told her that she didn't really need her ovaries anymore, so she might as well have them removed along with her uterus. "That way," they said, "you won't have to worry about ovarian cancer."

This woman told me that two or three weeks after the procedure, she came down with symptoms that were suggestive of lupus. She got spinal taps and magnetic resonance imaging (MRI) screenings. Then she got optic neuritis and is now 50 percent blind in her right eye. They also thought she had multiple sclerosis. She is convinced that all of these immunologic problems came secondary to having had a total hysterectomy and bilateral oophorectomy. I agree. What were they thinking, taking out her ovaries for no reason?

There are studies on women who have had breast cancer and decide to go on hormone replacement. Their overall mortality is decreased by 30 percent. For women who have had hysterectomies, bioidentical hormone replacement keeps them healthier, and by that, I mean everything is in balance. Bioidentical hormone replacement has been shown to decrease C-reactive protein in the body, a marker of inflammation. Progesterone and testosterone decrease the risk of breast cancer, provided it is given in the correct amounts and individualized for that person. Everybody is different, and everyone needs a dosage prescribed just for them.

There is literature to support that bioidentical hormone replacement boosts the immune system, improves neuromuscular function, and decreases cytokines (proteins that can inhibit immune cells). Other research indicates that women who are predisposed to rheumatoid arthritis have a four times increased risk of rheumatoid arthritis without hormone replacement therapy.

Every day in my practice, I see that the women who are doing well are taking bioidentical hormones in the right amounts for them. On the other hand, women who are taking synthetics are not doing well. Suddenly their clothes don't fit anymore because they've gained so much weight on synthetic hormones.

Desperate, they all come in with the same complaints, including weight gain or low libido. I explain to them that the average forty-five-year-old woman has lost 6.5 pounds of lean muscle mass. Then I review her symptoms. I explain which estrogens we are going to replace. Sometimes women are so desperate for relief, they don't want to get blood work right away. If they have been menopausal for a while, I know by their symptoms that they need replacement.

SS: So you start dosing them right away?

DP: Yes, I give them a prescription and tell them to call me in a week. I have been through so many different pharmacies, and I can't tell you what a difference the right pharmacy can make. And then there are issues with labs; so many don't get good blood levels, and we have to retest. So through trial and error, I have found the labs and pharmacy that I like to work with and that I can trust.

Once I am able to get blood work done on these women, I also check their FSH (follicle-stimulating hormone) level. This is a very important number for me because if that number goes above 100, it will lower all your other hormones and lead to premature aging.

For a menstruating woman, if her FSH level is between 5 and 7, she generally feels good, though it varies. If her FSH is high, it is the pituitary screaming to make more estrogen. I was always told you can't lower FSH. Not true. You can lower FSH with bioidenticals. I see it all the time.

Also, I wasn't even adding pregnenolone until recently when I found that 90 percent of all women over fifty had undetectable levels of pregnenolone. Their DHEA levels also need to be around the 300s.

SS: What about bleeding? A lot of women complain about heavy bleeding.

DP: I first make sure a woman has a transvaginal ultrasound just to determine that there are no fibroids and that her endometrial lining is at least 5 mm or less, then I feel comfortable in proceeding. Then there are a number of avenues I can take. I can give the woman a little bit of estriol with a tiny bit of testosterone inside the vagina. Then progesterone to shrink the mucosa. That's one route, and it helps with libido. The progesterone gets around the G-spot, increasing the blood flow to that area. If a woman is cycling, I will add an extra 50 mg progesterone at night, and then in the next two weeks, I further increase her progesterone.

SS: When a woman is on that much progesterone, is she going to gain weight?

DP: Personally, I am estrogen-dominant and therefore difficult to balance hormonally. Since turning thirty, I have menstrual migraines four days a month, very debilitating. My husband used to say, "Go to a neurologist." I would answer, "I'd just be put on a beta blocker because he or she doesn't know hormones. This is menstrual."

When I added extra progesterone, I did not gain weight. As a matter of fact, it helped with my water retention and I lost weight.

SS: This makes sense because progesterone is a diuretic. But headaches are usually a sign of not enough estrogen getting to the brain—at least that's the way it works with me.

DP: That could be also. Everyone is so different. But progesterone will not make you gain weight. However, we know that those on progestins, the synthetic progesterone, tend to gain weight, but not women who take bioidentical progesterone.

As for estrogen, if a woman is apple-shaped or obese, she has probably an estrone level of 90 to a level of 10 of estradiol. That makes me very worried, since it sets up an environment for weight gain and other problems. I usually put a woman such as this on indole-3-carbinol, a plant compound that blocks the conversion of estradiol to estrone. I have the patient come back shortly after that to check her levels again to make sure it is a ratio of two to one.

SS: What kind of delivery system do you prefer?

DP: Based on my experience, the best one is a gel that I put in a syringe. You just put a little pea-size on your arm. Because the skin is transdermal (through or by way of the skin), the hormone gets right into the bloodstream for better absorption.

I like working with estriol, the major hormone in the body. Numerous studies have shown that it doesn't cause cell division in the million breast valves or cause hyperplasia in the uterus. When we are menstruating, 80 percent of the estrogen in our bodies is in the form of estriol. When we are pregnant, the highest level of hormone that is secreted is estriol. So I put estriol in with the estradiol, and I don't use any estrone. Until I did this, I couldn't get my patients feeling good. When I did fifty-fifty, they felt fantastic. Also in the gel, I put a little bit of testosterone for some women. I have been getting great absorption with gels, and they are very easy to use. The great thing is that it costs them $50 for everything: melatonin, natural progesterone, pregnenolone, DHEA, and estriol with the estradiol.

SS: Is this all in one application?

DP: No, just the estriol, estradiol, and testosterone is in one application. If I add progesterone, there are too many molecules and they don't absorb. I get terrible results. I give the progesterone orally because it's been shown to give better blood levels, increase HDL, increase bone density, and give women more antianxiety benefits. The gel is cost-effective, too—priced at about $50.

SS: What are the ramifications on the liver of taking estrogen orally?

DP: It is important to detoxify the liver. It is such a busy organ, dealing with so much toxicity from the environment, and until you detoxify, too much of the estrogen is lost, and you do not get relief. This is why the gel transdermally is more effective.

SS: Let's talk more about testosterone. Do you feel that testosterone is the greatest brain food?

DP: Yes, it does increase short-term memory, but we don't know about long-term memory. It decreases waist-to-hip ratio (an important indicator of your overall health risk), it increases lean muscle mass, lowers hemoglobin, and improves insulin resistance.

I get asked by colleagues, "Aren't you afraid that testosterone replacement will raise the risk of prostate cancer?" I say no. There is no literature that shows testosterone replacement increases the risk. However, if there is an existing cancer, it may increase the risk of that cancer to grow.

SS: Tell me about your philosophy. How do you feel about your work?

DP: Since I started working in antiaging medicine, I have been gratified. I know am doing something beneficial. I do believe with all my heart that I am not only going to extend their life span, but also improve the quality of that life span. I know what I am doing; I have researched enough to know that I am not going to be increasing their risk of any cancers or immunologic disorders. I know that I am going to boost them up as much as I can with hormones. I do explain that preventive medicine is not holistic but that it is real medicine. The rest is then up to the patient. I can give them perfectly balanced hormones, but if they eat pizza all day, hormonal treatment is not going to work as well. Good nutrition, exercise, stress relief—these are measures that will uplift their lives.

I also tell my patients to not watch sad, terrible, gruesome programs on television. I tell them instead to listen to motivational tapes. Pamper yourself with daily bubble baths; use aromatherapy. Attend a house of worship, find joy in happy things, watch programs that are uplifting. I have even been known to prescribe a dog for lonely seniors. I put on their prescription: Go to the Humane Society and adopt a dog. Do whatever it takes to build yourself up physically, emotionally, and spiritually every day.

When patients on antidepressants come in and say these drugs are not working, I tell them that they will never, ever find happiness from a pill. There is no magic cure. You have to have balance in everything.

I am always trying to improve myself so I am able to give more to my patients. I feel honored to be in a position to have people come to me to help them and be involved in their health. There is nothing more intimate and precious than a person allowing you to help them with their health. I take that very seriously, and it gives me a great deal of pleasure. My patients have my cell phone number so they can call me anytime with questions or to let me know how they are feeling.

SS: Your lucky patients.

DR. PAUNESKY'S TOP FIVE
ANTIAGING RECOMMENDATIONS

1. Bioidentical hormone replacement therapy helps boost your immune system. Work with your doctor to obtain a regimen individualized just for you.

2. Talk to your doctor about adding the hormone pregnenolone to your bioidentical hormone replacement therapy, if you are a woman. About 90 percent of all women over age fifty are low in this hormone, which is a precursor to other hormones in the body.

3. Talk to your doctor about whether you need extra testosterone. It improves sex drive in women and improves brain function in everyone.

4. Even if you have perfectly balanced hormones, you cannot afford to eat junk food all the time. This will negate the benefit of bioidentical hormone replacement therapy.

5. Live an uplifting lifestyle—no exposure to gruesome, violent shows in the media, regular pampering, regular attendance at a house of worship, and listening to motivational tapes, among other measures.

CHAPTER 11

T. S. WILEY:
RHYTHMIC CYCLING.

T. S. Wiley is an anthropologist focusing on evolutionary biology and environmental endocrinology in molecular medicine and genetics. She is a member of the New York Academy of Sciences and has been a guest investigator at Sansum Medical Research Institute. She is the author of two books, Sex, Lies, and Menopause and Lights Out: Sleep, Sugar, and Survival. She is also the creator of a unique form of BHRT called the Wiley Protocol. T. S. Wiley understands the hormonal system from the inside out and has been a great inspiration for me to continue to study and learn about the inner workings of our physiology. I believe you will be fascinated by the depth of her knowledge of how it all works.

SS: Women of our generation from ages forty to seventy are now considered the sickest women in history. We have cancers of the breast, ovaries, and uterus. Our doctors perform approximately 1 million hysterectomies a year in this country alone. Do you think this was caused by the pill?

TSW: Well, I believe that's certainly where it started. At this point, it is my concerted opinion that bioidentical hormones are the answer, versus synthetics. But how you should take bioidenticals is a huge question. I mean, we know that synthetic hormones were in the pill. And we know the dosing rhythm the pill made was more like a bad TV screen than the normal rhythm that occurs in the body of a young woman.

So the pill's synthetic hormones and dosing regimen derange the original HPA (hypothalamic-pituitary-adrenal) axis, which is sort of a global positioning system, to tell your systems the time of day and year based upon your location to the planet. Unfortunately, whether or not the axis ever rights itself depends upon **childbirth.** If you have babies after the pill, that's a start, that helps. Whether or not this axis can stay righted as you continue to reproduce depends upon lifestyle. How late you stay up, how much sugar you eat, how old you are inside. But once the HPA axis is deranged, you need a jolt, like cardiac paddles, you know, when they jump-start your heart to get your hormones back in sync with the planet. You can use bioidenticals, if you use them in rhythm and use them the right way, to make peaks that feed back to the brain, and then the brain talks to the lower half. You have to make up the part of the song that is missing. Make sense?

SS: Yes. But if the pill was really synthetic hormones, which means that we women were not fully ovulating all those years, then all of us in this generation were in hormone imbalance. That's disturbing.

TSW: Well, that's why in my research, I went all the way back to the beginning of modern time. That's what scientists do. I wanted to know what it was to be a woman, and I wanted to know what had changed. I wanted to know what the lies were that made us all so desperately sick. So I had to look at what had changed for women in the last 150 years. The pill was the major factor. The pill was not mimicking nature, and whenever you do that, there's going to be trouble.

But the pill gave women a new kind of freedom. At the turn of the century, women were fighting for the right to vote. We were fighting for equality, but we forgot that men and women are different biologically, physiologically. The pill led us to believe that we could have sex without pregnancy, but nobody consulted our bodies about this premise. We were pressured to pursue higher and higher education, because we had to wait for men taking advantage of the GI Bill after World War II to marry and have children, leading to careers that put us in competition with biologically different creatures—men. What no one ever thought to ask were the real questions: Is it more dangerous to have a first pregnancy after thirty than it is to have no children at all? Or could delaying childbearing until we "couldn't" have children make us sick in ways we could never have imagined?

You see, the birth control pill was the first powerful drug prescribed to normal healthy women for long-term use. The pill was low-level estrogen (synthetic, not real), plus progestins, dosed in an abnormal rhythm, and it put the body into a sort of controlled menopause. Since menopause is the beginning of the end healthwise, this was a tragedy to perpetrate on eighteen-year-old women.

SS: Those of us who were on the pill were then in a controlled menopause, because we were unknowingly using the same hormones that the Women's Health Initiative told us to discontinue, meaning the synthetic hormones. Could this be the reason for the rise in breast cancer?

TSW: By 1962, research stated that there were 132 reports of blood clots and 11 deaths. Pill users were beginning to show abnormal glucose tolerance and some diabetes from altered metabolism. Today we know, from the Women's Health Initiative 2002 involving 103,027 women in Norway and Sweden, that even users of the minipill have a 22 percent increase in breast cancer versus childless women who haven't used oral contraceptives. When the pill came on the market, it contained even larger doses of hormones, far more than are found in today's diverse and still effective array of birth control pills. The early pill was as dangerous as today's pill, yet women whose doctors prescribed it received little or no warning of risks and complications, such as blood clots and strokes, et cetera, because since it had never really been tested in the way drugs are now, no one knew how destructive synthetic hormones could be to natural rhythms such as fertility, mating, and sleeping.

The Women's Health Initiative was abruptly curtailed when it was found that a common hormone replacement drug, Prempro, actually seemed to increase women's risks of breast cancer, stroke, and pulmonary embolism.

Women's bodies were designed to breed early and often, breast-feeding each child for years and thereby building up enough hormones to insulate themselves from later diseases. There's the pill, and the other reason women get breast cancer these days is that they don't have babies early enough, don't have enough babies, and don't breast-feed them long enough.

SS: Then where is the outrage, why don't we know this?

TSW: I try to get mad enough for all of us in my books.

SS: I delivered my baby as a teenager. No one ever talked to me about breast-feeding. The nurse brought my son to me and said that mother's milk had germs and that it would be better for the baby to give him baby formula. It was a decision I have regretted all my life. Further, they gave me a shot to dry up my milk. What was in that shot?

TSW: Yeah, that was very common in the seventies. It was probably DES in that shot.

SS: You mean tamoxifen? The cancer aftercare drug?

TSW: Not the same drug, but the same effect. Both of them are synthetic "superestrogens." Tamoxifen has the effect of destroying estrogen receptors over time, but DES is what causes cervical cancer in offspring generations later. If you force estrogen, you turn off prolactin (a pituitary hormone that induces lactation and prevents ovulation); that's how you dry up milk. Today they use something called Pariodel, which is a dopamine agonist that will also block prolactin reception. They think that this is safer, which is nonsense because it is not nursing that will hurt you.

SS: I'm beginning to see my history. I started having bad Pap smears early in my twenties. I had two D&Cs in those years. At that time, I was too young to ask what and why. I imagine now it was because I had the dry-up shot. I was then put on birth control pills for twenty years.

TSW: Oh my God. That is a long time to be on birth control pills. There are fifty-nine different versions of the pill on the market today, as well as a contraceptive patch called Ortho Evra that you can "preview" by tearing out a dud sample in women's magazines. Right now, 16 million women are on the pill in America. Approximately one-third of those women are on it for perimenopausal symptoms. The pill can in no way ameliorate the real and present dangers to health before, during, and after menopause. Our evidence shows that, at best, it masks the real symptoms of impending disease and enhances low-level estrogen-driven cell proliferation in the breasts, liver, and cervix. Birth control pills contain higher doses of synthetic estrogen than regular standard of care hormone replacement therapy. The very same progestins' thrombotic action [forming of blood clots] in birth control pills has been seen to be caused by the "Pro" in Prempro in the recently canceled HRT heart trials in the Women's Health Initiative. We in America have taken almost five times the amount of birth control pills as all the other countries in the world combined. For our health's sake, this is all very, very bad. We don't breast-feed the ones the pill prevented us from ever considering having. Contraceptives have been the key player in our lack of childbearing and, by degree, our subsequent lack of breast-feeding, so this starts to round out the picture of why breast cancer is an epidemic.

SS: Why is breast-feeding so vital to our health?

TSW: Breast-feeding immunizes the baby against death from the outside . . . germs and the like. But breast-feeding immunizes you, the mother, against death from breast cancer. In July 2002, the British medical journal **The Lancet** concluded that a woman's risk of breast cancer **decreases** by 7 percent for every birth she experiences; 3 percent more for each year under twenty-eight years old she is when that child is born; and most important, another 4.3 percent for every twelve months of her life that she breast-feeds. Add to that another 23 percent for whether or not she was personally breast-fed by her mother.

SS: So what are women to do? It's too late to go back. We've taken the pill. We didn't breast-feed our babies. And we postponed having babies so we could pursue our careers.

TSW: You're right . . . you can't breast-feed babies you never had, so that protection is gone, but you can put natural hormones back in a normal rhythmic fashion so your brain believes you might still be making them. With any luck, that may be all it takes to fool all of your systems into staying healthy for that potential. Young women should exercise all of the options when they are biologically capable of them before it's too late. It's hard to exercise your options when you're on chemotherapy or have Alzheimer's disease. Biological choice must come first before lifestyle choices. As a researcher into women's health, someone needs to tell our daughters what no one told us: that first-trimester abortion increases breast cancer by an overall odds ratio of one to three. Unfortunately, at this late date, for some of us, it seems biology **is** destiny.

Molecular biology makes it look very promising that we can stop the epidemic of breast cancer with rhythmic natural hormone replacement. Now that we have the knowledge of why breast cancer takes the lives of those we love, let's not repeat the same mistakes. The **Lancet** study and literally thousands of others like it make clear that the pill, lack of breast-feeding, and menopausal cancers are inextricably linked and no one ever told you.

Reproduction is an elemental force that you can use wisely or that can destroy you.

SS: But we're dying of breast cancer, heart disease, and dementia. Can bioidentical hormone replacement truly be the only answer for us?

TSW: There is another study, from the **Journal of Proceedings of the National Academy of Sciences** from October 2001 that says full-term pregnancy early in reproductive life is protective against breast cancer in women. Pregnancy also provides protection in animal studies against carcinogen-induced breast cancer [the environment]. Pregnancy shows the same protective effects for heart disease and dementia, and I believe these effects can successfully be mimicked by using natural hormones estrogen and progesterone.

In other words, I think it's going to be all right; just call your doctor and tell him what you want. Tell him you've done your homework, considered your options, and you want hormone replacement— natural bioidentical transdermal creams in a natural rhythm, probably for the rest of your life.

SS: One of the biggest obstacles in turning women on to bioidentical hormones is having a period at the end of the progesterone peak in your protocol. But what about doctors who give women a choice to have a period or not?

TSW: I sat with one doctor recently who said, "If a woman comes in and says she doesn't want to have a period, how can I argue with her?" I said, "I don't agree. I think women need to be informed. And they're coming to you for information. They have not been educated into understanding what normal and natural is. It's your job as the doctor to say to that woman, "I highly recommend you have a period." And he sat there with his mouth open.

SS: What about hysterectomies? My uterus was removed this year because of severe hyperplasia. It wasn't cancer or even precancer, but with my history of breast cancer, I was warned that this hyperplasia could become cancer. I felt there was no choice.

TSW: Cancer doesn't mechanically move like that. Women with breast cancer look to their lymph nodes as the next place it goes. But there was an article in the **New England Journal of Medicine** in 1991 or 1992 that stated that when you have a pinpoint-size lesion, like the end of a pen, in your breast, you already have breast cancer cells in the bone marrow of your shin or your leg. Now, realistically, it didn't travel there.

SS: I've never heard this.

TSW: I believe what is happening is a bodywide phenomenon of a change in stem cells. The stem cells in your breast made some wonky cells, and we'll call them cancer. But the stem cell in your leg can make breast cancer because a stem cell anywhere can make anything. That's how **I** believe metastasis occurs. That's why with a woman's uterus, I would first try a lot of estrogen and progesterone to reprogram bleeding before removing it, because once they perform a hysterectomy, all they've done is remove the evidence, but you're still not protected, you're still not in a normal rhythm. Does that make sense? I'm being candid with you, not trying to scare you.

SS: Yes, but what about excessive bleeding?

TSW: Actually, using the Wiley Protocol, we fix that problem with more estrogen. Doctors know that in a hospital setting, they "cure" hemorrhaging with high-dose Premarin intravenously. I'm saying you save your uterus with rhythmic cycling. You must put back the estrogen and progesterone in a template that is recognized by the brain and the stem cells. You can't just throw it in haphazardly. You can't give a static dose, either; it has to be given rhythmically just as it happened when you were a young woman still making those hormones. Putting back hormones is a huge question. Obviously they should be bio-identicals. The only logical conclusion I came to in the eight years of research was that you absolutely had to put them back the way you originally had them.

Women have hysterectomies routinely, but if women were given hormones rhythmically, I believe very few would need to have their uteruses removed.

SS: But what about repairing the damage of years of birth control pills? Can it be done?

TSW: Birth control pills have certainly exacerbated the situation. But taking a static dose of BHRT, the same dose every day, whether it's high or low, further deranges brain rhythms. You can't receive progesterone to stop the bleeding unless the estrogen makes a peak on day 12 and then comes down, because your brain and all cells in the body make a progesterone receptor at that crescendo point of estrogen. If you have a steady dose of estrogen and it's low, you just keep building and building the lining and that causes excessive bleeding, because even if you use progesterone, you can't "receive" it. Everything that happens to a cell happens at the receptor level through gene activity, and the rhythm of the hormones creates those receptors.

SS: I have to say this goes against many other doctors I have spoken with. They say that it is excessive estrogen that builds the lining and creates this excessive bleeding.

TSW: Sorry, they're wrong. The premise that in hemorrhaging, estrogen production is "excessive" is a misleading characterization. While the estrogen pours **continuously,** chronically, in a nonvarying way, the fact that it never reaches a peak of production means it never provokes a progesterone receptor. Is that "excessive"? Not exactly. It's dysrhythmic. I've done the science. What you want to reach is normal apoptosis—that is, death of the cells, the release of them (menstruation), and the birth of them again (rebuilding the lining for the next month to get ready to make a baby). Every woman goes through this process each month while she is still making hormones. This requires estrogen peaks and progesterone peaks. When this doesn't happen, cancer cells can proliferate.

We are about reproducing. That is what the brain knows. That is our job as members of the human species.

Let me tell you how powerful the human brain is. I was talking to a woman in Washington where we have group meetings. And this woman said to me, "I have nipple tenderness," and I said, "How many months have you been on the Wiley Protocol?" Because in the first three months of using that rhythm with bioidentical creams, you can have breast tenderness, like you're in puberty again. Your body wakes up. She said, "Three months." And I said, "Well, it should end at the end of this month, because that's what I see in group diagnosis. And she said, "I don't have breasts; I've had a double mastectomy."

SS: What's that about?

TSW: That's the morphic field. Your brain doesn't know once it has hormones and the right rhythm that your breasts are gone or that your uterus is gone. Just the brain talking to those organs makes them appear to exist again. The hormones actually, if they're taken right, change your personal reality. The women on the Wiley Protocol who've had hysterectomies can have cramps right before their periods if the estrogen's off, and they don't have a uterus. This proves [biologist Rupert] Sheldrake. You know, Sheldrake is the guy who does morphic fields. His last book was about how your dog knows when you're coming home.

SS: Because the brain doesn't know that the uterus isn't there?

TSW: Right, if the hormones are right, your body thinks you're intact. Do you know what that means? This is a huge deal in psychoneuroimmunology, in physics.

SS: So how exactly does a woman trick her body into believing she has a uterus?

TSW: We need to figure out when the first day of your last period was, even if it was abnormal bleeding. Because the brain was a part of a rhythm. So many women on the Wiley Protocol are missing their uteruses and can't tell me the first day of their last period, so we also use the lunar calendar. For women who have had cancer, I usually start them on day 14, because if they have any tumors, by starting them on progesterone and estrogen on day 14, they get a blast of progesterone with estrogen first, so we don't get tumor flare.

SS: But what about blood tests?

TSW: We draw blood in month 3, and we look at blood work on days 12 and 21. Looking before month 3 is not useful because in the first month that we give you this estrogen, you're not going to have enough receptors to use. It takes receptor turnover for a couple of cycles to get a full complement of receptors for both hormones. This way you receive enough estrogen to make a progesterone receptor. It can take two months. So on the third month we measure your blood and look at your symptoms and then raise the dose or lower it depending upon what you need.

SS: Cream as a transport system is controversial. Some doctors don't believe in creams.

TSW: The problem with troche or drops is that they peak in your body in two to three hours, and then it's gone. With cream we are making a depot in your fat base so that you get the "pulsatility" that is the hallmark of a hormone. Your brain doesn't receive hormones as hormones unless there's a beat. By putting it in your fat base in cream form, every time your heart beats the blood goes through you and you get a little pulse of hormone. This way nobody has highs or lows. The fat base as a delivery system works really well. A lot of women are very thin, but most of us have a little fat on the backs of our arms. By escalating and descending the dosing schedule, we recreate the "amplitude," also a hallmark of endocrine function. We justify this premise by measuring hormone levels in the blood on days 12 and 21 to see if they match twenty-year-old levels.

SS: Do you believe rhythmic cycling will keep women from getting cancer?

TSW: There's no cure for cancer. There is an understanding of cancer, however. If you give it what it wants, it stops, and it wants hormonal balance mimicking the way your body once made it. And when you understand cancer and give it what it wants, it stops bothering you. It stops trying to be a third thing, another life form that's not you. So in understanding proliferation and apoptosis, you aim for relative rates. You get the hormones right enough, then you get apoptosis, which is balanced hormones.

SS: This is a lot of information. If I smoked, I'd go have a cigarette. Thank you for being so forthcoming. I am fascinated.

TSW: I just want women to know what I know, and then they can make their own decisions on how to live their lives and how to take care of themselves.

SS: One more thing: In your book **Lights Out,** you explain that going to sleep early (between 9:00 and 10:00 p.m.) lowers cortisol and insulin. Could going to bed late be a major factor in women's inability to lose weight?

TSW: Yes. It's really very simple. This is something we can't sell or bottle; you just need to go to bed.

T. S. WILEY'S TOP FIVE ANTIAGING RECOMMENDATIONS

1. Use bioidentical hormones, but use them in rhythm and use them the right way. You can't give a static dose; it has to be given rhythmically, just as it happened when you were still making hormones. Call your doctor and tell him or her what you want. Say you've done your homework, considered your options, and you want hormone replacement—natural bioidentical transdermal creams in a natural rhythm, probably for the rest of your life.

2. Bioidentical hormones, given in this way, are one method of reversing the damage a woman has unknowingly done to her body by delaying childbirth, not breast-feeding, having dry-up shots, and taking birth control pills. That may be all it takes to fool all of your systems into staying healthy for that potential. Women should exercise all of the options when they are biologically capable before it's too late. It's hard to exercise your options when you're on chemotherapy or have Alzheimer's disease.

3. Natural bioidentical transdermal creams are the most effective delivery system. With cream, we are making a depot in your fat base. Your brain doesn't receive hormones as hormones unless there's a beat. By putting it in your fat base in cream form, every time your heart beats the blood goes through you and you get a little pulse of hormone.

4. There's really no cure for cancer. There is an understanding of cancer, however. If you give it what it wants, it stops, and it wants hormonal balance mimicking the way your body once made it. And when you understand cancer and give it what it wants, it stops bothering you.

5. One of the best but most overlooked ways to lose weight is to get to sleep early (between 9:00 and 10:00 p.m.). Doing so lowers cortisol and insulin.

PART TWO

MEN AND THEIR HORMONES

Aging equates to disease.

Energy equates to health.

—Dr. Michael Galitzer

CHAPTER 12

MEN AND HORMONES: IT'S NOT ABOUT ERECTIONS (WELL, NOT AT FIRST!)

As men age and lose their testosterone, an "all-nighter" means not getting up to pee!

If men could understand the joy of replacing their declining hormones with real hormones, they would be flocking to their doctors' offices. Most men are wrapped up in the thought process that testosterone is only for guys "who can't get it up"! Not only do men experience the male equivalent of menopause—andropause—they also experience fluctuations exactly like women from environmental stresses and the stress associated with being a man in a very competitive world.

As men hit forty (and sometimes younger), hormonal changes occur that inhibit physical, sexual, and cognitive function. The first telltale sign of a typical middle-aged man is increased abdominal fat and shrinking muscles, which is a hallmark of declining hormones. Once broad shoulders begin to shrink and droop downward, there is a loss of well-being, sometimes manifesting as depression, fatigue, alterations in mood and cognition, decreased libido, erectile dysfunction, prostate disease, and heart disease. All of these conditions are directly related to hormone imbalances that are correctable with diet, exercise, and bioidentical hormone replacement.

Even though a solution exists for men experiencing this hormonal decline, most still hide, run, and shrink from the therapy because somehow it is all tied up in their "manliness." I feel bad as I watch older men regularly suffer the effects of hormonal decline because it doesn't have to be this way. They lose their thoughts, run to the bathroom to pee constantly, lose their physiques, and quietly begin to fade to black rather than admit that all is not well. These men are in a state of hormonal decline, and it is correctable.

ANDROPAUSE IS REAL

Andropause, or male menopause, is finally becoming increasingly accepted. Andropause refers to the gradual but significant loss of testosterone, DHEA, and growth hormone: There is a slow and relentless decline of testicular function and, as a result, testosterone production.

We women lose our hormones (90 percent over a two-year period), and it's so "in our face" that most of us would do anything to relieve the symptoms. But it takes men ten to twelve years to completely drain out; in fact, it's so gradual that they do not attribute these "symptoms" to anything but aging. Most men have not realized that aging is declining hormones and that the decline can be slowed down and in some cases reversed with BHRT. Just as menopause is the change of life for women, andropause is the change of life for men. Every hormone has a "pause." Andropause is becoming increasingly accepted by the medical community, yet there are still many doctors in this country and around the globe who don't buy this premise. But look around you—men are falling apart, and it is happening younger and younger.

Other andropause symptoms to watch for include

- low energy
- fatigue
- loss in height or osteoporosis
- enlarged prostate
- depression
- anxiety
- less strong or less frequent erections
- impotence

Once men understand the benefits of real hormone replacement, once they "get it," they'll be as enthusiastic as the women who are on BHRT. Most women I ask say they would never give up their bioidenticals. The improvement in quality of life is so drastic, and so enjoyable, that life without them would be unthinkable. Men who have gotten turned on to real hormone replacement feel the same way. All of those symptoms men start to experience can be slowed down, and in most cases reversed, with bioidentical hormone replacement of the following hormones.

TESTOSTERONE

Testosterone is the hormone that gives men their strength and size. Most doctors don't realize that testosterone starts dropping for young men in their early thirties, and it's a long, gradual decline over the years. By the time a man is seventy, he typically has half the testosterone he had when he was thirty or younger.

Most guys think that as long as they can "get it up," all is well, and for most men the erection is indeed the last thing to go. Way before that, you experience a general loss of vitality . . . just a tired, worn-out feeling. Your belly starts expanding, your doctor starts telling you things like "Watch your cholesterol," you are put on statin drugs or blood pressure medicine. Your joints start aching, and your confidence begins to wane. It is crucial that men understand that testosterone loss is serious stuff, that low testosterone increases the risk of heart disease, prostate cancer, and Alzheimer's disease.

Testosterone is an "anabolic steroid," meaning that it builds bone and muscle. The heart is the largest muscle in the body, therefore testosterone is vital to keep the "heart muscle" strong and pumping. Testosterone also protects the heart by keeping cholesterol and blood pressure down. Age-related decline in testosterone closely parallels the increase in heart disease as men get older. Testosterone helps with heart conditions such as angina, and it increases blood flow to the heart.

The desire for sex as well as sexual sensation and performance is promoted by the stimulation of testosterone receptor sites in the nerves, blood vessels, and genitals.

Testosterone is also vital to the male frame; without it, the muscles begin to wither noticeably. A man who is experiencing testosterone loss can work out all day long but without results. Building muscle is impossible without testosterone. In fact, this factor alone is enough to get many men to consider replacement. No man wants his muscles to shrink. Testosterone also keeps your bones strong. Without it, a man can be prone to osteoporosis, which is not just a woman's disease.

Testosterone protects your heart in other ways. For instance, it helps to prevent angina (pain or discomfort due to lack of oxygen to the heart muscle). Interestingly, age-related decline in testosterone closely parallels the increase in heart disease as men get older. This should tell you something.

The desire for sex, as well as sexual sensation and performance, is promoted by the stimulation of testosterone receptor sites in nerves, blood vessels, and the genitals. Low testosterone can lead to atrophy of the male genitals but can be reversed with testosterone replacement.

Testosterone is part of the template that tells the brain "All is well"—that this man is still reproductive (young). By now you know that bioidentical hormone replacement therapy is the secret to keeping your insides young and disease-free. It's hard to understand why men are not jumping on this bandwagon, but I believe a big part of the problem is that the doctors do not understand the male hormonal system any better than they understand the female hormonal system.

Of all hormonal declines, loss of testosterone is the most common deficiency in men over age forty. Remember, a low or nonexistent sex drive is usually the last symptom to show up. Before that happens, the following changes in a man's physical and emotional self make themselves known:

- shrinking muscles
- weight loss
- decreased stamina

- weaker erections
- fatigue
- depression
- irritability
- gallbladder problems
- enlarged breasts

Testosterone levels are established by blood and saliva tests. For men, the optimal range for total testosterone is between 6,000 and 9,000 pg/mL—the level you typically see in young, healthy men. According to Dr. Philip Lee Miller, men feel their best when their ranges are in the upper part of the normal range. Up to 99.7 percent of the total testosterone in circulation at any given time is bound up with proteins and is not in an active form. The amount of free, or available, testosterone should ideally be around 25 to 35 pg/mL.

If your numbers come back low, a qualified doctor can prescribe bioidentical hormone replacement therapy in the form of patches, creams, gels, and sublingual tablets or lozenges, or even injections. All testosterone products require a prescription. Proper treatment can restore your levels to a normal range so that you can experience reversal of a symptom.

This hormone decline is not going to stop. You really can't ignore it. Every year, you go into further hormonal decline, so it makes sense that your hormone replacement needs would increase each year or more often depending upon your health and lifestyle. If you find that you are irritable or "testy," testosterone can help, just as estrogen helps women who become "bitchy." With hormones, too much or too little and you don't feel "right." Seemingly from out of nowhere, those seven dwarfs pop up again: Itchy, Bitchy, Sweaty, Sleepy, Bloated, Forgetful, and All-Dried-Up. They are real, and they visit men and women alike. The goal with balanced bioidentical hormone replacement is to send those dwarfs packing.

TESTOSTERONE AND PROSTATE HEALTH

After about age fifty or sixty, you may experience enlargement (benign prostatic hypertrophy, or BPH) or inflammation of your prostate gland, whose job is to contribute to the production of semen. The prostate is the male equivalent of a female breast; it has ducts just as in a woman's breast, and in these ducts, testosterone makes food for the sperm. Without testosterone, prostate problems begin. No testosterone, no food for the sperm; no food for the sperm, no semen; no semen, no sex! Younger men don't run out of sperm. Younger men don't get enlarged prostates, and they rarely get prostate cancer. Why? Because their bodies make a full complement of hormones, including testosterone.

Prostate disease is so common that men expect it to catch up with them at some point in their lives as they age. But it doesn't have to. You can head off prostate problems by beginning bioidentical testosterone replacement as soon as you become the slightest bit symptomatic.

Once the prostate has begun to age and wither, prostate disease has an opportunity to occur. It's time to get your prostate checked if urination is painful or more frequent at night. This is your body talking to you . . . it's a warning. An enlarged prostate is just the beginning of a downward slope. It's another sign. I'll say it again—young men don't get enlarged prostates. Young men don't run out of sperm; young men rarely get cancer. Because they make a full complement of hormones, including testosterone. Their ratio of estrogen to testosterone is in balance.

Testosterone replacement will make you feel young again, and you will enjoy the amazing health benefits: protection against heart disease, mental decline, prostate disease and prostate problems, loss of libido, and deteriorating muscles.

Mainstream medicine believes that an enlarged prostate is exacerbated by testosterone. If a man has an elevated PSA test, he is immediately taken off testosterone or is given a hormone ablation drug to stop all testosterone production. Did this happen in nature?

Enlargement of the prostate is caused by excessive proliferation of the cells in the prostate. While many doctors believe that excess testosterone aggravates BPH, numerous studies show that high testosterone levels are not a risk factor. In fact, the latest research suggests that it may actually be high **estrogen** levels that cause excessive proliferation of the prostate cells. New-thinking doctors are questioning this standard of care. Testosterone is your life force. When you were young and fully hormonally productive, you did not have prostate problems. It is only in testosterone decline that problems occur. Does it make sense to take your testosterone away as a means to correct the problem? Doesn't it seem that this would make the problem worse? The absence of testosterone takes away quality of life, and it also signals to the brain that all is not well . . . that you are no longer a reproductive person (remember, biologically speaking, we are here to perpetuate the species, and this includes men; otherwise we are not necessary). The "new thinking" is that you want to "put back" what you are losing in the aging process to perfect balance and stop the decline.

In his book **Life Extension Revolution,** Dr. Miller writes, "Evidence shows that prostate disease increases precisely as natural testosterone levels decline in the aging male and that the incidence of prostate dysfunction is at its lowest at the time when lifetime testosterone exposure is peaking." Dr. Miller goes on to say, "Maintaining healthy testosterone levels is one of the most important things a man can do to protect the health of his prostate. The newest research suggests that low testosterone in combination with increasing estrogen may be the true culprit in prostate dysfunction."

Prostate cancer is a serious concern. Most researchers agree that high testosterone is not itself a risk factor for this cancer. However, if cancer is present, it is thought that testosterone can fuel its growth. For that reason, many antiaging doctors are reluctant to use testosterone replacement in the presence of prostate cancer. Yet in Europe, where medicine is more progressive, testosterone is actually being used as a treatment for prostate cancer with great results. Obviously more research is needed, but it makes you think: Young men make buckets of testosterone all day long, young men don't get prostate cancer as a rule . . . so it doesn't make sense that taking away testosterone in an older man would be the way to go (as many doctors interviewed in this book have concurred).

ESTROGEN

For a man to be a "man," he must have estrogen. A male has more testosterone than estrogen, but it is the correct ratio that makes him a "man." As men age, they lose testosterone, and in doing so, they overproduce estrogen. When there is more estrogen than testosterone, the man is no longer a male. He really can't "get it up" at this point. Now it really is all about erections! His body becomes feminized; he develops a flabby stomach and small breasts; his voice becomes higher and softer; his vitality diminishes and his energy dissipates; he appears to give up on the world and drop out. You've seen this decline in men you know or in your fathers. They just aren't the same guy anymore. To stay in the game, correct bioidentical hormone replacement is the answer. Frequently, men over fifty have estrogen levels that are even higher than those of women of the same age. Too much estrogen in the male body can increase the risk of heart attack and stroke and lead to inflammation of the prostate. To make matters worse, too much estrogen can also suppress testosterone production in the testes.

Estrogen is as important a component of a man's hormonal makeup as it is of a woman's. It is important to have the correct ratio of estrogen to testosterone. If a man is overweight, he can become estrogen-dominant just as a woman can, because fat cells produce and store estrogen. What's more, exposure to estrogenic chemicals in the environment such as those commonly used in pesticides can also create an estrogen imbalance in men. Many researchers link these chemicals to the rising rates of infertility and impotence in American men. Estrogen dominance in men stimulates breast cell growth and benign prostatic hypertrophy (enlarged prostate). It is extremely important to work with a qualified doctor to replace testosterone in the correct amount with bioidentical hormones. A knowledgeable doctor will know to not only check testosterone levels through labwork, but also to get estrogen levels.

Some symptoms of estrogen dominance or excess in men include:

- hair loss
- headaches
- breast enlargement
- weight gain
- irritability
- bloating and or/puffiness

Excess estrogen in men can be corrected and rebalanced. Helpful changes for men with excess estrogen include proper diet, regular exercise, and, of course, bioidentical hormone replacement. Sometimes a natural testosterone/estrogen blocker such as indole-3-carbinol might be advisable.

PROGESTERONE

The male body also produces progesterone, although in tiny amounts in the testicles and in the adrenal glands. Even though the amounts are small, progesterone is vital to a man's hormonal health and helps balance the estrogen that builds up in his body.

Progesterone is a precursor, or building block, to cortisol, testosterone, estrogen, and other hormones. All hormone levels drop with age, and so does the level of progesterone, causing more depletion of other hormones. Being under stress further depletes progesterone, because stress increases the demand for cortisol. If progesterone is low or missing, you can experience symptoms such as:

- low energy or fatigue
- decreased libido
- increased body fat
- enlarged prostate

To counterbalance the effects of excess estrogen, natural progesterone is often recommended for men over forty years of age or even younger, especially if there is a history of prostate cancer or BPH.

THYROID

Thyroid imbalance is common in men and women of all ages. A qualified doctor can correct this imbalance with T3, T4, a combination of both, or a natural thyroid extract. Diet and exercise are also a vital part of keeping the thyroid in balance.

Here are some of the symptoms of low thyroid:

- stiffness of the joints
- intolerance to cold or heat
- fatigue, lack of energy
- weight gain or difficulty losing weight
- low body temperature
- fluid retention
- constipation
- pale, dry skin
- puffiness in face, hands, and feet
- depression

- anxiety
- irritability

HORMONAL BALANCE

The good news is that andropause can be treated successfully and safely. It is so much easier for men to become hormonally balanced than it is for women. Men don't have a cycle, so it's a matter of determining the correct amounts to replace. Too much estrogen and not enough testosterone, plummeting DHEA levels, and low HGH levels are all correctable. Loss of testosterone in middle age can leave men feeling as if their life force is draining out of them, and depression is often the result.

Just as with women, the object is not to push hormone levels higher blindly, but rather to mimic the body's healthiest prime. You don't want hormones that are normal for your age . . . your age is in decline. You want the hormone levels when you were feeling your best and were at your healthiest. That is the great news. Men in their forties, fifties, sixties, seventies, eighties, and beyond can maintain a hormonal environment similar to that at their healthiest physical peak. It's like stopping the clock. The results are spectacular.

Men's hormone levels need to be established by blood and saliva tests. When increased estrogen levels accompany low testosterone levels, it will show up in the blood. This testing information is important to ensure testosterone replacement is appropriate for men.

Just as with women, there is no "one amount fits all"; every man is different. It takes the skill and perception of the doctor to access the clinical picture by looking at the patient and asking how he feels. Hormone therapy is a creative collaboration between doctor and patient using not only science, but also the powers of observation, intuition, and insight that no test tube can replace. When the physician is not measuring the estrogen simultaneously to get the correct ratio, for example, testosterone can be aromatized into estrogen, thus creating the opposite effect. So do not do this on your own.

This is why you must find a qualified antiaging physician. If testosterone is not administered correctly, testosterone replacement can be useless or can drive the testosterone/estrogen ratios even lower. In an effort to get the desired effect, some men will increase their dosage to harmful levels. Unfortunately, this will not work and may even backfire. Remember that hormones must never be played around with. Too much is too much, and too little is too little. You have to find the levels that are just right. You will know when your levels are in the right balance. Your body will feel better than ever, and you will have the energy you had as a youth.

I have simplified this information for you, but I'm

sure you have now gotten the message that the best friend you can have regarding your health is a qualified doctor. No matter how far you have to drive or fly, it is worth it. We're talking about your life and your health. Hormone replacement is not a "do it yourself" proposition. You need to work with a doctor who understands the complexities of testing, hormone balance, and interaction. By reading this information, you will be armed with enough knowledge to be an informed patient and have the ability to question when something doesn't feel right. Your doctor is not a god. Ask your doctor to please be honest with you, and when he or she doesn't know the answer, to let you know so you can continue your search for the solution to this tricky passage. If it were only about feeling better, a lot of people wouldn't bother, but it is the combination of feeling great and the incredible health benefits that make this effort worthwhile. This is your chance . . . this is new medicine; it has never been available before in the history of man. You can actually slow down the aging process. Most men are rejuvenated by this therapy, essentially feel young again. This is a true gift you can give yourself.

I look at my husband every day. He is now seventy years old and has been on bioidentical hormone replacement therapy for seven years. The turnaround in his health and vitality has been astounding. He went from being an aging man to a man with the energy of a thirty-five-year-old. His skin is thick and unwrinkled. His muscles are defined. His weight is better than it has ever been, and his waistline has returned to its youthful measurement. He has vitality, energy, charisma, sexuality, and happiness and is in perfect health. In other words, he is a "hunk." This true fountain of youth is available for all men. It is cutting-edge, and those who jump on this bandwagon will be the winners.

Let me close this chapter with a letter from a man, Larry G., who did jump on this bandwagon. This is the kind of enthusiasm I hear on a regular basis from people who are tired of feeling tired. Those who take the leap and decide to embrace the new medicine have this kind of passion for life and their newfound health. I think you will enjoy what this man has to tell you. His results speak for themselves. And I must say I enjoyed the compliments he gave me.

Dear Suzanne,

I had just turned 65 and was feeling old and useless. I couldn't remember who I was calling when I picked up the phone. I couldn't remember why I walked into a particular room in my house. I couldn't remember the stuff my wife told me to pick up on my way home. I couldn't remember anything, not even the names of close friends.

And I was loving my bed too much, sleeping in because I was up and down all night, sweating during the night for no reason, napping a lot during the day. I was bitchy and short with colleagues and

friends. And my muscles were going away after all my exercise with weights, followed by a paunchy stomach, which I had never had.

I noticed the skin on my hands thinning and starting to look like my dad's hands. I snacked on simple carbs for energy during the day, which of course put on many pounds. I felt my libido waning, and my erections were not as dynamic or long-lasting. This is what really got me to take a good hard look at myself, my body, and my forgetfulness that I always excused with a laugh, "Oops, I am having a senior moment," which in retrospect is not funny. It is a warning of things to come down the line: senility, Alzheimer's, or any number of diseases of aging.

I decided to do something about it, so I picked up Suzanne Somers' book The Sexy Years, and read about not only me and my issues, but my wife's as well. She had just slipped into the forgetfulness thing, but not as bad as me. She was also experiencing the 7 dwarfs of menopause, but not as bad as Suzanne had.

And because my wife is my high school sweetheart, and we have a lifetime of great times, and we are very physical together, we both decided to take the Suzanne Somers' Sexy Years journey.

My wife started first with bioidentical hormone replacement therapy and felt good within a few days. I started with testosterone and then DHEA, followed by a handful of supplements and oral drops, and as of three months ago, human growth hormone.

How do I feel? I feel better physically than I have ever felt, ever! Even better than when I was in my prime. I feel biologically young, perhaps in my thirties. And I am able to do anything physically. My muscles returned. My libido returned with a vengeance, and my wife keeps looking at me with that what-happened-to-you look.

I have turned into a hiking fool and need to go straight up a mountain to get rid of this excess energy, and for the first time in my life, I am experiencing endorphins, which I love.

When I took my annual physical, which involved a stress test on the treadmill, instead of a slight decline over the previous years, which had been the case, I was 20 percent to 30 percent more fit.

My doctor is now reading The Sexy Years and recommending it to his patients.

I needed testosterone to build up my muscles, and my brain needed testosterone to function at peak performance. I don't know where all this is going, but I love hearing from my friends that I look fabulous. A couple of them have suggested that I had plastic surgery because my wrinkles have diminished, and my skin tone glows, and I appear to have more musculature in my face. Not bad for an old guy.

Most of my doctors told me not to do anything. "Let nature takes its course. We don't know enough about testosterone and human growth hormone yet. Most of those supplements you are taking are probably ending up in Santa Monica Bay. Why do you want to do this?"

I dumped all my doctors and found new ones who are young and forward-thinking. The new age of medicine is not the old school of doctors terrified to do anything other than what the drug companies tell them to do. The new age of medicine is Eastern-influenced and homeopathic and designed to heal rather than cover up, which is what most prescriptions do. Think about it: If the drug companies make something that actually heals, they will soon be out of business, and their many shareholders would be very upset.

I may not live one day longer than nature allows me, and I may not be able to avoid future disease, but I am having the time of my life, and I feel better than I ever have and a lot better than any of my friends, who are really a bunch of grouchy old farts who pooh-pooh what I am doing while they are losing their minds and their bodies.

Kudos for you, Suzanne Somers; you have entertained me for decades and you have provided me with the Fountain of Youth. For you nonbelievers, take a good hard look at Suzanne, who I believe is 60 years old. That's a hot-looking babe!

CHAPTER 13

BRUCE: A FORTY-YEAR-OLD IN PERIANDROPAUSE

For the sake of my readers, I will tell you right off the top that this is a conversation between me and my son, Bruce Somers (so the adoring tone will be noted, but I will try to keep it under control). Bruce has always been forward-thinking, long before I was. He is one of many young men who have experienced periandropause. His work and lifestyle are stressful. Additionally, I did not nurse him, which makes me wonder if other young men his age, born to mothers of the sixties who were encouraged to give their babies formula rather than breast milk, have experienced the same syndrome. If you are one of those mothers, Bruce's interview may give you some insight.

SS: So, Bruce, how old were you when you started taking vitamins?

BS: Thirteen.

SS: And you made me nervous.

BS: I know. But I had read Earl Mindell's **Vitamin**

Bible, and while most kids were reading **Lord of the Rings** and **Lord of the Flies,** I needed something more concrete. As relaxed as I seemed to be, I was already worried about living forever, so I thought, no better time to start than now.

At thirteen—that would have been 1978—I remember going to you and Alan and asking if I could get these vitamins I had read about, and there were a lot of them. You said, "How do you know that what you are doing isn't hurting you, and how much can it really help you?" But you relented and said, "All right, if you go to our doctor and he says fine, then we'll support you in this." The interesting thing is that our doctor at that time said, "Well, if you want to waste your money, go ahead and take all these vitamins."

SS: As in "expensive urine."

BS: Exactly, which I think is the common belief. But I do remember how sick I was as a kid. I was always getting a lot of colds, flu, and bronchitis. But do you realize that when I started taking vitamins is when I started saying, "Oh, I never get sick"?

SS: You know, you're right.

BS: I remember being kind of a sickly child.

SS: And you had the stress of my divorce when you were a toddler. Then you missed me when I had to take a trip. And then there were some unpleasant stepmoms, and it was also a time when there weren't many kids from divorced families.

BS: Absolutely. It was stressful, whereas today

there is not much social stress for a child to come from a divorced family, at least in metropolitan cities. So the sickness could have been partially psychosomatic. But my well-being today stems from the time I started taking vitamins right up until this very moment. I know there has to be a psychosomatic element, but I think psychosomatic positive thinking is part of wellness.

SS: The mind/body connection.

BS: Right. Studies have shown that when a patient has a strong belief in his or her medical practitioner, the potential for healing goes up about 40 percent.

SS: What do you think it was about you (besides the fact that you are incredibly smart, says the mother) that you would have such innate intelligence about this? Because it was very forward-thinking at that time.

BS: Being a child of divorce had a maturing effect on me, one that a child from a typical 2.3-sibling family doesn't experience. A part of you becomes a little adult, which is interestingly similar to being a child of an alcoholic or any other addiction. Other parts of you aren't so mature, of course. But being a little adult and being your best friend—you know, going out with you all the time and getting a lot of pop psychology early through the talks we'd have, or the talks I'd have with your friends—made me mature for my age. Your friends would talk about taking care of their bodies, for example.

SS: So way back then you decided to choose to take good care of yourself?

BS: Absolutely.

SS: So I guess it would follow that you would be the first one in your age group to start working with hormones.

BS: The first hormones I started taking were in a tablet—DHEA.

SS: How old were you?

BS: I was thirty-three. My doctor recommended I start taking it. I remember you and I shared a smile over it because Alan was also taking it, and it was strange that someone in his sixties was taking it, so why did I need it, too?

SS: Why **did** you need it?

BS: Quite simply from my blood results. My DHEA was low for my age.

SS: Do you think it was stress-induced?

BS: I think so. I guess I have always been stressed, but from the time I went to graduate school, and well into the birth of our two children, pulling all-nighters was very routine. You know, there's that dumb badge of honor of working harder than any-one, which is pandemic in our driving society.

SS: And also there are particular stresses on young men to achieve and "make it."

BS: That's true. You see, I was in my chosen field but not doing exactly what I wanted to be doing. I know this sidesteps the hormone discussion, but it is hard to understand when you are going through these passages that you are supposed to be experiencing this kind of stress for life's lessons. But somehow God or the forces protecting me steered me toward a career that enabled me not only to feed my kids, but to be there for them. I think my biggest guilt in life would be not being there for my kids and my wife.

SS: Your lucky family. Walk me down your hormonal path. What was the first sign that you needed something beyond DHEA?

BS: With the pressures of marriage with kids, my libido was suppressed because there was no time. If you do have the ability to sleep, you take it, because between work and kids, you're up every few hours, and that's universal. Something was "off" with me. My libido was low. I would feel sexual and feel stimulation, but I was just too fatigued to do anything about it. One of the questions my doctor, Dr. David Allen, asked me was: "If you see someone hot walking down the street, do you notice her and do you say 'hmm' . . . you know, if you could, you would?"

SS: And what was your answer?

BS: Yeah. So he said, "Okay, well, that's a good sign." Still, I just wasn't in the mood like I once was. But think about it: Sex for most people doesn't just happen. Jokingly you say foreplay, but it's long before foreplay where you have to set the mood. You know, gotta make sure you don't have a little argument.

SS: Yep.

BS: Gotta make sure you help with the dishes. You gotta make sure you're clean, and that was too much effort, let alone the physical act. You know, you gotta set the whole thing up.

SS: So you were fatigued; you were just tired?

BS: I don't know that I realized I was tired then. I've been tired, I mean, I've been trying to be cognizant of being tired in the last few years and not letting myself get burned out. I'm not good at it. You see, I have a mom who's a workaholic in everything she does. She's the best mom, the best nightclub entertainer, the best salesperson, the best at everything she does.

SS: I'm working on it. I left dishes in the sink last night, you'll be proud to know.

BS: Good for you.

SS: So what did Dr. Allen say?

BS: About three or four years ago, he said that he wanted to put me on testosterone.

SS: What was your reaction?

BS: I guess my reaction was "Really?" but he said my levels were very low. Interestingly, my testosterone has always been lower on the baseline than it should be. But it got to the point where the things we were doing that should help my body stimulate its own testosterone production like DHEA didn't seem to work. So he put me on testosterone, and my levels started to go up.

SS: In writing this book, I have learned about periandropause in men. It sounds like this is the phenomenon that happened to you. Are your hormone numbers now at optimum?

BS: Yes.

SS: So once you were on testosterone, did you feel any difference, even though your lifestyle hadn't changed?

BS: I felt a difference. My hobby is cycling. It's totally illegal to use testosterone if you're cycling when you're racing. Even on amateur races, you're not allowed to use it. First off, I would never hide it, so when I was on the bike, I'd tell everyone that I was trying to get to where I'm supposed to be hormonally for my health.

SS: When you were cycling after taking testosterone, did you feel a newfound strength that you hadn't felt before?

BS: Yes. With cycling, it is tough to hang in there with the other cyclists, even on training rides, fighting for the front and going toe-to-toe with people. I was nowhere near the strongest, but I was on the front line. I was in the big group.

SS: You're also the first person I knew to inject human growth hormone. Once again, you made me nervous.

BS: Right.

SS: How did you have the confidence to do that? Who recommended that you take HGH?

BS: Again, it was Dr. Allen, and it was based upon tests. A lot of the motivation for me was because of sports. You've always heard about HGH and athletes, and frankly, testosterone is considered a steroid. So when my doctor recommended I take HGH from looking at my blood work, I asked him about athletes. "How come it's okay for me, but it's not okay for athletes to do it?" He told me that a lot of these athletes are ten to fifteen years younger than me. Their testosterone and HGH levels are already through the roof, and they're topping off the tank, basically. They're trying to get that extra 1 or 2 percent, which frankly is what separates the gold medalists from the losers.

So basically he was trying to get me balanced yet better for my age level. He wasn't trying to make me a twenty-five-year-old. That would be weird and dangerous. Everything is about moderation. Dr. Allen has been trying to get me five to seven years younger on the inside. That will manifest on the outside. That's the benefit.

SS: Yes, but at the time you started, you were somewhere between thirty-five and forty.

BS: Right.

SS: Were you declining in hormones?

BS: Yes.

SS: Okay, so you were declining early?

BS: Yes, and he said that by thirty-five most people are declining. He's a very smart doctor. I hate to say we live in a vain world, but when you look good to yourself, your self-perception is better, you feel better, and you do things to keep that feeling. I attributed a lot of that good feeling to the testosterone, the HGH, and the sixty-five vitamins, minerals, and Chinese herbs I take twice a day. That good feeling motivates me to get up early in the morning. I like that. It's worth waking up early to go cycling or running or to go to the gym to lift weights.

SS: Do you feel any different on HGH? Do you feel the strength that they talk about?

BS: I go through periods where I might be training for the summer, so that requires that I spend all spring in training. As part of training for cycling, you climb mountains, and I know how fast or how slow I can do them at any given point of the year because I've climbed them so many times. Now, I am cycling better than I do during the summer when I'm at my peak, even better than I was five years ago.

SS: Could that be that you're a better cyclist, or is it a combination of your training and the regimen you're on?

BS: I think it's a combination. I'm certainly smarter. I certainly have more mental resolve. People think of hormones and vitamins as purely something to do to have an end benefit that is a physical manifestation, but it's equally important that it ends up being mind-empowering, meaning that it helps to control your attitude. By taking all of these vitamins and minerals, I believe I'm programmed to work harder when I'm on the bike. I have the mental acuity to sit there and say, "This is temporary." I can relate to Lance Armstrong when he says, "Pain is temporary; quitting is forever." It's a mantra I use when I'm climbing. With each year I seem to be able to have that much more resolve and focus.

A lot of people probably think that with HGH you just get bigger muscles and you go faster. I think your muscles are going to be leaner for sure, and you're going to drop fat. I did have a little love handle, but the HGH has recontoured my body in conjunction with the exercise that I do. I also think you are feeding that part of you that says, "Hey, I look good. My wife thinks I look good." So now I feel sexy, and I also . . .

SS: Do the dishes? (laugh)

BS: Yep. Now I do the dishes. I make sure we don't fight. I dim the lights. I think ahead. That part is great. But also, I have the mental resolve to focus, and I see it in my work as well. Whatever the task at hand, it gets done. It's that ability to focus and get to the bottom of whatever business challenge I have.

SS: Because you're not worn out and exhausted.

BS: That's right. Another thing Dr. Allen gives me is a bone longevity pack, which is specific to someone who is athletic. Interestingly, it is also specific to the elderly for walking. Before taking testosterone and HGH, if I had a particularly hard workout, I'd feel it. I'd have very sore calves. If I did something other than cycling, like running, it would be very painful to walk down the stairs the next day. Now I can throw a run in, and the soreness is actually diminished. The only thing different in my regimen now is testosterone and HGH.

SS: I find that, too. Maybe it's because I've done yoga regularly for some time, but I never feel any soreness, and we do rather strenuous workouts. I feel HGH helps my performance.

BS: The Tour de France is a great example of what we're talking about. It's like running a marathon on a bike every day for three weeks. I think one day when it's better understood, everyone will have a regulated amount of testosterone and HGH because that's the new medicine.

SS: I also think for superathletes like those who compete in the Tour de France, the stress of such a grueling schedule is blowing out their natural hormonal levels. If anybody would need supplementation, it would be these athletes, because of the kind of stress they're under.

BS: Lance Armstrong's strategy is basically about building your body up to the point of what is called the "edge of the razor." You get to the point where you've lost all your body fat. You've lost everything that is not enhancing your performance as a cyclist, but in doing so, your immune system gets fragile. In cycling, everyone pays attention to one another. When an opponent sniffles or sneezes, it gives you a psychological edge. You think, Oh, they're getting a cold. They're never gonna make it for three weeks.

SS: It must be very frustrating for someone like a Lance Armstrong to understand the benefits of hormone replacement and not be able to take advantage of it because of ignorance. What do your friends think about you and your hormones?

BS: One friend in particular who is captain of the cycling team started going to Dr. Allen when he was ill. I suggested to him that he just get an IV vitamin push, which to me is more powerful than any penicillin I could take. When my friend was talking with Dr. Allen, he said, "I don't know what you're doing with Bruce, but you know, I cycle more than he does and he always stays up with me." He jokes about it, but I can tell he wants to have this kind of energy. In sports, but also in life, feeling youthful is addictive.

SS: Yes, and the addictive part of feeling youthful is the internal youth. To know that my body is working great. It's not about having a brand-new outfit or having my hair done. If I don't feel good inside, all the cosmetic work in the world won't help. Bad health shows.

BS: Yes. All these vitamins and minerals are also helping so you can make the correct decisions in life. However, let's say you take two people who have identical lives and are about the same age and put them in a decision-making mode, be it business or social. One is on vitamins and minerals with balanced hormonal levels; the other is not doing any of this. I'm gonna put my money on the person who's been taking vitamins and minerals and hormone replacements to make the better decision more consistently. I don't want to put down Western medicine, however. If someday I have a heart attack or, as happened to me as a kid, get run over by a car, I'm thankful for Western medicine. Otherwise I wouldn't be here.

SS: Absolutely. Western medicine excels at surgery, pain, and infections.

BS: One of the issues I see with Western medicine, however, is regarding antibiotics. I think they are losing their effect. When I was a kid, we were given penicillin. Then penicillin stopped working for us, so we were prescribed amoxicillin. Today, it's Zithromax, but even it is running its course. And now it's Levaquin; that's got to tell you something.

Recently, I was sick, and so was my producer. We had identical symptoms—coughing, bad throats, dizzy, and a little bit of a fever. I don't like any sympathy when I'm shooting because I have to be the general on the set. I went to Dr. Allen to have an IV vitamin push to try to see if I couldn't nip the illness in the bud. I suggested to my friend that we go together to my doctor and get an IV drip. I went; he didn't. The next day I woke up and realized I felt good. I got to the set. He was coughing blood.

SS: And what was in your IV drip?

BS: I had 25 mg of vitamin C, directly into my blood.

SS: What a progressive way to heal yourself rather than with an antibiotic! You're feeling so strong and healthy, your brain is working great, and you're at the top of your game. What would you say to young men who are reading this book, looking at what you do as expensive urine, and thinking this is a kind of craziness?

BS: We live in a world where people want quantifiable data, and what doesn't lie is your blood work. Everyone respects a medical lab because it's a Western concept, so we get our blood drawn and have our levels checked. Now you have concrete numbers. Take it to as many doctors as you want. Take it to the full traditional doctor, take it to one who's halfway there, and take it to a purely holistic doctor. Or find an endocrinologist. Take it so that you can feel comfortable about the information you're getting. All you need to hear from them is what are the average baselines for each of these numbers? What do these numbers mean? Assess it. At least give it a try. We know that this stuff isn't toxic. If hormones are scary, start with vitamins, or start with something like DHEA, which is very controllable. I know a lot of people are nervous about testosterone, estrogen, and HGH. Don't jump right into that. Life is about moderation.

SS: You're a walking example of health. You glow, and you shine. I'm saying this not just because I'm your mother. Really, when you walk into a room, you look great, and what you radiate is health. You're in peak physical condition; you've got no excess body fat. You're a walking example of the fact that what you're doing really works.

BS: Thank you. Obviously, we are born with certain genes, and we can enhance our health if we choose to do so. I believe that following this regimen of vitamins, minerals, Chinese herbs, and hormones, and seeing the positive results, has been self-fulfilling.

BRUCE'S LIST OF CHINESE HERBS

Xanthium fruit—an herb with anti-inflammatory and antiallergic actions.

Magnolia flower—popular as a remedy for maintaining respiratory health.

Platycodon root—a principal herb in Chinese medicine used to treat respiratory disorders, intestinal disorders, diabetes, and injuries.

Schisandra—a tonic considered to be a youth-preserving herb, with benefits to the skin, brain, and sexual performance.

Angelica root—used to promote blood circulation and maintain healthy bowels.

Wild chrysanthemum flower—used to correct imbalances in liver and kidney function.

Siler root—used to treat cold-related headaches and body aches, diarrhea, and chills.

Schizonepeta herb—may promote the removal of toxins and help confer an overall feeling of well-being.

Astragalus root—a tonic for boosting the immune system.

Licorice root—included in many Chinese herb combinations to balance the other herbs and promote vitality.

CHAPTER 14

DR. EUGENE SHIPPEN: MEN AND HORMONES

Dr. Eugene Shippen is a board-certified family practice doctor who for ten years delivered babies and today has a big following of women and men he delivered in his early practice. As their needs changed, so did he. He realized that so many of the babies he delivered are now of menopausal age and that their requirements to feel good in this day and age needed to be understood. As a result, he has written the book The Testosterone Syndrome to help men and women through the difficult passage of declining hormones. He is a big proponent of bio-identical hormone replacement and continues to grow, learn, and keep up with cutting-edge ways of keeping the aging process at bay. You will learn about forward-thinking approaches to health and wellness in his interview. Dr. Shippen practices in Reading, Pennsylvania.

SS: Nice to talk to you again, Dr. Shippen. People are so interested in what you have to say. What are you thinking about these days?

ES: Well, selenium is on my mind . . . Selenium supplementation is definitely part of the framework of anticancer and so simple to supplement safely. Selenium supplementation should not be missing from anybody's program. Additionally, vitamin D (especially vitamin D_3 is absolutely critical as a strong anticancer, antiaging supplement. It's a health hormone for every part of the body, not just for your bones and calcium. Then there's iodine replacement. These are nutrients that I feel are absolutely essential for everyone's health routine, not just women but men as well.

SS: Speaking of nutrient supplementation, every time I hear RDA [Recommended Dietary Allowance], they never seem to be sufficient. Who is setting these guidelines? And why are they so underestimated?

ES: Well, the nutritional community is very conservative and has been for many years. Initially, the minimum daily requirement was established to prevent deficiency in the overt form. How do we prevent rickets? How do we prevent scurvy? How do we prevent thiamine deficiency? So the government developed the minimum amount that would relieve the overt vitamin deficiency diseases.

Later, the minimal daily requirement became transformed into the recommended dietary allowances.

The government figured if you get more than that, you're okay. They never really paid much attention to the huge individual variation that's genetically determined in people's requirements for vitamins. The scientific way would be to actually measure vitamin levels in people with or without supplementation and adjust their vitamins individually; but, of course, that's expensive and time-consuming. Nobody wants to go through that tedious process. So we supplement with levels above the RDAs, and sometimes these megadoses are too much for many people.

It's a very crude science when you start to talk about supplementing vitamins, where one individual might need ten times the amount of vitamin than the next person to achieve optimal levels. And, of course, just taking a blanket megadose of vitamins is not healthy.

SS: Why?

ES: Overloading vitamins downregulates certain enzymes. For example, an overload of vitamin B_6, which is very important in many functions, can actually cause neuropathy, and a deficiency can also cause neuropathy. There's a range for many of the vitamins, where optimal levels are healthy but excessive levels may actually do some damage.

SS: What's neuropathy?

ES: Neuropathy is a nerve impairment that causes symptoms such as numbness, tingling, or lack of sensation or weakness. Carpal tunnel symptoms in which the hands get numb are frequently a sign of a vitamin B_6 deficiency. Excessive vitamin D can cause carpal tunnel–like symptoms, too.

Most people might need 10 mg or 25 or 50 mg of vitamin B_6 in some cases; and some individuals might require 100 or more because of genetic defects. But if everybody took 500 mg, then many people, over time, would start to get numbness and tingling. So just taking a load of vitamins, although the body excretes it, may have some negative effects.

I'm cautious when it comes to supplementation. I think we should all take a basic multivitamin. Your doctor then should be looking at specific things that might require larger doses of certain vitamins like niacin, if you have problems with high cholesterol levels. We have found that megadoses of niacin actually have reversed arterial plaque. None of the statins that lower cholesterol will reverse plaque, but niacin will in large doses.

SS: That's interesting. Do you think calcium supplementation is important?

ES: If you get adequate vitamin D, you absorb calcium at a much higher rate. Vitamin D regulates the absorption of calcium. So if you're low in vitamin D, you may actually be downregulating the calcium you're taking.

SS: A lot of calcium supplements have vitamin D in them. The problem with calcium supplements for most women, as doctors have been telling me, is the side effects—namely, bloating and gas. And then that report came out a few months ago in the media about the uselessness of calcium, so you don't know what to believe.

ES: The amount of vitamin D that's in calcium supplements is not sufficient; 400 IU (international units, the typical amount in supplements) of vitamin D is minuscule. Neither calcium nor vitamin D is absorbed well in supplement form.

SS: What's a good calcium supplement?

ES: There are different forms. Liquid forms or calcium tablets dissolve and liquefy well. The best thing a patient can do is stick a couple of calcium tablets in a glass of water and see what happens. If the tablets are still sitting there the next morning undissolved, they're probably going out through evacuation the next day. We even see calcium supplements on X-rays.

SS: The whole supplement?

ES: Yes, right there in the colon—and they haven't broken down at all. The chewable calcium citrate seems to be the least irritating to the gastrointestinal tract and seems to break down better. The tablet forms compress the calcium too much, making it hard to break down.

SS: One of my neighbors here is Dick Van Dyke, you know, the comedian. He's around eighty, looks amazing, and is in great physical shape. He grinds all his supplements up every morning and takes them down in some awful, gaggy two to three gulps of some drink. But he told me that when coroners do autopsies on people, they find all these undissolved vitamins.

ES: He's right. If you get adequate vitamin D, your calcium absorption from food increases so much, you may not need very much calcium supplementation, unless you're really eating a poor diet. There is lots of calcium in all the foods that you recommend in your Somersize program, Suzanne. So if you add it up, you get between 700 and 1,000 mg a day of calcium in a good diet.

SS: Now let's talk about the brain.

ES: I did some research for a talk recently, and I spent four months researching the literature on the connections between the brain, the brain cells, the aging brain, Alzheimer's disease, and all of the different functions in the brain that are required to keep the brain healthy during your lifetime.

Only one in every ten cells in the brain is a neuron. The neurons do the work of the brain. They store memory, make memory, move our arms and legs, and so on. So it means nine-tenths of the cells are supportive cells. These little supportive cells repair tissue, repair the neurons, supply nutrients to the neurons, and generate their own hormones. They're called neurosteroids.

Most people don't realize it, but the brain can make all of the hormones that are present in the body. It can make its own cortisone, estrogen, testosterone, DHEA, and progesterone. These little supportive cells have the capacity to generate hormones within the brain structure itself.

These hormones regulate every major function of the brain, from brain repair, growth of new neurons, to the structural maintenance of the long axons, which connect different areas of the brain from one brain cell to another in different areas. In fact, the long axons go from the brain out to your fingertips. And these are myelinated, meaning they're coated with myelin. Myelin is the sheath around the neuron cells that protects it. And myelin requires progesterone.

SS: And the brain requires a template that it recognizes as reproductive, in the right proportions of the minor and major hormones, to operate optimally.

ES: Yes, and in the peripheral nervous system, the cells that coat and make myelin are called Schwann cells. In the brain they're called oligodendrocytes, and these require progesterone. What's fascinating is that synthetic progesterone does not help these cells make myelin.

SS: But bioidentical—

ES: But bioidentical does, and of course, regular progesterone that's either produced by the ovary or in males (we men don't have ovaries) is generated by the cells. Progesterone has a lot to do with maintenance of these long axons and the repair of the axons and the coating. Progesterone in both men and women can help in regenerating spinal nerves, because those are myelinated fibers that go up and down the spine. Some research is going on to show that progesterone is neuroprotective and neuroregenerative to repair myelin to make these connections.

SS: Let me understand—for male hormonal decline, it's not just a matter of throwing in testosterone. It's looking at the ratio of all of them together, and that men need to look at their progesterone and estrogen levels?

ES: Yes, those cells that make their own progesterone need to be healthy to keep **making their own progesterone.** So it's really a balance between maintaining circulating levels of systemic hormones and replacing those that are no longer being produced.

Looking at all the hormones requires a balancing act among all of them. As we age, the synchronous production of hormones becomes dissynchronous. The rise and fall during the day gets dysregulated and upset, so part of the skill of replacing hormones is trying to bring some synchronous side to hormones. DHEA, for example, is probably best given at bedtime.

SS: That's interesting, because I take mine in the morning.

ES: That's fine for your morning, but your brain regenerates at night. The night is not a sleeping, quiet period. The night is your regenerative period. The night is the most active regenerative time in your whole body for the entire twenty-four-hour period. Your body tears down during the day and rebuilds at night. There's a surge of hormones at night that helps to direct the replacement. So people with sleep disorders, who are not treating their sleep apnea, are having dysregulated production of hormones during this dysregulated sleep cycle.

SS: I understand the importance of sleep and the healing hormone work that happens during the night. We are sleep-deprived as a society.

ES: There's a lot of science that needs to be done by looking at the synchrony of hormones with aging in men. For example, testosterone normally rises at night, and then in the early morning hours, it peaks and then declines during the day.

SS: That is not a surprise to me. I have a husband who is on full hormone replacement.

ES: Yes, you're right. Other things rise in the early morning with men, and that's a sign of health. That early morning rise actually reflects testosterone. It's a very good biomarker for when testosterone is inadequate in men, because they lose that early morning erectile capacity, but when you replace hormones, you see that rise return. That indicates health, and it's not a sexual thing. Those morning rises actually aren't very useful. They're reflex erections that relate to the sensitivity of the vascular tissue and neural tissue in the pelvis.

When those tissues are healthy, nerve and vascularwise, they're much more responsive. The rise and fall has been documented, and it goes on all night long. Men just don't pay much attention to it until they wake up in the morning. But if testosterone is low, this rise disappears or is significantly reduced, and that is a good way to have some assessment of whether their testosterone levels are low and whether their treatment is adequate.

At any rate, going back to the brain and the importance of hormone replacement for regenerating cells, you need to understand that the immune cells in the brain are little cells that actually migrate. These little cells in the brain are called microglia, and they monitor for infection and help suppress excessive inflammation after injury. These cells are very sensitive to estrogen. When levels of hormones go down, these microglia can't do their job, and then brain inflammation goes up.

After a stroke, if adequate estrogen is present, it suppresses excessive damage—and the area of the stroke is much smaller and heals much greater. When estrogen is not present after a stroke, there's a greater widespread inflammation that causes cellular destruction.

So if women and men are on hormone replacement, including estrogen, and have a stroke, they will have much smaller areas of stroke and much greater healing of the area of tissue around the stroke.

SS: That's fantastic information.

ES: The studies are very clear. The damaging effects of stroke are controlled by hormones.

SS: This is a great argument for those women who

are toughing it out and going natural. I don't really believe they are doing themselves a service.

ES: Everything I say about estrogen is true for men, but we men get our estrogen from our testosterone and from our DHEA.

SS: But at some point, in testosterone decline, estrogen production exceeds testosterone, right?

ES: Yes, because if you look at the estrogen levels in aging men, the estrogen levels go down very slowly, but the testosterone levels go down much faster. Some men are very estrogen-deficient, and some men, because they became obese, have estrogen production that is still quite high, but no testosterone.

SS: And this has got to be at epidemic proportions because of the obesity problem in this country.

ES: Yes, it is. There are two kinds of testosterone deficiency. One is overt deficiency, in which the testicles aren't working and you don't have enough estrogen or testosterone. This can occur at any age from the forties on. If it's below age forty, it's probably related to other endocrine problems. But if you become completely deficient in testosterone, you don't generate enough testosterone to make estrogen. Add to that, if you get syndrome X and become centrally obese and/or obese late in life, then you generate these estrogens in the fat cells. And estrogen suppresses testosterone.

SS: So what's the prognosis for these men?

ES: We find that the men with higher estrogen have an increase in problems with heart attacks.

SS: Well, as I look around America, there are many men who fall into that category.

ES: This is why estrogen and testosterone have to be measured in men. I measure estradiol as a primary powerful estrogen in men. Some of the men are high in estrogen and low in testosterone, and some are low in both. So it really needs to be done on an individual basis. And those men who have middle-age spread are the high-estrogen guys. They have more risk factors for stroke and heart attack.

SS: When a patient walks into your office, in that first thirty seconds, do you pretty much know what's going on with them?

ES: You have to look at their life history to get a clear picture. Were they thin when they were young and now they are obese? Or were they obese all their life? Now, strangely, I've seen men who were obese all their life who have low testosterone, and some with high estrogen, and they are healthy as a horse. They have no sexual dysfunction, either. Their bodies have adapted to that balance.

SS: I didn't realize that the body can adapt to this condition.

ES: Yes, this condition is normal for this man. If a man goes from having a low estrogen/high testosterone ratio—in other words, muscular and athletically built—to becoming dumpy, fat, and centrally obese in his forties and fifties, he will have real trouble. His estrogen goes up and becomes a serious problem. A lot of men are being given aromatase inhibitors, which block the fat cell conversion of testosterone into estrogen to help control the problem. The problem with this is, yes, it may downregulate the estrogen, but what does it do to the brain?

SS: What **does** it do to the brain?

ES: We men get our estrogen in our brain from aromatase conversion of testosterone and DHEA. So when you give an aromatase inhibitor, you are downregulating one of the key hormones that causes the brain to be self-repairing and self-protecting.

Another factor is the use of Proscar to block DHT [dihydrotestosterone] conversion from testosterone to shrink the prostate. But there's DHT in the brain. And this medicine that blocks DHT formation is also affecting the conversion of progesterone into something called allopregnenolone, which is different from pregnenolone. Pregnenolone is a potent neurosteroid that's important in brain repair. So these men are being given DHT to shrink the prostate, and the prostate shrinks because you make it deficient in DHT, but **you're shrinking the brain at the same time.** I think more studies need to be done to see if this really makes sense. The drug companies that give us systemic-acting hormone blockers should be aware that these medications are going to have pervasive effects in other tissues that might show up in two, three years, five years, ten years.

SS: What do you think about statins?

ES: Statins inhibit the ability of your body to generate its own cholesterol. So if we lower cholesterol, there's a clear reduction in events with the studies on statins. There are reductions of stroke, and there is a reduction of heart attack of 20, 25, 30 percent, depending upon the study.

SS: Significant.

ES: However, long-term studies have failed to show any improvement in overall mortality rate. It's interesting that if you lower the major cause of death by 25 or 30 percent, you don't see an upside on longevity of an equivalent amount. So what's happening? We're becoming unhealthy in other ways. But they don't seem to report on what is causing these other people to die.

The brain itself makes its own little neurosteroids by manufacturing its own cholesterol in the brain. So if we inhibit the body's ability to make its own cholesterol, are we also inhibiting the ability of the body to make its own neurosteroids?

SS: So are you saying that ultimately statins could actually be working against us?

ES: Exactly. And those studies are yet to be done. Statins have some important positive effects on inflammation. So now drug companies are talking about maybe using them to treat Alzheimer's. Remember I said when hormones decline, the inflammation of the brain goes up? Well, they're touting the anti-inflammatory effects of statins to cut down the brain inflammation of Alzheimer's. That's the theory. Drug companies would love to have a drug that would go in and stop Alzheimer's.

The problem is, if you inhibit the brain from making its own cholesterol, you're inhibiting the brain from making its own neuroprotective hormones that control the Alzheimer's process. But if your cholesterol is very low, you have an increased risk of Alzheimer's disease.

There's a study called the Cache Study that showed that if you had lower cholesterol, you had a lower incidence of vascular dementia. Those are the strokes and heart attacks that come from ministrokes, or brain degeneration that comes from ministrokes.

But if the condition was high cholesterol, researchers found a lower incidence of Alzheimer's disease. So people with higher cholesterol have a lower incidence of Alzheimer's disease. Is it because they have more precursors to making their own neurosteroids? It's an interesting question.

SS: What do you think?

ES: It makes sense to me that the good Lord put our cholesterol-forming enzymes in our brain for a reason. And if He wanted us to make cholesterol in the brain, cholesterol is a great antioxidant. You know, it's not just a neutral molecule. It's not a bad guy that needs to be eliminated. It's there for a reason. Cholesterol forms the backbone of every single neurosteroid in the brain. Estrogen, testosterone, progesterone, allopregnenolone, plus pregnenolone that people are taking, are all based upon a cholesterol structure that the brain is able to make from cholesterol itself.

SS: Let me play devil's advocate for a minute. The standard treatment by cardiologists is to take heart patients and put them on statins and then eliminate all fat from their body. In light of what you're saying, zero fat intake to lower cholesterol . . .

ES: Not fat. We're talking about cholesterol now.

SS: Right. But the cardiologist takes the patient off fat so that the body can't produce the cholesterol, in order to keep the cholesterol at rock-bottom low.

ES: Well, that's true in a sense. Acetate comes from fat metabolism, and acetate is converted into cholesterol by enzymes that produce cholesterol, and that enzyme is inhibited by statins. So if we give a drug that causes that enzyme to be less active, less cholesterol is being produced by the liver and by other tissues in the body.

SS: But my point is that most men of a certain age are on statins, and their heart doctors have taken them off all fats. They look terrible. Is that healthy?

ES: No. There are good fats and bad fats. We are eating too many processed fats that are not similar to what the fats are in the normal diet.

SS: So this is that specialization: We go to individual doctors who are looking only at their little area of specialty. A diabetes doctor, for example, is just looking at diabetes, not the whole picture.

ES: That's right. The cardiologist's job is to ensure that you have a lower risk for either having a heart problem or attack or a recurring event. That's his or her concern. Statins do that. Cardiovascular disease is primarily an endocrine disease, and cholesterol only adds to the abnormal decline of the hormones. If your hormones are intact, cholesterol doesn't damage the arteries. So if you have adequate estrogen, your arteries are actually protected from plaque formation.

SS: Well, I can proudly announce I have zero plaque in my heart and arteries.

ES: And you're a high-estrogen gal. When they did primate studies, the research showed that if you took perimenopausal monkeys and put them on estrogen from perimenopause until old age, and looked at their arteries, they had almost no plaque. If you waited till menopause and looked at the primates that had their ovaries taken out at menopause and then started on estrogen, they had about 10 percent plaquing. So even in perimenopause, plaquing is starting.

If you waited five years, took the ovaries out, made them estrogen-deficient for five years, there's 40 percent plaquing in the arteries. So those doctors who tell women, "Well, let's wait and see how you do for a year," are telling women, "Let's see how bad your arteries can get before we add estrogen back in." It's the worst advice they could possibly get!

SS: Do you feel that men experience a type of perimenopause? Periandropause?

ES: What happens is a man in his forties begins to have testosterone decline. His tests look normal, but decline has started, and now in most cases his estrogen is also declining. This is serious because men start to get plaquing when their testosterone is declining well before they become deficient. So if you wait for a guy to be totally deficient before you treat him with hormone replacement, the plaques will be so bad that they won't reverse from HRT. Plaques don't form when hormone balance is healthy, except for plaques due to stress or that which comes from infection. What's more, there are many types of plaques that are unexplained.

SS: Then the message to young men who are in their late thirties or early forties is to start doing hormone panels. But young men don't think this way.

ES: Actually, the way to keep your hormones elevated is all the things you tell your women to do in your Somersize books. Eat right, keep your weight in check, avoid sugar, stay active, and exercise.

SS: Eat real food.

ES: Yes, eat real food, and your hormones will stay much higher longer in most cases. And positive stress helps, too. Being a winner will raise your testosterone levels. With the losing football team, for instance, all the testosterone levels are low after the game. The winners get a buoyant surge of testosterone from being on top, winning the battle, so to speak. So positive stress—from those things that drive us in our business pursuits or our lifetime pursuits that feed us positive feelings, those things we're happy about, such as having a job that you're happy with—all drive your hormones up. By contrast, having a job that beats you down every day will lower your testosterone and increase your cortisol levels. Cortisol, of course, is damaging to the system.

SS: So here's where the craft of the doctor comes in: being able to assess that a man who is happy in his life, happy in his marriage, happy in what he's chosen to do, or to understand that this is a guy who is just beaten down by all of it. That assessment allows the doctor to understand what needs to be done, right?

ES: That should be part of the assessment. Plus, the doctor should understand the effects of the environment, toxicity, stress, and all those factors that figure into it. It's much more complex than a simple weight reduction exercise program or a change in lifestyle. It's all of it combined; no single study is ever going to come out that finds one factor to be the primary cause anymore.

SS: That is what this book is about.

ES: All these factors are part of health and antiaging. The more you can be aware of lifestyle and hormonal factors, and how they change individually, is part of the picture. Studies that assess total hormone replacement will never be done, because hormone replacement will be different for every single person. You can't do a double-blind study on a test group that are all getting different amounts.

SS: So what do you do, personally? Everyone wants to know what his or her doctor is taking.

ES: I don't like to say because then everyone will want to do what I am doing, and it's individualized. But I do take vitamin D, and I take my hormones in a certain pattern now.

SS: In a rhythm?

ES: Yes. Taking hormones in a steady day-in-day-out pattern doesn't make sense. You must try to replace them with some pulsatility that reflects the natural pulsatility or rhythm that is there.

SS: By creating a peak?

ES: Yes, peaks and valleys. A resting phase. Just as you need it in your menstrual cycle.

SS: I so agree.

ES: There's a surge, and it needs to relax. Is that healthier than steady (static) hormones? Probably, but we don't have the studies to really show that it is a lot better. For most men, if they just take a very high dose of testosterone, they'll feel good for a while, and then it kind of wears off. The testosterone receptors should be fired up, but they aren't. When you ignite a receptor over and over and over again, it downregulates.

SS: I take my hormones in a rhythm to create a peak. What is the process for men? Do men reach a testosterone peak each month?

ES: No, thank God we don't have a monthly . . .

SS: There's nothing that simulates it?

ES: I believe there should be resting periods and surges. In other words, peaks. It's very much similar to how we treat diabetics. With diabetics, you need insulin replacement. We give them a baseline level of insulin, long-acting insulin, and they take that. It lasts all day long. Then every time they eat, they take a dose of insulin to rise and fall with the meals. So with testosterone, there are a number of ways that you can take testosterone that will give you a peak-and-valley effect. When we're young, in our teens and twenties, there's a peak of testosterone every ninety minutes. It's a rapid cycle up and down. So testosterone's bouncing off the ceiling and off the floor. While on the ceiling, it's activating the receptors and firing us off and making every coed look wonderful. And then it relaxes a little, thank God, and recharges, then it surges again. So all day long, we're distracted every ninety minutes.

SS: I always say to my husband, "All men think about is sex, isn't it?" And he always goes, "Yep."

ES: He's got that right. Those receptors in men and women are made to activate and deactivate. So treatment should be aimed at trying to have some activation and deactivation. That's why the typical injections really don't work very well.

SS: It's a big bang, and then it peters out? (Excuse the pun!)

ES: That's right. So for a while, you have far too

much testosterone, and then you don't have enough. Then you have far too much. The testosterone receptors weren't made to fire up over a two-week period and then decline. They were supposed to be pulsating all day long.

SS: I have male friends who tell me that their doctor has told them they "have more than enough testosterone" or "too much" and that they don't need testosterone replacement. But at age sixty-five and seventy, they would have to be in decline, right? Does this mean that the ratio is off somewhere else?

ES: Well, I'll tell you what is usually the problem: It's sex hormone binding globulin, and they don't measure it. Sex hormone binding globulin goes up as men get older, and in some men it skyrockets. Sex hormone binding globulin is a protein that binds testosterone and keeps it from being useful. So when you measure total circulating testosterone, you can have a very high level. But if you're at a level that sex hormone binding globulin is high enough, it completely negates it. I had one seventy-five-year-old guy who came to see me. He had lost his wife, and he had a new girlfriend who was very voluptuous. And he just couldn't rise to the occasion. I did his testosterone. He had read my book, and he said, "Oh, I'm jumping out of the pages of your book." He had his testosterone done, and it was over 900.

SS: So what was the problem?

ES: I did his sex hormone binding globulin, and it was off the charts—very high. In other words, there's a normal range, and he was 50 percent above the normal range, but he had very little free testosterone.

ss: And the free testosterone is the available active hormone, right?

ES: Right. So with this guy, his testicles were fine. He was pumping plenty of testosterone, but wasn't going anywhere, so he started having problems in parts of his body that no one realized or attributed to sex hormone binding globulin. There are some natural products to lower sex hormone binding globulin, and there are also drugs that we know will lower it. What I did with this man was to treat his sex hormone binding globulin to lower it, and his overall testosterone levels dropped. His sex hormone binding globulin dropped to the middle of the normal range, and his free testosterone came back. Now it's well in the normal range, and he is happy because he is firing bullets again.

ss: With the voluptuous babe.

ES: He is a happy camper. Yet he is now running a lower total testosterone. But his free testosterone is normal, whereas at a higher testosterone level he was deficient, but his numbers looked like they were off the charts. That was a revelation to me, because most doctors would have said, "You're producing too much. There's nothing wrong with you," it's organic or psychological or something, and written it off.

ss: And when testosterone is imbalanced like that, is that a dangerous place for a man to be?

ES: Well, in the sense that this man is symptomatic in that the blood vessels in his pelvis are not dilating. So if his free testosterone is low enough that he's not able to get dilation of the blood vessels in the pelvis that give him a good erection, he's two to three times more likely to have a stroke. Or a heart attack.

SS: Okay. So it is dangerous.

ES: That means the arteries in his brain and the heart are not dilating. You see that on the Viagra ads or the Levitra ads that say that if you have erectile dysfunction, you have a two- to threefold increased chance of having a stroke or a heart attack, and this has been well documented. But what's the connection? Well, testosterone is a major vasodilator for the heart, brain, and pelvic vasculature. Not the peripheral, not the arms and legs, but the central critical arteries that are very hormone-sensitive.

SS: Let's talk about ministrokes. Men and women don't seem to realize that they are having them. It is just attributed to aging, momentary confusion, or forgetfulness. I know what ministrokes look like. I remember my father, before he had the big one, was having these little ministrokes. Could it be caught in time and reversed through hormone replacement?

ES: Well, we know that men with lower testosterone have more severe strokes with more damage, just like the model I told you about estrogen. And all I can say is, if you take testosterone, you'll immediately improve the circulation of the heart. We know that because you can put a man on a treadmill who has heart disease, give him a shot intravenously of testosterone, and he'll last a minute longer before any of the vascular changes occur. So it does work quickly to restore nitric oxide, which is the basic vasodilator in the arteries of the heart and the brain. So whatever you say about circulation of the heart and the pelvis, you can also relate to circulation for the brain.

SS: That's important for men to know. Now, let's talk about iodine.

ES: The linkage between hormones and iodine is fascinating. Iodine is trapped and concentrated in the thyroid, so most doctors are focused only on the iodine relationship to the thyroid gland. But the second and third most concentrated areas are in the breasts and in the ovaries. Our glands concentrate iodine, and the breast tissue is very, very sensitive to iodine. You can mimic the model for fibrocystic disease in animals by making them iodine-deficient. They'll get fibrocystic changes in breast tissue just like the women today with fibrocystic disease. Dense breast tissue will go away with iodine, and so will cystic tissue.

SS: Is iodine something you would supplement daily?

ES: Yes. The Japanese, who have one-eighth the prostate cancer and nearly as little breast cancer and bowel cancer, have iodine levels about eight to ten times the American levels.

SS: I remember when we were kids, our mothers

bought iodized salt. Did they know the importance of iodine replacement back then?

ES: Yes. Iodine deficiency was associated with goiter, so at that time they thought that putting a little iodine in the salt would be the end of it. And again, they set the RDA level . . .

SS: Let me guess, very low?

ES: Way low. But the daily intake of iodine of the Japanese is eight to ten times higher than ours from eating a lot of miso, kelp, seafood, and other foods very high in iodine. In our country, we get less than 1 mg a day.

SS: So do you think iodine, as we age, is a must?

ES: Yes, it's absolutely critical to get more iodine. We are depleted of iodine in many ways. For instance, our water contains fluoride, and our swimming pools contain chlorine, so we are surrounded by "iodinelike molecules" that get brought into the body by these chemicals. If you don't have enough iodine, these iodinelike molecules build up in the various tissues, causing a buildup of larger levels of bromine, fluorine, and chlorine where there should be iodine. These chemicals won't activate the cellular functions the way iodine does. In fact, they lock it. Every single hormone receptor in the body has iodine residue in it.

SS: Naturally?

ES: Yes. There is an amino acid in every hormone receptor, insulin receptor, androgen and estrogen receptors. All of these hormone receptors have tyrosine residue with amino acid. Tyrosine is the building block for thyroid hormone. Tyrosine becomes iodinated very easily, and tyrosine residue is in every receptor researchers have ever studied. So we really need trace amounts of iodine in all of our hormone receptors for our hormones to work right.

SS: So when you supplement iodine, how much do you give to a person on a daily basis?

ES: You take a 50 mg dose. If your body needs it, you will latch on to that iodine, and it's not going to come out in your urine. You can get an accurate reading from a iodine-loading test that will tell you if you are deficient and by how much. This test also measures the excretion of bromine, which is clogging up the iodine residue. You've got to get rid of the bromine and put iodine in. It takes a long time. It takes six months to a year to get rid of the buildup of all these other compounds and to get iodine back in your system. But people will start feeling better within days, weeks, or months of going on iodine supplementation.

SS: Why are we feeling so bad? Why do we need to do all this?

ES: It's from our poor diets and the chemicals in the environment.

SS: Are we living too long?

ES: No, it's not that we are living too long. We are living past our hormonal health. Hormones are the cornerstone to preserving age-related decline. I don't think they reverse aging. They just make the landing a lot softer with more working parts.

Preserving age-related decline is not for everyone. It takes commitment. There are so many experts and so much misinformation that only a few people will ever really find their way to the doctors who are thinking this way. This is an evolving area of specialty. People ask me what I specialize in. I'm not an endocrinologist. I'm not an internist. I'm a doctor interested in the endocrine changes of aging. That's a separate health specialty that has never been designated.

How do you best take care of aging people with different drug demands and different physical and nutritional demands? Not to denigrate the specialty of geriatrics—it's very important—but the geriatricians are really just modifying and helping people who have degenerative disease.

Those of us in the antiaging movement—the doctors who are coming to the surface and studying aging—will really have a chance at intervening at early enough stages to prevent many of the age-related declines and diseases.

SS: What I love about you and the other doctors in this book is that you are excited about what you are doing.

ES: I'm more excited now about what I do than ever before, and I am doing my best work because I have more tools at hand. But there is a learning curve. I find it fascinating that in the next seven years, the total knowledge that we have from the beginning of time to now will be doubled. That means that there is no specialist who can keep up with his or her own specialty.

There is no multispecialty doctor who can possibly keep up with all of the interactions that are going on in different parts of the body. The problem with traditional medicine as we know it is that the specialists are getting more specialized and focused and less integrated in their thinking. They are dealing only with the kidney or the heart or the brain, or they are neurologists or renal specialists or cardiologists. They do a great job focusing on their one organ, but they are missing the forest by focusing on the trees.

SS: I agree.

ES: The specialty of the antiaging community says that if we really do integrative medicine and start looking at all the systems of the unit, it becomes a total endocrine system integrated with the immune system, integrated with the cardiac system, circulatory system, and neurological system. They are all one system, but with different instruments in the symphony that all have to be tuned together to play the music properly.

SS: Well put. And if people embrace this new medicine and take steps in their lives to replace declining hormones—focus on iodine, vitamin D, and functioning of the brain, eat right, avoid chemicals, and exercise—can they expect to live and die healthy?

ES: I'll tell you this: They'll know in their heart of hearts that they are healthier. They will not want to go back to where they were. Would you want to go back to where you were?

SS: Never. Wouldn't consider it.

ES: It's a pervasive sense of health that you know intuitively. Unfortunately, so many sit and listen to the lady next to them at the hair salon who says estrogen causes cancer and all these horrible things, so she throws her hormones away. Or somebody else who says testosterone causes prostate cancer so that person immediately stops hormone replacement. These messages can come from a specialist or layperson, but one comment can destroy the confidence a person has towards moving in this area.

But once you experience the positive effects of this new medicine, when you get really fine-tuned on your hormones, you won't ever give it up, because you'll know intuitively that you are healthier. It's not as though you are going to be healthy for a short time and then pay a horrible price with things exploding at the other end of the line.

The vast majority of studies show that with balanced hormone replacement, there is improvement in overall mortality. When those hormones are in their best balanced levels, you are your healthiest. Will you live longer? I think so, but I know for sure that you will certainly feel better while you are alive.

SS: Well, let's end it there. That's fantastic. Thank you so much.

DR. SHIPPEN'S TOP FIVE ANTIAGING RECOMMENDATIONS

1. Four important antiaging supplements to include in your regimen are selenium, vitamin D$_3$, iodine, and a multivitamin/mineral supplement. Speak with your doctor about exact dosages for your situation.

2. Certain structures of the brain require adequate hormones, particularly progesterone and testosterone. Bioidentical hormone replacement can keep the brain young and healthy.

3. In men, estrogen and testosterone have to be measured. Some men are high in estrogen and low in testosterone, and some are low in both. High-estrogen men are at greater risk for stroke and heart attack.

4. Sex hormone binding globulin increases with age, resulting in a decreased concentration of free testosterone. Testosterone deficiency is likely to be a primary contributor to erectile dysfunction. Talk to your doctor about the connection, as there are some natural products to lower sex hormone binding globulin, and there are also drugs that will lower it.

5. In addition to bioidentical hormone replacement, the way to keep your hormones elevated is to eat real food, keep your weight in check, avoid sugar, stay active, and exercise. Being a winner will raise your testosterone levels. Winners, whether in sports, business, or personal life, get a buoyant surge of testosterone from being victorious.

CHAPTER 15

DR. JOE FILBECK:
MEN AND THE EFFECTS
OF AGING

An eloquent and passionate proponent of antiaging medicine and its marvelous rejuvenating effects on the human body, Dr. Joe Filbeck works with men and women of all ages. His patients are profoundly changed by his approach to medicine. Dr. Filbeck has a biography pages long, with accomplishments including line officer in the U.S. Navy; BA and MA in psychology; MD of surgery at Huntington Hospital in Pasadena; anesthesiologist at L.A. County Hospital; medical director of Longevity Life Extension, West Lake Village, California; and medical director of the Palm La Jolla Medical Spa, San Diego, California, where he is currently seeing patients. His passion for antiaging medicine is infectious, as you will see in this interview.

SS: Good evening, Dr. Filbeck. I appreciate your time. I know you are very busy, but please tell me about your kind of medicine.

JF: For twenty-five years, I was an anesthesiologist. About ten years ago, I decided to specialize in what I call "quality of life medicine" because I felt there was a gap between disease-based medicine and medicine that focused on optimizing health as a first line of defense against disease and degeneration. The gap is wide, too, since the methods and treatment are quite different from what traditional medicine would consider to be appropriate.

SS: Do you find yourself at odds with other doctors who have not chosen to embrace antiaging medicine?

JF: Yes, I do. Take me as an example. I'm sixty-nine years old. Let's say I went to a urologist and had my testosterone levels checked but was not taking testosterone at the time. Suppose my results came back low but fit into the range for a man my age. The doctor would probably say to me, "There is no way under the sun you are going to get testosterone because it would put me at too great a risk for a malpractice lawsuit."

However, at age sixty-nine I like to continue to fly my plane, sail my boat, chase my wife, and do all the wonderful things that I do because I have restored my testosterone levels to that of a gentleman who is probably thirty to thirty-five years younger. This is critical. I see changes like that which occur every single day, thanks to the presentation you made in your book **The Sexy Years.** That book didn't affect just women; it drove a lot of men into my office as well—men who never really got introduced to the concept of bioidentical hormones for men until you included that information in your book.

SS: Thank you very much. I know men are vitally interested, but they need a little prodding to go to the doctor about aging. Once they get there, they become wildly enthused.

JF: Yes, men want to get their lives back. But here is the big problem: They go to their physician and are often dismissed as hypochondriacs or unqualified for the kind of treatment that you and I know is absolutely essential to improve the quality of life. That's sad. On the other hand, I can happily say that 45 percent of my practice is composed of men. They are coming to me because they watch their buddies do so well in the gym, and they are impressed with that.

SS: Do you ever find a wall with men who see testosterone replacement as an assault against their manhood, as in "I have no problem there"?

JF: It's a delicate balance, but a lot of my patients come in as couples. Thankfully, they are able to discuss their sex life with me quite openly, and as a rule, that gives me an opportunity to be able to address the issues that are important to them.

It's also great for a couple to come in together because they can act as advocates for each other. There is so much new information being thrown at them during an office visit or checkup. If one is sitting there with a notepad and writing everything down, it helps a lot. Now they are in this together. I talk to them about the opportunities and where I see their deficiencies, plus their strong points. They begin to see the possibilities. That usually puts an end to "manhood" issues.

While I am getting their hormones back in balance, I am able to offer them not only testosterone replacement, but also Viagra, which has opened up men's eyes to a whole new world. It allows men in the second half of their lives to enjoy the same sexual satisfaction they had in their youth.

I can then explain to them that they really need testosterone to drive their libido and increase their desire so that Viagra can be more effective. In time, when I get their hormones in complete balance, Viagra isn't as necessary as it was in the beginning.

SS: That's interesting. If you are balancing testosterone, you **do** need Viagra to jump-start things?

JF: For some men, yes. Other men are deficient in growth hormone, which has amazing results when replaced. I have worked out all my life, but I could never do anything about my belly. I could never get to a six-pack. But when I first tried growth hormone, suddenly my rectus abdominis starting coming into view. Talk about a motivator. I was back into the gym before you knew it. It wasn't until I became more sophisticated about hormone replacement that I began to see the changes. But I had a hard time talking my buddies into taking it.

SS: Because hormone replacement is all tied up with menopause in women?

JF: To an extent, but it has more to do with psychological issues. People start to rationalize if their sexual behavior becomes a problem. I've had women say to me, "Please don't give me testosterone because I don't want my sex life to come back. John and I have reached a point where we are happy with the fact that we don't have sex anymore." But you see, it is a part of your life that is missing.

SS: But also it means that you are imbalanced and then subject to the diseases of aging.

JF: Absolutely. My goal is to enrich and extend the quality of a patient's life. If you are willing to work with me, watch your diet, exercise, take supplements, replace lost hormones, add to your regimen growth hormone, then I can help you reinstate a lifestyle that makes every day worth getting up for.

SS: What can a man or woman who decides to take you on expect for the rest of their lives?

JF: Men on testosterone can expect the following advantages. First, they will now be able to sustain muscle mass, whereas men who aren't on testosterone will lose muscle. I see these men in the gym every day—men in their thirties and forties who are round little guys with very pale color; being on testosterone corrects this pale, pasty look. Second, testosterone increases red cell count, which is absolutely critical for delivering oxygen to the tissue. My patients who are on testosterone are well oxygenated, and they are able to sustain muscle mass, whereas before, without testosterone, they were replacing muscle with fat. So I see a leaner, healthier, better-oxygenated individual at this stage.

Third, a man can regain his bone health. Men lose estrogen in the aging process. When estrogen is lost, bone density declines. This process can be rectified by getting the right ratio of testosterone to estrogen. This will rebuild his bones and restore the integrity of his bone density. Without the correct ratio, that won't happen; a man needs testosterone and estrogen in balance.

SS: Because testosterone is an anabolic steroid?

JF: In a sense, bioidentical testosterone is both anabolic, meaning dedicated to building muscle, and androgenic, meaning promoting the development of secondary sex characteristics such as sperm production. The anabolic benefit leads to a more muscular physique; the androgenic benefit leads to more virility and an improved sex life. In short, we increase his testosterone, we build his muscle mass, we restore the integrity of his bone density, and we reinstate his sex drive.

SS: If men only knew this kind of treatment was available, they would be running to your office. Every aging man would like to get back his energy, muscle, and sexuality. What is the first thing you do when a man comes into your office?

JF: I check his hormone levels first, then his PSA so that we know that this man's prostate is okay. A male's estrogen level should be around 50, ideally, and if this man's levels are around 32, we've got room to play. If his PSA is .2 or .5, that is great. Anything below 4 is great. Now we can add some testosterone, and we can add it to the point that his performance begins to increase and the safety factors are not violated. On the next series of tests, we look at his estrogen again. Has it gone up? No. Has his PSA gone up? No. Such results tell me that he is responding very favorably to treatment. We need to establish those values for every single one of the hormones that we are trying to administer, and that is a long, hard process for traditional medicine. However, in my kind of practice, we can do it because we have time, and we can do it repeatedly.

SS: As women get older, reaching orgasm gets more and more difficult. No one seems to know why. Is the same phenomenon true for men?

JF: It is exactly the same. Not only do men find that it takes longer to reach orgasm, but they are very concerned about the volume of their ejaculations—not as much of it, or the force of it. We get into delicate issues here because how the sexual act is performed can be so emotionally charged.

SS: This approach to treatment is catchy. You see someone in their forties, fifties, sixties, or seventies who is hormonally balanced, and their youthful way of being in the world is very appealing. You say to yourself, I'd like to feel like that, too.

JF: I am in this practice because my mother had Alzheimer's disease, and all of my aunts and uncles had it. Mental attitude is a critical issue. All of the things we do tend to reinforce our neurochemistry to the point where we can accept the idea that there is a brighter future. It is possible to optimize our health; we do not have to accept the degeneration of previous generations.

SS: In recent years, there has been lot of talk about perimenopause in women. But what about men? Do they go through a "periandropause"?

JF: Yes, they do, but the difference is much more subtle, and it is usually much lower in onset. When a young man comes to me with low libido and low energy, I check him to see if he has primary or secondary hypogonadism.

SS: Please explain.

JF: Primary hypogonadism means that the testicles are not producing enough testosterone. Secondary hypogonadism is the result of problems with the pituitary gland or the hypothalamus, meaning that his testicles are not stimulated enough to produce testosterone. In either case, normal performance of the testicles is compromised.

This is a fascinating aspect of medicine. If you took my growth hormone cells (somatocytes) out of my pituitary and stuck them in a petri dish, they would produce growth hormone like there was no tomorrow, like I was fifteen years old. But if you take them out of the petri dish and stick them back in my pituitary, they wouldn't produce 10 percent of what they produced when I was a young man. It's as though there is some kind of genetic faucet gradually cranking down. We don't yet know what it is. We can rectify this with testosterone replacement and growth hormone injections.

This is incredibly rewarding work. I've now got patients in their eighties who sit there and smile as a couple. They both look at me and say, "Yeah, Doc, we're doing it maybe once or twice a week."

SS: How great . . . and they have the time!

JF: Absolutely. They also have the energy and the desire. This line of medicine doesn't pay a tenth of what I was making as an anesthesiologist, but the personal rewards are huge.

I put my aunt with Alzheimer's disease in a convalescent home. Once, I looked down the hall, and there were about thirty people sitting there in wheelchairs. One yells and then they all start screaming. If anybody walks into my office and says, "I want to stay healthy," I will bend over backwards to help them because I don't want to see anybody end up like that, least of all me.

SS: What do you want people to know so they won't be terrified of stepping into this new realm of medicine, into this new approach to living your life?

JF: Life itself is an experiment. We weren't asked to

be born, yet we were thrown on this planet and now we are experimenting with opportunities placed before us. Up until now, we have accepted that the second half of our lives would be one of degeneration and disease. Now we need to turn our attention to the fact that the opportunity exists to be able to use medications that were previously reserved for disease to produce a kind of optimum health that becomes the first line of defense against degeneration and disease, and that those medications are available and they are natural (bioidentical). Everyone should have the opportunity to experiment with those to make sure (within the safe parameters) that they can enrich their lives much beyond what they ever thought possible.

When I was a little boy on the farm, somebody said something to me about the year 2000. I remember thinking to myself that I would never live to see that time. Yet here I am, and I see no end in sight. This is an incredible change in my life, and I love sharing it with people and living it by example. It gets me out of bed in the morning and keeps me in my office until late at night in order to continue setting a positive example for others.

SS: As a father of four, do you find that your children are following suit?

JF: Absolutely. They are wonderful people and very, very hip on all kinds of nutritional things. They all exercise, and they all believe in what I am doing, and they follow my example.

SS: Thank you so much. You are inspiring.

DR. FILBECK'S TOP FIVE ANTIAGING RECOMMENDATIONS

1. Testosterone replacement is important for sustaining and building muscle mass, delivering oxygen to the tissues, regaining bone health, and reinstating sex drive.

2. Testosterone replacement can be accompanied by an erectile dysfunction (ED) drug such as Viagra, although in time the ED drug won't be as necessary as it was in the beginning.

3. If you're a young man experiencing low libido and low energy, have your doctor check you for primary or secondary hypogonadism. Primary hypogonadism means that the testicles are not producing enough testosterone. Secondary hypogonadism is the result of problems with the pituitary gland or the hypothalamus, meaning that the testicles are not stimulated enough to produce testosterone. In either case, normal performance of the testicles is compromised.

4. Definitely consider growth hormone replacement if you are deficient.

5. Bioidentical hormone replacement is for men, too—it can enrich their lives much beyond what was ever thought possible.

PART THREE

THE THREE S'S: SEX, SLEEP, AND STRESS

Every stress leaves an indelible

scar, and the organism pays for its

survival after a stressful situation

by becoming a little older.

—Hans Selye

CHAPTER 16

SEX, SLEEP, AND STRESS

> A ninety-seven-year-old man goes into
> his doctor's office and says, "Doc, I
> want my sex drive lowered."
> "Sir," replied the doctor, "you're
> ninety-seven. Don't you think your sex
> drive is all in your head?"
> "You're darned right," replied the old
> man. "That's why I want it lowered!"

SEX

Hmm . . . wasn't sex just a given? Didn't you think
that this one life pleasure was just something you
never even had to think about? You want it . . . you
have a partner . . . bingo. There it is.

I think the one subject that comes up more often
than any other when I am speaking to a group is sex,
or I might say the absence of sex. "The feeling is just
gone," I hear from so many women. "It's not that I

don't want to 'do' it, it's just that I can't feel anything."

And what about men? How many times a day do you see commercials on television for Viagra or the blue pill? Or the one that really cracks me up, which warns, "If your erection lasts more than four hours, call your physician"? What a sales pitch. I can feel men running to the phones to get that one. Four hours! But what has happened to both sexes that suddenly nature's most primal urge has become problematic?

Well, let's first look at stress. Stress is the biggest romance killer that exists. But the other reason is hormones. Remember, stress blunts hormone production. Both women and men will lose their sex hormones in the aging process, and the negative effects are more prevalent today than at any other time in the history of mankind. Why? We are living longer, and we are living more stressful lives.

For women, loss of hormones takes away their feeling. It's not just that their testosterone is low; it's that everything is low, and the ratio is off. Without hormones you have no feeling. The sex hormones are your minor hormones: estrogen, progesterone, testosterone, DHEA, pregnenolone. When you are low or missing your sex hormones . . . guess what? No sex! No feeling! Research shows that testosterone levels in women in their forties are half the levels of women in their twenties. A similar decline is seen in the levels of DHEA, the primary precursor to testosterone. DHEA peaks at age twenty-five, slips to half that level by age fifty, and may be totally absent in the elderly. Since DHEA is a precursor to testosterone, any reduction in DHEA results in lower testosterone levels. Testosterone increases genital blood flow, which increases sensitivity and responsiveness of the clitoris. Hormonal balance, including testosterone replacement, will reawaken a sleeping clitoris. This is a good thing. This is quite a simple problem to fix if you have a doctor who gets it. I know this from experience. I lost my sex hormones, and I experienced this awful dead feeling (my sleeping clitoris). I love my husband deeply, and we have always enjoyed each other sexually very much, then all of a sudden . . . nothing. I could "do" it, but I would rather be reading a magazine. In fact, the best sex for me during this time was when the TV was on because then I could still watch the program and "get it over with." But this is not the way I wanted it.

I had never been one of those women who "wanted to get it over with." I was always a willing participant. I loved it.

I was embarrassed to tell my husband; I was embarrassed to tell my doctor. I didn't understand hormones adequately at the time to understand that what I was experiencing was not emotional but physical. My body was not working correctly. I was experiencing severe hormonal loss. The vagina must have adequate amounts of estrogen. Low estrogen levels decrease vaginal lubrication and thin the vaginal lining, which results in vaginal dryness, itching, burning, and painful intercourse. Low levels of estrogen also reduce vaginal blood flow and impede nerve transmission, which impairs sexual function. If I'd understood the syndrome better at the time, I also would have noticed that I couldn't sleep more than two hours at a time, that I was sweating all night, my body itched from head to toe, I had headaches, I was depressed, I would cry, my stomach was always bloated, I was gaining alarming amounts of weight even though I was eating less, my usual cheerful mood was becoming downright bitchy, I couldn't think, I was so forgetful that I couldn't remember who I was calling on the telephone, and then my sex drive dried up. What was wrong? I felt like I needed a psychiatrist. The life I had had left me, and I didn't like the new one that had taken over my body. No one had prepared me, and my doctors didn't know what to do. Antidepressants were suggested, so were diet pills, sleeping pills, fat farms, synthetic hormones, and nonfat foods. Nooo! I thought.

There has got to be an answer. As you know, I found it in bioidentical hormone replacement. It was not easy. I went from doctor to doctor, and I was horrified at the way menopause was being treated. There was a complete and total lack of understanding of this passage.

In the defense of the doctors, we were not meant to live this long, so menopause was something hardly thought of in medical school. Then the pharmaceutical companies seized the opportunity and handed out synthetic hormones like candy to the doctors. Finally, the doctors had something to give their female patients to calm them down: synthetic hormones that took away the nastier symptoms, like hot flashes, but did not restore sexuality (or their hormones, since synthetic hormones are **not** hormones). But what the heck, we're just women.

For the men they had Viagra, which gave them back humongous hard-ons, so the men thought, Whoopee! This is better than ever. What men have never known is that even though the blue pill gives them erections, the testosterone loss they are experiencing is part of their ongoing body failure. Little by little, these men are falling apart internally, and eventually the symptoms will show up as either cancer, heart attacks, or Alzheimer's (or all three).

It became clear to me that we women were "on our own." There was no little blue pill developed for us. And that is probably the good news. If we had a "sex pill," we might not be so driven to find balance with our hormones. This search for a solution will ultimately save our lives. We don't have to fall apart and get sick if we find balanced BHRT. Of course, the answer for me was not synthetic and not a drug . . . the answer was bioidentical hormones, and they have clearly changed the quality of my life.

To regain your sexual feelings, it's simple. You need to replace your sex hormones with real bioidentical sex hormones (estrogen, progesterone, testosterone if you need it, maybe DHEA, maybe pregnenolone), mimicking the time in your life when you were your strongest. That is usually about thirty-five years old or even younger. Isn't it wonderful? You get to be as sexy as your thirty-five-year-old self. You don't want to replace your hormones to normal status for a woman your age, do you? A woman your age is in hormonal decline; that's your problem. So if your doctor tells you that you are "normal," tell him or her you don't want to be normal for your age. You want to be restored to your healthiest prime. If your doctor just stares at you, thank him or her and leave. This is not the right doctor. You want the "good old days" to come back. Remember when sex was on the kitchen counter or in the bathtub, or when you were on vacation how you would try to sneak it under the blankets on the beach? Remember those fabulous, vibrant times? That's when we were alive, ready, excited! Bioidentical hormone replacement gives it back to you. I'm giving you extravagant examples, and just because you are not doing it on the beach anymore is not the issue. You just want to feel in the mood and have a good time with it.

For me, today, my life has returned to how it used to be. There are times of the month when I am "more in the mood" than other times, although with a little encouragement I am a willing participant almost anytime. It makes me feel that I am part of the universe again. When I had lost my "feeling," I felt as if I were on the outside looking in; I felt it was a cruel trick. I finally had the time, I had raised my children, I had put aside my own needs to take care of my family, and now I no longer had the inclination . . . in other words, the well was dry.

Young women whisper to me constantly that they have no sex drive; women my age just roll their eyes, like "Forget about it"; older women have given up. Did you know we can remain sexual until the very end?

How many of your friends are now sleeping in separate bedrooms? How many of your friends who once had fire in their eyes are no longer touching and joking with their partner anymore? Sex is our human gift. It is our most intimate act. It is how we communicate with our partner. Sex makes us feel alive and young. When my sex drive diminished, it was the only time I started to feel old. I have nothing against getting old; believe me, each year gets better and better for me. The wisdom that is starting to permeate at sixty gets me to thinking how incredible my thoughts will be at eighty and ninety and a hundred. Think of what I will know and will have seen. My goal is to get to each of these stages healthy and with vitality. That's the mission and goal of antiaging medicine.

If BHRT is not working and you can't seem to jump-start your libido, find a good sexual urologist to make sure there isn't a physical problem that is impeding your sex life. A sexual urologist is someone you and your partner can talk with in frank terms, someone who deals with sexual issues all day long. In my book **The Sexy Years,** I interviewed Dr. Jennifer Berman, a sexual urologist (her address is listed in the Resources section of this book). If there is no issue physically, then find a good antiaging endocrinologist. He or she will take blood or saliva tests to determine your deficiencies and prescribe a bioidentical hormone regimen especially for you, and it won't take long before "that old feeling" comes back. You must be clear with your doctor that this is one of your issues. He or she is not a mind reader.

If your lack of sexual feeling is psychological, you might want to read Dr. Laura Berman's book **The Passion Prescription.** It is loaded with helpful information. A good therapist or sex therapist can help you through issues that might have kept you inhibited or turned off your inner light. Often, overbearing fathers or mothers or religious schools made sex unmentionable or, worse, a "bad thing," so it might be necessary to get your head screwed on in a different way about it. The services are available, so take advantage of these professionals.

Often, after a woman gives birth, the nerves get cut during the common episiotomy (the cutting of the vagina to make room for the baby to come out), and the new mother is sometimes left with no feelings because the nerve was severed and blood flow to the genital area has been damaged. Couple that with the fact that often after giving birth, a woman suffers from such low progesterone that she experiences the common postpartum depression, and you have a recipe for disaster. Along with the "blues" and depression comes a loss of sexual feeling or appetite. Most doctors don't know or realize that temporary restoration of natural bioidentical progesterone will not only take away the depression, but will also restore the woman's sexual feelings. Think about the positive effects of that. Having a new baby in the house is wonderful, but we all know it is a very stressful time. Add the mother's depression and weepiness, and the poor new father feels completely left out and alone. If there has been nerve or blood flow damage, a sexual urologist can help.

As much as I know and like Brooke Shields, I disagree with her doctor's treatment. This is a criticism not of her, but of her doctor. Perhaps an antidepressant was her only option, but it made me wonder whether by giving Brooke an antidepressant, her doctor, like so many others, was demonstrating that most likely he or she didn't understand the hormonal system.

Once the umbilical cord is cut, all the progesterone **whoosh**es out of the mother into the baby. The mother is left in a complete state of hormonal imbalance, which we all know wreaks havoc on her emotions. Depression is often the result. A qualified doctor who understands the hormonal system and how it works would take a blood test to get a hormone panel, replace the missing progesterone to appropriate levels, and possibly replace some estrogen short-term until the woman's body can rev up again and start producing a full complement of hormones.

Unfortunately, most doctors go the pharmaceutical way. Why would you take a drug when you could take an exact replica of what your body makes and replace what is missing? Besides, if a woman is nursing, she most probably has to stop nursing if she is taking a drug. You wouldn't want your baby to be getting antidepressants from breast milk. And as you have read earlier in this book about rhythmic cycling, nursing is the greatest thing you can do for the mother's immune system and the baby's. The longer you nurse, the more eggs you save, and the healthier both mother and baby will be.

Also, there is always the danger that once on an antidepressant, it's hard to get off. Antidepressants make you feel good unnaturally. The object in BHRT is to get to a place of such balance that no antidepressant could ever compete.

As you become more informed about bioidentical hormone replacement, you will understand that lack of a sex drive is not an imposed sentence on menopausal women and men. Men can get their testosterone brought back into peak range through replacement. Sometimes men are also low in DHEA, which is another hormone present in both men and women that works in concert with testosterone.

Women can also restore their hormonal systems to balance when they are with the right doctor. Sex does not have to become a distant memory as we age. It can be a vital and satisfying part of life and bring much pleasure and closeness to a relationship.

I truly believe that marriages break up during menopause from lack of understanding. Women who are not hormonally balanced can hardly stand to live with themselves, and it is very difficult on the other members of the family. If the man of the house is getting dumped on day and night because of hormonal imbalance and then on top of it is not having any satisfactory sexual contact, after a while even the nicest guy will say to himself, What do I need this for?

Getting your hormones balanced with real bioidentical hormones can bring you back to the woman or man you used to be.

THE IMPORTANCE OF SLEEP

Sleep . . . glorious sleep. You never appreciate the fact that sleeping is a daily function until you can't sleep. Without hormones, it is really impossible to sleep. Without sleep, prolactin keeps escalating. Prolactin is a pituitary hormone that induces lactation and prevents ovulation. Prolactin is the domain of nursing mothers. A mother with a new baby needs to be awakened many times during the night to feed her baby . . . thus the high prolactin. Nature has provided this phenomenon for the new mother.

A young healthy reproductive woman has a full

complement of hormones, and if she goes to bed early, sleep is a given; but as we age and begin to lose our hormones and develop bad sleeping habits, the body gets confused and prolactin keeps escalating.

T. S. Wiley writes in **Sex, Lies, and Menopause,** "At the end of perimenopause, cortisol soars and estrogen and progesterone hit bottom . . . just as they do during labor and delivery. At this point in the template, your immune system revs up so high that it may attack your cartilage and mucous membranes, and that scenario creates joint pain (arthritis), allergies, and an autoimmune disease called Hashimoto's thyroiditis can also happen. Once your immune system has attacked and halted thyroid function, with the insulin resistance from sleeplessness, you just keep getting fatter" [and more and more tired].

Wonderful things happen in the night if you go to sleep early enough. Early is between 9:00 and 10:00 p.m. I know, I know, nobody goes to sleep that early; it is one of the reasons we are in such poor health in our country. As a nation we are sick because we don't sleep. In fact, sleep loss is the new American deficit. We are fat and diabetic from lack of sleep. We are dying from cancer and heart disease from lack of sleep. Our healing hormones have no chance to do their work without sleep.

When you lose sleep, you really can't catch up. Your hormones don't spring back like that. Sleeping less than you need affects at least ten different hormones, not just melatonin. That's just the tip of the iceberg. Sleeplessness causes shifts in all these hormones and changes appetite, fertility, and mental and cardiac health.

The National Institutes of Health concludes that six hours of prolactin production in the dark is the minimum necessary to maintain immune function like T-cell and beneficial killer-cell production. But you can't get six hours of prolactin secretion on six hours of sleep a night. It takes at least three and a half hours of melatonin secretion before you even see prolactin. So if you don't go to bed two or three hours before midnight, there won't be enough time for this hormonal action to happen. Remember, if you sleep enough each night, you will lose weight as a result of your cortisol going down. Now you're listening, aren't you?

If we go all the way back before electricity, we had to go to sleep when the sun went down. There was no light—at all—so there was no choice. During the night healing hormones would go to work. Going to sleep early caused cortisol levels to drop, and when the cortisol levels were lowered, insulin levels lowered. We had no choice but to sleep until it was light the following morning. When the sun came up, cortisol and insulin levels would rise. Nature had it all worked out beautifully. Plenty of sleep, increased vitality and energy, controlled weight because the lowered insulin at night helped to keep weight at optimum. This is the way it is supposed to work.

Did you ever think that going to bed early was a

component of weight loss? If you are eating correctly, exercising in moderation, and going to bed at 9:00 or 10:00 p.m., you are ahead of the game.

I tried this experiment on myself this year. I do eat correctly almost all the time, I do exercise in moderation regularly, my hormones are balanced, but there was some extra weight hanging around me through the middle that I just couldn't shed. I have a lot of stress in my life, and I tax my adrenals regularly as a result. I know that if one hormone is out of whack, they are all out of balance.

So for the past year, I have been going to bed at 9:00 and 10:00 in the evening most nights. Guess what? Without trying, without changing my eating program or changing my exercise routine, I lost ten pounds . . . from sleeping!

And one more thing—you must sleep in complete darkness. Even the smallest bit of light keeps your cortisol from lowering. Put tape over the computer lights, and the light on the phone, and the light from your digital clock. These tiny bits of light will all affect your sleep and keep your cortisol level high. There was a study done where they put people in a completely dark room except for one tiny pin light on the backs of their knees, and their cortisol stayed high as a result.

In **Lights Out,** T. S. Wiley says that "an avalanche of peer-reviewed scientific papers supports our conclusion that when we don't sleep in sync with the seasonal variation in light exposure, we alter a balance of nature that has been programmed into our physiology since day one." The National Institutes of Health confirms that it is a scientific "given" that light and dark cycles turn hormone production on and off and activate the immune system. According to T. S. Wiley, "If the lack of prolactin at night doesn't get you, the lack of melatonin ultimately will. Melatonin is the most potent antioxidant known. Less melatonin and more free radicals mean faster aging even without chronic high insulin racking up a 'clock time' of four years for every one you live."

Now here's the problem: When you are losing hormones and cannot sleep, your doctor most likely will prescribe antidepressants and/or sleeping pills. If your hormones were balanced, believe me you would not have trouble going to sleep. Once you get on the antidepressant merry-go-round, you'll have a hard time getting off. Why take an antidepressant when balanced hormones and a regimen of proper sleeping will do the same thing, but more effectively and naturally? Because it's easier for the doctor to give you a pill, and you **will** feel better. You will sleep better with an antidepressant; you will stop complaining to your doctor. He can go on about his business without having to do the work of trying to get to the bottom of why you seem to need an antidepressant. In essence, you are allowing your doctor to give you a Band-Aid instead of fixing the problem. Then the problem will continue to get worse and worse. He will up your dose, then give you sleeping pills. Your emotions, which were originally calmed down by the antidepressants, will get harder and harder to control. Doesn't this upset you? But you keep taking the pills because you are feeling so much better . . . for a while. Then you are going to be bothered by the fact that even though you are enjoying your drugged sleep, and your drug-induced daytime calmness, you will start asking yourself, Why am I gaining so much weight? And you **will** get fat on antidepressants. The reason is that you haven't addressed the underlying cause of the problem, which is hormonal imbalance. It happens to everyone—all of us experience hormonal decline as we age. Shockingly, it is happening at earlier and earlier ages. It is not uncommon for women in their mid- to late thirties to start perimenopause because of the stressful lives they are living. Stress blunts hormone production.

Now the antidepressant scenario continues. Guess what—you will lose your sex drive, you will continue to get more and more depressed, and you will eventually get sick because the antidepressant has been a Band-Aid masking the underlying problem, which is hormone decline. Without hormones, the internal "you" starts to decline, then the diseases of aging begin, among them heart disease, cancer, and Alzheimer's.

The good news is that bioidentical hormone replacement therapy can rectify this entire scenario, along with sleeping, eating right, and managing stress. It's a little tricky and will need constant "tweaking" from your doctor because of your surging hormones. But a good qualified doctor will know how to handle this. Remember, sleeplessness and stress will change your hormone levels, and the fact that the surges come and go will change your hormone levels. This is the exciting part of this new medicine; when you are working with your doctor to balance during this tricky phase, you would call when you have even the smallest symptom, because every symptom is an indicator that things are not in balance . . . and balance is the goal.

STRESS

As we get older, we tend to produce less DHEA and at the same time more cortisol. I've already discussed the dangers of living with high cortisol. Everyday stress blunts hormone production: the argument you had with your husband this morning, the gardener and that damn blower he uses, highway traffic, daily schedules, convincing your teenage daughter that she can't wear **that** to school!

I'm also talking about the big stressors in life: a death in the family, a serious illness, that near miss in the car yesterday, divorce, sick children or spouse, money problems, an abusive home, an abusive boss, the daily news about the war and trouble on the globe, 9/11 and the fear of another attack. These are just some of the stresses most of us are living with on a daily basis. Cortisol was originally designed to give us energy to run from saber-toothed tigers, but our bodies never expected that we would be running from the saber-toothed tiger many times every day. We are all under too much stress, and it leads to chronically elevated cortisol levels.

Young people have career stress, middle-aged people have stress from fear of being marginalized, senior people are stressed from ill health and money instability. Stress, stress, stress! No wonder we are all so sick. No wonder we are all on different forms of drugs.

I saw a documentary on one-hundred-year-old people recently, and they were asked, "What's the secret?" Each one of them (unrelated) said the same thing: Avoid stress and confrontation, and get used to change quickly (by the time you get to be a hundred, you have lost everybody in your life, and if you get dragged down every time someone dies, the stress will eventually get you). We can learn from these wise old (young) people . . . some of whom claim they are still sexually active!

Stress is the great aging accelerator. All those things you are letting "get to you" are making you old. Calm will keep you young. Stress will literally age your body both inside and out. The danger of continued high cortisol will eventually lead to heart attack, stroke, and/or diabetes. People with diabetes have high insulin, and when you have high insulin you automatically have high cortisol. As I have said and will say over and over in this book, hormones are an internal symphony. When one instrument (hormone) is off, the whole concert is discordant. You can't keep eating sugar, which raises your hormone insulin, without affecting all your other hormones. Why do you think people get cranky after they have eaten a lot of sugar? Because their insulin went sky-high, and now all the other hormones are "off," throwing that person into hormonal imbalance. We are a walking, talking symphony of chemicals. That is why diet and nutrition are so key to successful aging. When we were younger, hormones were pouring into us at all times, so we could binge on French fries, milkshakes, hamburgers, candy, and cookies; or when we were in college, we "drank till we puked" (remember that one? ugh!). Nevertheless, our bodies could bounce right back because of all the hormones filling our "tanks" at all times.

Here is where bioidentical hormone replacement and a qualified doctor are your best friends. For women of perimenopausal and menopausal age, putting back your hormones to your healthiest prime can calm you down, get you off drugs and antidepressants, help you get a good eight to nine hours of sleep at night, and keep you rational. Just sleeping soundly each night will lower your cortisol, but if you are already so stressed that you don't sleep more than four or five hours a night, you need to have a blood test and put your hormones back in balance. For men, just slapping on that testosterone patch each day (or whatever form your doctor chooses) can mean the difference between 100 percent vitality or no vitality at all, or between "getting it up" on demand or "shooting pool with a rope." (Sorry!)

STRESS AND YOUR LIFESTYLE

Things are different now, and that is why aging takes some work. You have to find a way to change your lifestyle to eliminate stress. When you become perfectly hormonally balanced, these things will "roll right off your back."

Of course, **lifestyle** is an overused word. We tend to think of it as the kind of houses we live in, the cars we drive, the vacations we take. These are all just peripheral things—little bonuses for our hard work. True lifestyle is how you manage your work, the time you allow for play, and the routine you find that is best for your system.

I have found that the one thing I must concede with aging is that my body will no longer take the abuse I once hurled at it. I am watching the young actresses who are in the gossip magazines going to constant parties, up late every night, drinking, drugging, not sleeping, not eating properly, driving their hormones out of whack, all of which creates the imbalances in their moods, screaming at photographers and their "people." We read about them or see them on the gossip TV shows and get exhausted just thinking about their lifestyles. There is no envy watching from this vantage point. Who would want to be that chaotic at this time in our lives? By the time the TV gossip shows are over, I am pretty much ready for bed and sleep.

But it wasn't always like this. I used to think that nighttime was when I could really get to work. Many nights I would wait until my husband went to sleep, and then I would get up and sit in front of my computer until around 3:00 in the morning. I liked it. I could speak with you, my readers, without interruption. The silence of the night freed my brain. Around 3:00 in the morning I would fall asleep, and then the alarm would go off at 7:00 for a full day's work, whether it was running to the studio or business meetings during the day. Once a month, I would fly to Florida to be on the air on Home Shopping Network for twenty-five hours, getting very little sleep. As soon as I got back home, I would be into it again, and the craziness would continue. It seemed normal. It was my lifestyle. I thought I knew what I was doing because I was on bioidentical hormones, eating real food; I loved my life and my husband; I loved my work. But something was still wrong. I couldn't put my finger on it, but I was feeling blue, kind of depressed, exhausted. Occasionally, I would take a Sunday and lie around in bed all day, but that didn't seem to be enough.

Then, Christmas Day five years ago, I woke up in tears. Tears, on my favorite day of the year! Nothing had happened to make me feel this way. The kids were coming over, Alan woke up and told me how much he loved me, it was all perfect. I called my endocrinologist and apologized for bothering her; she said it was okay, she was Jewish and didn't celebrate Christmas. I asked her what was wrong with me. I had balanced hormones, and my lifestyle was perfect. Silence. Then she said, "Perfect? What a joke! How long do you think you can keep this up? What did you expect?"

I couldn't believe her cold, hard reaction. "I keep telling you, Suzanne, that you have to change your lifestyle or face very serious consequences. You can't keep breaking down your biochemicals through overwork and not enough sleep, along with constant stress, and then not give yourself equal time to build back up." Then she said the clincher: "The next call you make to me will be that you've had a heart attack!"

"Heart attack!" I exclaimed. How could that be? I have zero plaque in my heart and arteries, I eat properly. She said, "How much sleep do you get? You get so little sleep that your cortisol is soaring and your adrenals have finally flatlined. You are a recipe for a heart attack. You are burning it at both ends. No hormone replacement or dietary program can possibly compensate for the burden you put on your body by not resting it. The stress you are under at all times is fighting against all the good things that you do for your life."

This silenced me. Meekly I asked, "What can I do?"

"Sleep," she said. "Sleep, sleep, and more sleep; daily vitamin B injections. Change your lifestyle if you want to live."

I heard her. I suddenly realized the craziness of what I was doing.

I have always gotten some perverse pleasure from "outworking" everyone. I think it comes from being called a lazy good-for-nothing by my drunken father as a child. But it was deeper than that. I realized it had to do with my self-esteem. If I had self-worth, I would not treat my body with such disregard.

I started on a regimen of sleep and vitamin B injections. At first, sleep was impossible. I had so screwed with my internal clock that dopamine (a brain chemical linked to energy mood) was pouring in at all times, making sleep impossible. My cortisol levels were sky-high, and it was Dr. Galitzer who gave me tinctures and drops to start the process of lowering my cortisol. I put myself on a schedule. I went to bed at 9:00 and did my best to fall asleep. At first, my doctor gave me a prescription for two weeks' worth of 50 mg trazodone, a mild sleeping agent, to try to retrain my body to sleep. After two weeks, I took melatonin (6 mg) before bedtime along with two Tylenol PM caplets. Melatonin is an important hormone that triggers the sleep mechanism. Read about it in chapter 2. Soon I was falling asleep on my own.

Then I changed my daily schedule. I told my office I would take phone calls only between 11:00 a.m. and 1:00 p.m. Before or after that was off-limits, and they were to send e-mails that I might or might not answer that day. This new schedule allowed me to write my books during the day. My office was suddenly quiet because the phone wasn't ringing. I had all my doctors' appointments scheduled for only one day a month so I wasn't driving into town several times a month. Business meetings were scheduled the same way. Television appearances were all cleared through my husband, who is very protective with my time and vigilant about not wasting it. At the end of each day, I stopped working at 6:00 p.m. and made a beautiful healthy delicious dinner for Alan and me.

Guess what? A calm came over me. I woke up happy, grateful, and well rested every day. My libido increased. The extra five pounds I had been carrying around disappeared. I looked fresher, younger. People noticed.

All my blood work improved. Dr. Galitzer kept using words like "perfect." I knew it, too. I had made such progress in my life, but I think without constant vigilance it is easy to slip back to old negative habits. I had had a slip, just like an alcoholic. I had to ask myself some hard questions. This kind of work is agitating and upsetting. I realized that in addition to overwork, lack of sleep can contribute to feelings of depression because of the hormonal imbalance from raised cortisol. Sleep and a determination to change have paid off. It was a change in my lifestyle that did it.

I wake up pretty happy almost all the time these days. But I have learned never to get cocky. The body needs tender loving care. Without it I am the loser.

One of our dearest friends and my husband were business partners for many years in the early 1970s. I watched the schedule my husband's partner has been on with awe for years: flying back and forth to New York each week, then back to L.A. the next day to run the production company; late nights, early mornings, diabetes that I never knew about. My husband and I had dinner with him and his wife regularly over the years, and we all loved being together. This intense schedule went on like this for years. He was a "wonder, invincible, successful," enviable.

Then came the phone call: "My husband has had two major strokes," said his wife. Both Alan and I felt numb. How could this be?

In my grief for him, I started to think about the craziness of his lifestyle. In understanding physiology, I know that cortisol could never have had a chance to go down with all the flying and late nights. When cortisol doesn't go down, insulin doesn't go down, a very dangerous scenario for a diabetic. Because he didn't carry weight, he didn't appear to be diabetic, but most likely his adrenals were so revved

up that he couldn't put on much weight. Eventually
he would have, but the stroke got him first.

Today, he is in the fight of his life. He has the will
of a soldier, and in one year he is walking slowly and
speaking well enough to go to work. I know where
he came from with the stroke, and his progress is
nothing short of a miracle.

I tell you these two stories so you might see yourself in the big picture. The body is not invincible.
The chaos of your youth will kill you in your later
years if you do not make a change in your lifestyle.
Nobody is above it. No hormones can fight it. You
have to understand the toll that stress takes and care
enough about living to realize that changes have to
be made.

You hear stories of fifty-year-old-men suddenly
dropping dead from a heart attack. It is usually followed by "He had just been at the doctor's and was
told he was fine." These men and women who drop
dead suddenly are usually A types, "superworkers"
who burn it at both ends. They don't see sleep as anything other than a nuisance. It catches up . . . even
big strong "he-men" can fall. Learn from these stories. All the vitamins, supplements, injections, hormones, and vegetables in the world can't fight
biochemical breakdown (exhaustion). The body can
do only so much, and then it breaks down, and the
picture is not pretty.

Lifestyle is a choice. Choose to live well, manage

your stress, eat healthy, value sleep, and think good thoughts. Avoid stress and confrontation, adjust to change, maximize your energy, and enjoy your life. This is the only life we're sure that we have. Don't waste the opportunity.

CHAPTER 17

DR. HERB SLAVIN: SLEEP, SEX, AND ANTIAGING MEDICINE

Dr. Herbert Slavin has been in private practice in south Florida for twenty-five years specializing in internal medicine and has helped thousands of patients regain their health and vitality through natural methods, including nutritional therapies, bioidentical hormone replacement, and chelation therapy. Dr. Slavin has been on the radio since 1990 and currently hosts the talk show Healthline on WLVJ (1040 AM) at 11:00 a.m. Mondays, Tuesdays, and Wednesdays. The show can also be heard live online at www.wlvj.com. Dr. Slavin is a dedicated doctor, a good guy. I sent my best friend, Susie, to him because I was so impressed with his forward-thinking, cutting-edge approach to medicine.

ss: How did you become interested in antiaging medicine?

HS: Years ago, I had heard about the American College for Advancement in Medicine (ACAM), a not-for-profit medical society, and I learned that a large group of doctors worldwide were treating the underlying causes of their patients' problems rather than just prescribing medications. One of the events early in my medical career that really motivated me to look for a better approach to illness occurred at a meeting of the utilization review committee at a hospital that I was attending. They were reviewing the hospital records of two ninety-year-old female patients who had died as a complication of bypass surgery. When I heard that, I started thinking to myself that these patients would probably still be alive if they hadn't had surgery, but what other treatments could we offer them for their coronary artery disease? This is a national problem, but especially here in Florida where we have so many old people who get overtreated in my opinion.

SS: I never thought about the retirees being in the majority.

HS: Right. You see, in the rest of the country, physicians would typically look at a ninety-year-old and weigh the risks of the operation versus the risk of not having it. After all, you're supposed to do what's best for the patient. But in Florida that's the age group that makes your practice. I mean at ninety years old, other treatment options without the risk of dying have to be explored. So this was when I began thinking about ways to implement alternative medicine into my practice. At about the same time, there was a doctor on the radio talking about chelation therapy. I had never heard of it, but he was interviewing patients on the radio, describing a condition caused by poor circulation in the legs that causes calf pain when walking. I thought, They never taught us that in medical school, or even in residency training. They never even mentioned chelation therapy except for the treatment of acute lead poisoning. My initial impression was he must be paying people to say these things because mainstream medicine has no cure for this condition. They have treatments for it, and when the pain gets bad enough, they might try surgery to improve the circulation, but they never recommend anything to reverse the problem. This doctor on the radio was also interviewing people who were cured of their angina without surgery. But I still was skeptical. Around this time, by coincidence, I learned that one of the nurses in my office had formerly worked with this doctor. Naturally, I asked her what she thought about what she had observed. She said she watched these patients have amazing results. One example she gave was of a patient who had had a stroke and required a wheelchair to get around. After the chelation therapy treatments, the wheelchair was no longer needed. I had heard enough and started my own research into this seemingly amazing therapy. I attended a seminar on chelation therapy where before and after pictures were shown showing marked improvement never achievable with drugs or surgery. It was recommended that I read a book written by Dr. Elmer Cranton, called **Bypassing Bypass.** And that's where I heard about ACAM, which I've now belonged to for fifteen years.

This type of medicine is not based upon a patient's complaint to be treated with a drug. In ACAM, we ask the question "What caused the dysfunction in the patient?" Once you know the cause of a problem, your focus shifts to removing the cause rather than just prescribing drugs to treat a symptom.

SS: So yours is holistic in its approach rather than a Band-Aid?

HS: Yes, but it's real medicine. Taking drugs to correct the problems of aging today is useless in so many cases, because drugs do not address the cause of the problem. If you don't address the cause, the problem won't really go away. In medical school, doctors are taught "Don't treat abdominal pain until you know what is causing it." In other words, you don't want to mask appendicitis or colitis or a gallbladder attack until you know what is causing the pain. So in that particular case in medicine—treating abdominal pain—we don't mask the symptoms, yet we do that in every other phase of medicine. If someone has high blood pressure, which is not a disease but a symptom, we mask it with a medication. We also do that with cholesterol issues, diabetes, and just about everything else

SS: So if someone has high cholesterol, how do you treat it?

HS: I look for the underlying causes of high cholesterol. In the vast majority of people, high cholesterol is usually adult-onset hyperinsulinemia, a condition that most of these people didn't have when they were younger, and it's associated with insulin resistance. In other words, patients with insulin resistance have high circulating insulin levels, which, in turn, raise their blood pressure, cholesterol, and triglycerides. Therefore, taking a cholesterol-lowering drug only masks the problem and doesn't address the underlying cause, which is insulin resistance and elevations in circulating insulin. The drug is not going to make the problem better; in fact, it will make the problem worse.

SS: How much of our illness in later life is caused by diet and bad lifestyle habits?

HS: These have a tremendous effect. But so do drugs. It is estimated that the United States uses more prescription drugs than the rest of the world **combined!**

SS: I believe it. I lived in Europe for many years. When you get sick there, European physicians first treat you homeopathically. Drugs are the last line of defense. How did drugs become the first line of defense in the United States?

HS: This issue has to do with the influence of the drug companies. They have taken control of health care in this country. It actually dates all the way back to about 1910, when the Flexner report was published.

Abraham Flexner was either directly or indirectly representing the Rockefellers and the Carnegies. His job was to go around to all the schools that taught health care, which back then included chiropractic, osteopathic, naturopathic, homeopathic, whatever schools they had. But what they did not have was allopathy, which is what we practice today, essentially the use of drugs and surgery to treat disease.

Flexner was hired because both the Rockefellers and the Carnegies owned pharmaceutical companies, and they had to figure out how they were going to market their products. They came up with this idea that the best way to market pharmaceuticals was to teach the doctors to use them. So Flexner went around to various medical schools such as the Mayo Clinic and Johns Hopkins and offered financial incentives to these institutions to change their curriculum to educate their doctors on the use of pharmaceuticals. The schools received a huge influx of money and changed their curriculum so that now today when patients come into their doctor's office with a chief complaint (which is a symptom), they are given a prescription for a drug or drugs.

SS: And we, the patients, got used to this fast reaction.

HS: That's the problem. So in medical school today, you are taught when you go into your clinical years that everything starts off with a chief complaint. If there is no complaint, health care (the way it is practiced today) has nothing to offer the patient.

What has been lost in this approach is the understanding that a patient can be very ill yet still be walking around with no symptoms.

SS: So when patients come in to see you who are in their forties, fifties, or older and are just not feeling their usual vitality, what are the first things you start thinking about?

HS: Their complaint might just be that they are tired or not as sharp mentally, or they have gained weight (that one is universal), or there is a loss of libido. So I start thinking outside the box: How can I reverse the underlying disease? I check to see if their cholesterol is high or if their blood pressure is high. As I mentioned before, high circulating insulin levels, which is known as syndrome X or metabolic syndrome, is common. Although this syndrome has received much notoriety in recent years, physicians do not routinely test for it because you must do a glucose insulin challenge test to identify an insulin problem. Those people may have a normal fasting blood insulin and normal fasting blood sugar; when challenged, they will show a very high insulin level even though other indicators appear normal. Unless you challenge those people through testing, you don't detect it. But it's so often the explanation for weight gain, high cholesterol, or high blood pressure.

As a doctor I have to ask myself: What has changed in these people? It is usually a decline in their hormone levels that is associated with an increase in insulin resistance. In other words, their bodies need to keep churning out more insulin in order to keep their blood sugar under control.

SS: Insulin is a major hormone, one that is very important to keep under control. So what do you do for them at this point?

HS: I measure their hormones—estrogen, progesterone, testosterone, and DHEA. I also check their thyroid levels to establish a baseline for future comparison, because thyroid problems cannot be strictly identified from a blood test. Thyroid is tricky; the blood test may say normal, yet the patient may have a whole list of symptoms that can be attributable to the thyroid. Testing has some value, but you also have to ask patients about their symptoms. Patients typically tell their doctors that they are gaining weight inappropriately and are unable to lose it or are troubled with constipation. Most of the time, doctors will treat each of these complaints with a symptomatic treatment. If you're constipated, take this laxative, for example.

Or physicians might dismiss a lot of the symptoms such as thinning hair or dry, scaly skin and go strictly by a blood test. If the blood test is normal, then all those symptoms that could be caused by a malfunctioning thyroid are missed because the blood test is normal. See how so many diagnoses can get confused?

Let's say the patient is depressed, or has moods

that change easily, or has difficulty concentrating, or has no sex drive. All of these could be thyroid driven, but the blood test says normal so the patient gets treated for the wrong thing and usually with a drug.

SS: Having no sex drive is a big one. I hear that from women all the time.

HS: That applies to men also, but they won't admit it as easily.

SS: Women are disturbed, but also troubled because the low sex drive is more related to having no feeling left rather than not being in the mood.

HS: But I also believe that if a woman has gained weight and her hormones are off, she is probably not happy with her appearance. This mood state may also make her a little less comfortable with having sex.

SS: I agree. What about environmental effects on the hormonal system and our health?

HS: It has a big effect. Thyroid is a big issue. Well, think about this: Thyroid disease or dysfunction is a very prevalent problem. One reason is that we are constantly being exposed to two substances that undermine thyroid function: chlorine and fluoride. The environment is loaded with these substances. Fluoride is known to suppress thyroid function. Some municipalities are still putting fluoride in their drinking water despite the fact that studies show that fluoridation has no bearing on tooth decay and dental cavities. Fluoridation is about money. It's an industrial waste product, and companies have found a way to get rid of it by selling it off to the unsuspecting.

SS: What about chlorine in swimming pools?

HS: I believe that it can have an effect on the thyroid gland, as does chlorine in drinking water. Some cities have both fluoride and chlorine in the drinking water.

SS: I even taste chlorine when I buy shrimp. In a restaurant, very often the shrimp tastes like chlorine.

HS: It is common practice to put chlorine, bleach, or antibiotics in shrimp to keep the bacteria count down so the shrimp doesn't spoil.

SS: What about cortisol? If your patients are old, they must not be sleeping; therefore they must have high cortisol.

HS: You're right. The best thing for cortisol regulation is sleep. Just getting enough sleep is so essential, yet most people are not sleeping well due to the loss of hormones and to stress in their lives.

SS: Sleep is the magic potion, so simple yet so abused. Many people try to sleep as few hours as possible at night, thinking they are doing themselves a favor. They believe by "not wasting time sleeping," they can get more done the next day

HS: Our bodies were originally intended to sleep and wake up according to the cycles of night and day. Yet one of the major changes that has happened in our modern society is the opposite: not falling asleep with the sunset and not getting up with the sunrise. Instead, people now turn the lights on and stay up for extended periods in artificial light and then wonder why they can't sleep when they turn the lights out.

SS: You mean that we have messed with the internal biological template originally within us?

HS: Exactly. Our bodies have become confused as to how to function correctly.

SS: Speaking of interfering with our natural biology, I have some questions about the birth control pill. In my generation, the pill gave us permission to have all the sex we wanted without worrying about getting pregnant and that we could put off childbearing until later. Yet in my generation, the breast cancer rate is astounding. The hormones in those original pills were synthetic, just like the hormones that menopausal women have been taking. We weren't truly ovulating when on that pill. Was it too good to be true?

HS: You can't mess with nature. The pill today is not as strong as the ones you were on. But there are broader issues as well. Increasingly, we are exposed to hormones everywhere, including in meat and poultry, all having a major negative effect. For example, you have probably read the reports that the age of menarche is beginning much younger than ever before. Consider the fact that in primitive societies today, where people are still eating a natural diet, the age of menarche is still around fifteen or sixteen. But in "civilized" countries, our little girls are starting their periods at ages nine and ten. Part of the problem is the highly processed carbohydrate diet (which elevates insulin) that our children are eating. Here in south Florida even female alligators are reaching maturity before the males, according to reports. This all has to do with estrogen in the environment.

SS: That's trouble when animals are affected.

HS: It's a serious issue. When I test women, I'll often see in older women (meaning very post-menopausal women), and even in younger women, estrogen dominance. These women just don't seem to make enough progesterone to keep the estrogen properly balanced. It's not about one hormone being good or bad; it's about the balance of all the hormones together.

SS: Older women get irritated by the subject of balancing hormones naturally. I often wonder if it's because they have been on synthetics so long, and no one wants to feel that they didn't get the best advice. I frequently hear, "So our hormones are imbalanced. So what?" My instincts tell me that these women feel it is too late for them, and they are irritated with me for stirring up the subject. Leave it alone. Who cares? But what is more important to women and men than being able to replace lost hormones with real hormones and not synthetic hormones? Is it too late for older women? Do you feel that anyone can experience a reversal?

HS: Absolutely. When an older woman gives me a list of her symptoms, I explain how this symptom is associated with hormonal imbalance. Frequently, she has no hormone production left (I mean extremely low), or her body is making estrogen disproportionately to her progesterone—which is why she has an imbalance. I am then able to show her what I can do to make her feel better. We will address the underlying cause, which is usually hormonal imbalance. Getting older is a reflection of a decline in hormone levels. You get old and your hormones fall off.

SS: Are you able to return patients to their healthiest prime?

HS: I'm not talking about being eighteen again. What I'm talking about is raising those hormone levels off the ground floor, balancing them, and giving them that little extra support. It makes a world of difference in their complaints.

I also check for biological age using computerized equipment to gauge flexibility, strength, cardiovascular fitness, along with measurements of cholesterol, triglycerides, fasting blood sugar, and body mass index. I do calipers of patients' skin thickness. This information gives us a real sense of a person's strength, flexibility, and energy. Some eighty-year-olds have amazing strength—a sign of youthfulness—and others have no flexibility left at all. When we know this, we can design treatments to improve their energy and flexibility. The problem with so many older patients is that they are not addressing their physical fitness. They're busy taking lots of pills to make sure their cholesterol is okay, but they are not doing anything to make sure their body is functioning correctly.

SS: Do you recommend detoxification in your practice?

HS: Yes, with very seriously ill patients. But I explain to my healthier patients, "If you're living a healthy life and eating properly, your own detoxification systems are working all the time for you. Just make sure you are moving your bowels at least once a day, if not more. You have to drink adequate amounts of water and not put artificial substances in your body." Artificial colorings and preservatives are harmful. In fact, a study demonstrated that after people die, their bodies are not decomposing as quickly as they used to because we are consuming on average eight pounds of preservatives a year in the food we eat.

SS: So you're saying that lifestyle habits, exercising, sleeping well, eating good foods, and managing stress are all key to successful aging?

HS: You must pay attention to everything. Sometimes I ask people, "What is the most important nutrient?" Answer: The one you're lacking. The most important component of a healthy lifestyle is the one you're not including.

SS: It can be difficult to be a patient and sort through all of this. One doctor will say this, and another doctor will say that.

HS: As a patient, you must be responsible for your

own health and just keep questioning your doctors until you find one who resonates. You also have to keep educating yourself. Breast cancer is a good example of an area in which women can better educate themselves. For example, many women get yearly mammograms. I feel that mammograms are a waste of time because statistics show that they miss 15 percent of the tumors; this probably happens more among perimenopausal age women because of breast density (dense breasts make tumors difficult to view). Mammography emits radiation, and radiation is carcinogenic. If you have a cancer and you compress it in the mammography machine, this is like compressing an egg. You crack the eggshell, and the contents may leak out. One study showed that sticking needles into breast cancer increases its chances of spreading.

I feel a better testing option is thermography because it measures only heat. Heat is a sign of increased blood flow, and a cancer cell cannot grow without increased blood flow, or angiogenesis, through it. Before a tumor can start growing, it has to establish its own blood supply. The blood supply obviously will be a source of heat.

An abnormal thermogram probably represents estrogen dominance, shown by the heat and the blood flow. You can work to correct that imbalance by giving the patient progesterone. If it did suggest the presence of a tumor, I would follow up with an MRI of the breast. That way, you avoid radiation and compression and yet get the information you need.

With my own practice, I try to intervene as early as I can so we don't have to deal with those hard decisions of "Now you've got cancer, what do you want to do?" Overall, you reduce your chances of getting serious illnesses by balancing your hormones, metabolizing them properly, keeping your vitamin D level high enough, and supplementing with nutrients in which you are deficient. This approach is the best you can do.

SS: It is largely up to us. Thank you, Dr. Slavin.

DR. SLAVIN'S TOP FIVE ANTIAGING RECOMMENDATIONS

1. Have your hormone levels checked on a regular basis—estrogen, progesterone, testosterone, DHEA, thyroid, and insulin. Keep the estrogen properly balanced. It's not about one hormone being good or bad; it's about the balance of all the hormones together.

2. Getting adequate sleep is the best way to regulate high cortisol levels. Chronically elevated cortisol can lead to high blood pressure, heart disease, and other serious illnesses.

3. Move your bowels at least once a day, if not more.

4. Drink adequate amounts of water, and do not put artificial substances into your body. Be careful about drinking water that contains fluoride and chlorine. Both can have harmful effects on thyroid health. Both are found in drinking water.

5. Mammograms may be a waste of time because statistics show that they miss 15 percent of the tumors; this probably happens more among perimenopausal women because of breast density (dense breasts make tumors difficult to view). Mammography emits radiation, and radiation is carcinogenic. A better testing option is thermography, followed up with an MRI.

CHAPTER 18

DR. PHILIP LEE MILLER:
HORMONES AND STRESS

Founder and medical director of the Los Gatos Longevity Institute in Los Gatos, California, Dr. Miller—author of The Life Extension Revolution—**has been a practicing clinician for more than thirty years. He is a diplomate of the American Academy of Anti-Aging Medicine and serves on the medical advisory board of the Life Extension Foundation. Dr. Miller is convinced that by embracing antiaging medicine, your health will soar even though you are aging chronologically. Dr. Miller's website is www.antiaging.com.**

SS: As women and men start to feel bad from hormone loss, they feel that there is no way out. Is there a solution for this stressful time of life?

PM: Definitely. The women I see are largely professionals because my practice is located in Silicon Valley; so not only is this an issue of quality of life, feeling good, and feeling rejuvenated, but it's also often an issue of being competitive and youthful.

These are women who, even though they might be sixty-five or seventy, want to hold on to their job. They don't want to be told they can't work any longer. They want to look, act, and feel younger and stay mentally sharp. What we do here at the Longevity Center is prolong or restore their careers, along with quality of life.

Some of them have been on synthetic hormones, and they tell me, "Listen, I still want to be on hormones, but I want something safer. I want something that is individualized." So I put them on bioidentical hormone replacement, and it gratifies me to see these women who look and feel like they are fifty-five or fifty-eight, even though they may be seventy-two. They have a kind of spirit, an excitement; they have that look in their eyes. Their skin quality is improved. It has been a real joy for me knowing that I can help this expanded population of women.

SS: What is the number one complaint you hear among your patients?

PM: They mainly say, "I don't feel right. I want to feel better than this."

SS: What do you do for them?

PM: I spend at least an hour doing a thorough history. I give them their physical and go through the usual formalities of making sure I haven't missed anything. What things have you tried? What worked? What didn't work?

Then we sit down and talk about the general approach of what I do, and I try to figure out by clues and questions and certain repetitive patterns that I see over time. Does this sound like a thyroid problem, or does this sound like an estrogen problem or a progesterone, or adrenal, or testosterone problem?

SS: What I hear mostly from women is the loss of sex drive. Are you getting that complaint?

PM: There is a myth in our society that when women get to their late forties and fifties, they are no longer interested in sex. But that is not true at all. I have patients say to me all the time, "Fix me up. I used to really enjoy myself. My partner and I were once little bunnies, but I'm finding I can't enjoy it anymore."

SS: Hormonal loss takes away the "feeling." It's like being dead inside. What do you do for a woman who has lost her sex drive?

PM: First, I ask her a series of questions: "Do you love your husband? Is he still attractive to you? Has he gotten fat? Do you two fight? Do you enjoy any time together? Do you turn off your cell phones?" When she responds, "Yes, I love my husband," that's when we can get to work. I need to explore whether hers is an estrogen, testosterone, or progesterone problem and look at all of these levels and their relation to one another. So many women want me to put them on testosterone immediately, but I need to see how all of these hormones are related to one another to restore the correct balance.

The same is true with men. I have seen guys with

really high testosterone levels, but they're not interested in sex. Then I see other men with low testosterone, and they have a high libido. It's not just about testosterone; it's about ratios and balance.

SS: What have you encountered lately relative to hormone replacement?

PM: High cortisol is a huge issue in today's world. People are so stressed out. I think 9/11 had a lot to do with it, in particular, and so has lifestyle in general. Elevated cortisol leads to adrenal burnout, and adrenal exhaustion takes away a person's stamina and happiness.

When your adrenals are exhausted, you have no bodily reserves to deal with inner stress. Consequently, you get illnesses such as colds or bronchitis, or you experience psychological stress that shows up as depression or personal stress, at home or on the job. What happens then is you start to eat a lot more sugar.

SS: What are we doing to ourselves in this country?

PM: I would rephrase that question: What's being done to us? I believe fear is being manufactured in this country—fear of outside forces, 9/11 fears. Over the past few years, I have seen the cortisol levels of my patients soar. People are spinning out of control from both the political climate and environmental problems. It also has to do with the type of lives we are leading; we are just doing too much. Cell phones, for example, are destroying people.

SS: Because they are never by themselves?

PM: Exactly. It seems as though if they're not talking to someone, they get nervous. I see women in the supermarket line on their phones or a mother and daughter walking down the street who are both on their cell phones.

My advice to them would be: Pay attention to your life. Here you are with your loved one or your child, yet you are on this inanimate phone talking to someone in space. I do believe this constant in-touch technology is really stressing people out—and it's one of the main reasons chronic disease is on the rise. You know, the number one cause of breast cancer is stress. Frequently, it's a combination of physical, social, and economic stress.

SS: Isn't stress a result of hormonal imbalance?

PM: It can be. Stress affects the thyroid and adrenals first. So if your thyroid is depressed, your immune defenses can be weakened, since your immune system is connected to your thyroid functioning. Now perhaps you're a candidate for a disease.

Stress can lead to cancer, diabetes, and cardiovascular disease, to name just a few. But no one takes this seriously. Men think it's fixable. I tell them that stress not only will lead to serious illness or death, but along the way it's also going to alienate you from your kids and your wife, and you could lose your sex drive, unless stress is managed.

SS: So you deal with all of this from a mind/body/spirit connection?

PM: My approach is a fully integrated program, with five steps. In the first step, I deal with metabolic issues, focusing on exercise, supplements, and a raw diet, if necessary. Many people have gastrointestinal problems, so I look into that initially, because resolving these problems sets the stage for hormones to work better.

The second step is hormonal modulation, but it's not "here's your prescription; have a nice life." It doesn't work that way. If a patient wants his or her hormones to work effectively, they must do some basic nutritional, exercise, and supplementation routines.

I deal with bioidentical hormones only—not just estrogen, progesterone, and testosterone, but also DHEA and thyroid.

The third stage is cognitive. Now that we've got your hormones working better, your mood is improved; I can start fine-tuning your cognitive abilities. This is where it gets really interesting. For example, how do we affect mood without using psychoactive drugs? How do we get the mind functioning to get you as mentally sharp as you can be?

SS: How do you do this?

PM: It boils down to the balance between dopamine (a brain chemical) and choline (a B vitamin), which are stimulating, and GABA and serotonin, two brain chemicals that are sedating. Most people need a little more choline, along with a drug called

Deprenyl, which is a brain enhancement agent, to get them sharper. I will ask my patient, "If you're in a meeting with a lot of people and events to remember, are you able to keep on top of everything, or do you have trouble keeping up?" Their answer helps me to determine what needs strengthening.

SS: We've gone through the first three steps of your program. What's next?

PM: The fourth step is stress reduction. At this point in the program, my patients are eating better, their hormone balance is better, their cognitive abilities are better, and their ability to withstand the vicissitudes of daily life is immensely improved. But they are really still in the eye of the hurricane. Everything is circling around them at 175 miles an hour, but in the eye it's only 25 miles an hour. They haven't yet reduced all their life demands, but they have improved their ability to cope with them.

Part of this step involves yoga and meditation; both are important ways to reduce stress. Yoga is also good for stretching because it keeps us limber. It loosens our ligaments and tendons, which thicken with age, and helps our bodies become more elastic. Beyond that, yoga teaches you to slow down and breathe.

SS: And number five?

PM: Step five is the mind/body/spirit connection and involves coming to grips with where you are in life. How do you relate to the universe and the people around you? What or who are you? What are you doing? Where are you going? For me, this is the most satisfying work I have ever done.

SS: How great! If you could change anything, what would you change in the lives we are all living today?

PM: I would like to see more people realize that you've got to take responsibility for your own life. It's not someone else's fault; it's not someone else's responsibility. The life you lead is up to you. We are all buffeted by things we can't control, but the life you live is determined by you. You are in charge of your choices. You have to be motivated to make changes in your life that are positive and life-giving.

SS: Thank you so much for this wonderful information.

DR. MILLER'S TOP FIVE ANTIAGING RECOMMENDATIONS

1. Loss of sex drive in a woman can be related to a decline in estrogen, testosterone, or progesterone. Your doctor should check your levels and restore the correct balance.

2. If you want your bioidentical hormones to work effectively, you must do some basic nutritional, exercise, and supplementation routines.

3. To enhance your brain function, talk to your doctor about supplementing with choline or a drug called Deprenyl.

4. Definitely consider yoga and meditation; both are important ways to reduce stress. Yoga is also good for stretching because it keeps us limber. It loosens our ligaments and tendons, which thicken with age, and helps our bodies become more elastic. Beyond that, yoga teaches you to slow down and breathe.

5. Take responsibility for your own life and your choices. We are all buffeted by things we can't control, but the life you live is determined by you. You are in charge of your choices.

CHAPTER 19

DR. GORDON REYNOLDS: STRESS

Dr. Gordon Reynolds spent thirty years in obstetrics and gynecology and then returned to school to get a PhD in nutrition. His interests today lie in reproductive endocrinology, and he is a sought-after speaker on the lecture circuit. He is currently part of the faculty at the Green Valley Spa in Utah.

SS: Let's talk about the effects of stress on aging.

GR: We've accelerated our lives considerably. We're in a state of constant compulsive thinking about making money, obtaining more things materially, and trying to do so many things—a state of turmoil that almost creates a collective disease. Stress is responsible for the majority of the processes we experience. Stress increases cortisol levels, which, in turn, can interfere with hormonal balance and inhibit thyroid function. In a postmenopausal woman or even in a premenopausal woman, usually the progesterone has already dropped out. Stress speeds up this process. In fact, 50 percent of women over thirty-five are no longer producing adequate progesterone. That may or may not influence testosterone or DHEA, but as soon as progesterone drops out, the rest of her hormones are now imbalanced.

SS: You obviously feel that stress is a major factor in today's world, and it interferes with our hormonal system. I require enormous amounts of estrogen to think straight, and I believe in mimicking normal physiology, meaning having a period. If we need estrogen and progesterone in balance, or in the correct ratio, shouldn't we try to achieve the same balance we had at our strongest and healthiest?

GR: It depends upon the individual. If she requires more, then we replace more. But I differ with you in that I don't demand that a period occur if all the criteria are met. However, if a woman wants a period, if it makes sense to her as it does to you, then we can make that happen with bioidentical hormone replacement.

The reason I feel so strongly about replacing hormones is that I didn't start at sixty-four, I started much earlier. When I speak to a group, I say, "Let's draw a line down the middle of the board, fifty on this side and fifty on the other. Let's look at the things we did when we were younger and what your hormone balance was then." I show how DHEA peaks at twenty-five and then fizzles out at 2 percent a year, then testosterone drops off, and then progesterone stops production.

Then we look at the other side, and I ask what we can learn in these next fifty years from what we garnered from the past. If you understand that your peak health was in your reproductive years, can we safely increase these hormones by keeping them in balance on the other side of the fence without problems? I say we can. It's been shown. There have been enough studies by the antiaging society medical groups and enough published worldwide literature to say that this is not hazardous.

Twenty-five percent of all women go through menopause pretty well; another 25 percent have a terrible time; and 50 percent are just all over the board. Those who go through it well, without a lot of stress, are the ones who have a good nutrition and exercise program in place.

Interestingly, most women in third world countries don't have a problem with menopause. It's not even in their vocabulary. Most of them don't have hot flashes or any of the typical symptoms. What's the difference? Stress!

SS: So American women who are trying to be everything are paying a price?

GR: Absolutely. You've got to get off the treadmill. It's killing us. By contrast, we have more than fifty thousand people in this country who are over a hundred years old. When asked the secret of their longevity, these people say that it is attributable to a good diet. Moreover, the ones who lived the longest are insulin-sensitive; they have not had insulin resistance. In addition, they have a very positive outlook—they don't think negative thoughts—and they are consciously positive.

Some of them might say staying away from doctors and hospitals (**laugh**). In actuality, the third or fourth common cause of death in this country is iatrogenic.

SS: Meaning?

GR: Induced by surgery or medicine.

SS: That's scary. So it goes back to diet and lifestyle?

GR: Absolutely. Hormone imbalance is a very significant factor, which is why women should be having hormone panels done in their mid-thirties for the first time. Men should start at forty. But the number one factor is diet. Without a good diet, you get insulin resistance, type 2 diabetes, and all the problems that accompany these conditions. When I started practicing back in the 1950s, we were prescribing diets high in carbohydrates and low in fat. That kind of diet can lead to these conditions. It's very tragic, and physicians played and continue to play a part in this.

SS: Don't get me started; I have written several books on that subject. It all started when President Dwight Eisenhower had his heart attack in the 1950s. His doctor put him on a low-fat, high-carb diet, and that turned the tide to become the trend.

GR: The American Medical Association says that 50 million people in the United States have coronary artery disease. The sad thing is, heart disease is preventable, but it's hard to get that across.

SS: You and I both agree that bioidentical hormones are a big missing piece of the health puzzle. Why is it so difficult to get the rest of the doctors to come along with this thinking, and how long is it going to take?

GR: Having been a physician for fifty-five years, I have certainly seen how slowly it does change. I believe it will take another twenty-five years for this concept to be accepted. It will take a long time because there is a kind of animosity toward physicians who follow the bioidentical protocol.

The thinking is: How dare you do something different? But it's really fear of criticism by their peers, so the majority of doctors go along with the "standard of care."

But you must have hope. I attend meetings that combine alternative and functional medicine. The discussion of menopause and bioidentical hormones is a topic of discussion. So slowly, it's happening.

I also see the pressure put on the doctor by the patient. Patients are standing up and saying, "Hey, Doctor, I want more of an answer."

SS: A lot of the women I have interviewed talk about estrogen dominance, bloating, and inability to lose weight, water, and fat. Explain estrogen dominance.

GR: It's the loss of balance with progesterone. Estrogen is a growth hormone; it's also an excitatory hormone, so it's responsible for insomnia and many of the mood changes as well, whereas progesterone is a very calming hormone that balances it.

The number one reason I would see patients as a gynecologist would be women in their forties complaining about weight gain in their lower abdomens. They were exercising and eating well but still gaining weight.

That, of course, was a major clue. It just told me that they were not producing progesterone anymore. They had estrogen dominance. It's not being in balance—and, of course, estrogen likes to put on fat in the middle area. But more important, estrogen dominance inhibits thyroid. It inhibits the conversion of thyroxine, or T4, to T3 at the cellular level. T3 is by far the most potent of the thyroid hormones, and it's seldom checked. Even when it is checked, it's not that accurate, but it does give us a clue if we check.

The tiredness women experience, plus the fat deposition, are both probably due to a change in the thyroid as well. You know hormones all work together; if one hormone is off, then they are all off.

SS: Let me ask you again: Doesn't cycling make sense?

GR: Absolutely, cycling. I just don't necessarily subscribe to the fact that menstruation has to occur. That would depend upon the patient. During perimenopause or early menopause, the amount of estrogen needed to build the endometrium may be enough to have a period, and that's fine because we're using progesterone on a fourteen-day cycling basis. So if there is an increase in the endometrium, it will slough off at that time.

As time goes on, you continue to produce estrogen either from the ovaries or the fat cells, and studies go all the way up to eighty years of age that some women may still have enough estrogen. And if progesterone is in balance, it will enhance the receptor sites.

You don't have to have as much estrogen to build the lining of the endometrium to make the brain feel good. I don't think it was intended that way. I mean, when we didn't have any medicines and women went through menopause, I don't believe they were intended to fall apart.

SS: Yes, but we didn't live as long as we do today. This long life is no fun without quality of life. What about the antidepressants prescribed for stress and anxiety? Most woman my age are on some kind of antidepressant.

GR: I don't like them. I have never prescribed them, and I won't prescribe them. A big problem in medicine today is the HMO. A doctor is given approximately eight minutes per patient. What can you do for a patient in eight minutes except write a prescription? That's the kind of medicine we are practicing today. A prescription mill. Doctors no longer have time to sit down with their patients to find out what's really going on.

The system is not working. I hope it has hit bottom, but I don't know how it is going to straighten out. We have the government handling our health. I don't know any agency in the government that is really helping people.

SS: What do you tell audiences in your lectures?

GR: To take responsibility for your own health and challenge whatever your doctor tells you to do. Verify and feel comfortable with what he or she is prescribing. When doctors have only eight minutes per patient, they have no time to make new discoveries or make changes. Doctors learn more today by reading lay magazines!

The reason I'm still doing at my age what I am doing (I'm eighty years old) is that it isn't happening with the doctors. They don't have the time. When I first started my practice, I talked to my patients and taught them how to stay healthy. Very few doctors do that anymore.

For instance, men need to know that testosterone levels are dropping about a decade earlier than they used to. Coronary heart disease is associated with low testosterone levels; it's not just erectile dysfunction and libido. To stay healthy, a man has to have adequate testosterone levels. If estrogen dominance is an issue, then he may get cancer of the prostate, because that is likely to be caused by the estrogen rather than the testosterone. But who is going to tell people in the community these things when the doctors are too busy? This is why I say you've got to take responsibility for your own health.

How do you educate everybody? When you get hooked on sugar, how do you get off it? You can't eat sugar every day and be healthy. Sugar should be a treat, a reward. There are some school systems that are taking junk food out of the school cafeterias. They are trying to educate kids in school, but it's a drop in the bucket. But that is where it has to start, because I don't think enough parents are into this. Parents are so busy that a good many of them really aren't paying attention until something happens. I mean, 40 percent of today's meals are eaten in restaurants and fast-food takeouts.

We have so many health problems, from bacteria overgrowth to inflammation to acid reflux, I'm hearing more and more about esophageal cancer probably as a result of acid reflux. Our whole medical system is in a big mess.

But I see little signs of hope. If people are educated and exposed to the new information, they will want it. Little by little, step by step, we'll get the information out, and change will happen. This is what I dream about.

SS: Thank you for your wisdom.

DR. REYNOLDS' TOP FIVE ANTIAGING RECOMMENDATIONS

1. The number one factor in managing health is diet. Without a good diet, you get insulin resistance, type 2 diabetes, and all the problems that accompany these conditions.

2. Testosterone levels are dropping about a decade earlier than they used to. Coronary heart disease is associated with low testosterone levels; it's not just erectile dysfunction and libido. To stay healthy, a man has to have adequate testosterone levels. If estrogen dominance is an issue, then he may get cancer of the prostate, because that is likely to be caused by the estrogen rather than the testosterone.

3. As for menopause, those who go through it well, without a lot of stress, have a good nutrition and exercise program in place.

4. Women should be having hormone panels done in their mid-thirties for the first time. Men should start at forty. This is a different world.

5. Take responsibility for your own health, and challenge whatever your doctor tells you to do. Verify and feel comfortable with what he or she is prescribing.

PART FOUR

DETOXIFICATION AND THE EFFECTS OF THE ENVIRONMENT ON YOUR HEALTH

A study demonstrated that after people die, their bodies are not decomposing as quickly as they used to because we are consuming on average eight pounds of preservatives a year just from the food we eat.

CHAPTER 20

ANTIAGING MEDICINE

> Reporters interviewing a 104-year-old
> woman: "And what do you think is the
> best thing about being 104?"
> The woman simply replied, "No peer
> pressure."

Aging is a part of life. Each cell in the body has a function to perform. Heart muscles have to function for our hearts to beat. The nerve cells in our brain have to function so we can think. These functions are fed by the hormones in the body. If you have read this far, you know that hormone loss is the hallmark of aging. By replacing the hormones lost in the aging process, we can substantially stop the clock. As several doctors in this book have stated: **Our hormones do not decline because we age, we age because our hormones decline.**

The second component would be the effects of our damaged environment and the toxicity all around us that are aging us prematurely. Our bodies are under an assault unlike anything the human species has ever before endured. Our environment is polluted, our food has been poisoned, our water is contaminated, the stresses of our daily lives are killing us, and we are taking too many pharmaceuticals that are making us sick.

Antiaging medicine understands this assault. In fact, antiaging medicine is a relatively new specialty brought about by Western doctors who realize we are living in a changed world, a polluted, stressful world. We are living longer, and traditional medicine has for the most part not kept up. In other words . . . it is not working. Like medics on the battlefield, these doctors work to heal the aging, environmentally wounded body and then reverse the damage through detoxification, hormone replacement, energy replacement, supplementation, and real food.

Traditional medicine focuses on treating the **effects** of the aging process, while antiaging medicine concentrates on treating the **causes** of aging. This is functional medicine, restoring the body to optimal functioning levels. The only way to reverse or slow down aging is to prevent or attempt to reverse the diseases we expect to get in the aging process. We have to make a shift in our thinking. The way we are being taken care of at present is pharmaceutically based and, for the most part, is not healing us. Again, I am not antipharmaceutical—when we need them, they are godsends—but in general, as a society, we have become addicted to our prescriptions, and then that drug causes another problem, which creates another problem requiring yet another drug. It's a merry-go-round that never stops. Look around you . . . are your friends and family well and healthy?

Antiaging doctors work to stop the clock dramatically by slowing, preventing, or even reversing the diseases of aging that I talked about in chapter 4. These doctors take the environmental assault very seriously. Every day they work with people who once felt hopeless relative to their health and well-being and have helped them reverse their chronic, degenerative conditions. I've interviewed several of these doctors in the chapters that follow. Once you read what they have to say, I think you'll agree with me: This is exciting medicine!

This chapter provides important information on how the environment affects our health and provokes premature aging and chronic inflammation (the two are related)—and what you can do about it. Pay close attention to the sections on detoxification and ways to reduce inflammation. This information is cutting-edge and will help you clarify what you can expect on this journey to becoming ageless.

AGING, DETOXIFICATION, AND THE ENVIRONMENT

Every moment of every day we are exposed to thousands of toxic chemicals. They are everywhere, all the time. They are a big part of the reason we are getting sick. Yet it wasn't always this way.

When I was a child, my parents didn't have a cabinet full of chemicals stored under the kitchen sink. My mother washed her dishes with Ivory soap. If we had an ant infestation right before a rain, she washed down the baseboards and sink tops with soap and water. The food we ate wasn't labeled organic because the food **was** organic. We didn't spray our fruits and vegetables with pesticides. If my mother found bugs on the fruits and vegetables in her garden, she washed the leaves with soap and water.

Our milk came in glass bottles. Our babies drank their milk from glass bottles; our meat was wrapped in white butcher paper. We didn't drink our sodas and coffee from Styrofoam cups; they didn't exist. There were no preservatives in our food, nor were there hormones in our meat. The oceans were clean; our fish were not filled with mercury and other poisons. It was a simpler time.

Growing up, I loved root beer floats—my mother would buy a bottle of root beer and a carton of vanilla ice cream once during the summer to make this yummy dessert. Mmm! I waited all year for that one. We didn't have numerous six-packs of sodas and colas sitting around. Back then it was a once-a-year treat, not a sweet I ate every day as kids today might do. At mealtimes we drank milk—milk that wasn't loaded with hormones and additives that you can't pronounce. Now we walk around with giant plastic cups called Big Gulps filled with diet sodas loaded with aspartame or other artificial sweeteners. Aspartame is found in sugar-free chewing gums, cola drinks, sweets, and many other foods we enjoy every day, and it is made of chemicals. They say in America we consume a gallon of chemicals every year! And this is a conservative estimate.

Sweets are no longer a treat, they are an everyday occurrence, and our children are showing the effects. Adult-onset diabetes is now called type 2 diabetes because so many children are also affected by this disease. It now accounts for up to 45 percent of new cases of diabetes among youth. Fifteen years ago, type 2 accounted for less than 3 percent of all cases of newly diagnosed diabetes in children and teens. Also, children are eating so many sweets that they're now showing symptoms of heart disease—heart disease! This is a tragedy.

Who had ever heard of the word **phthalates** (the outgas that comes from the plastics so innocently used to wrap our food in today's world)? In fact, we eat so many plastics daily, unknowingly, that the government has established an average daily amount that we can "safely" ingest. Once inside our bodies, these phthalates, or plastics, hook tightly on to our cell parts, where they wreak havoc. They damage hormone receptors, leading to loss of sex drive and energy, or they damage brain chemistry, leading to learning disabilities and hyperactivity, or they accumulate in organs and trigger cancers of the prostate, breast, lung, and thyroid. We also find these poisons in industrial compounds used in everything from plastic shower curtains to lipstick. That "new car" smell, which is particularly strong after the car has been sitting in the sun for a while, comes from the outgas of phthalates volatilizing from a plastic dashboard. Phthalates have been known to cause kidney and liver damage and harm a developing fetus. Nice, huh?

Who had ever heard of dioxin, either? Dioxin is a man-made chemical that is now almost inescapable in our food. Created in part through the manufacture of plastics, pesticides, and other chemicals, dioxin is spewed from industrial smokestacks, taken up into the clouds, and then rained down onto the soil, where it is absorbed by the plants consumed as food for animals and humans. When you wrap your food in plastic, then microwave it, you create carcinogens from the dioxin in the plastic. Dioxin is one of the most potent carcinogens known to man. Toxic chemicals like dioxin and phthalates are everywhere—in the air we breathe, the water we drink, the food we eat, and the soil in which we plant our very future.

There is not a home, office, institution, or manufacturing site where plastics do not abound. They are used in construction materials, building products and furnishings, plastic baby bottles, baby rattles and teething toys, plastic crib bumpers, car seats, mattresses, kitchen appliances, shoes and sneakers, IV tubing, computer housings, automobile dashboards and undercoatings, electrical wire coverings and cables, carpet backing, cosmetics, notebook covers, clothes, dishes, tablecloths, shower curtains, toilet seats, gadgets, games, and much more. Not only do these plastics get into our food, they also get into our air, assuring an easy route to every one of our internal organs. Any chemical you can smell in the air makes its way into your bloodstream, eventually disseminating into all your organs.

Currently, there are about fifty thousand chemical compounds in production: Ten thousand different chemicals are used in the processing of food, and more than three thousand chemicals are added to our food supply. Our drinking water alone may contain over seven hundred chemicals. One of them is fluoride, an extremely toxic poison that is banned in nine European countries. A portion of the fluoride in the water we drink is deposited in our bones, where it has been shown in studies to weaken bones and increase the risk of hip fracture in men and women over age sixty-five who have been exposed to twenty years or more of fluoride in their drinking water. Read the label of your fluoridated toothpaste sometime: "Keep out of reach of children under 6 years of age. If more than used for brushing is accidentally swallowed, get medical help or contact a Poison Control Center right away." Why? Apparently, there's enough fluoride in that toothpaste tube to kill a twenty-pound child. That should tell you something! (Be sure to read Dr. Herb Slavin's interview and see what he has to say about fluoride.)

Heavy metals, particularly mercury, are another example of deadly toxins hidden in our foods. We can get mercury toxicity from contaminated fish, shellfish, and small fish that feed around the mouths of rivers. Large fish such as swordfish, mackerel, and tuna feed on those smaller fish and then stockpile those heavy metals in their own flesh. As if we did not have enough ways to contaminate our foods, there have been accidental spills that have led to silent yet serious poisonings. Add to this the highly polluting commercial shipping industry, incinerators, and others that have brought us to the place of existence we are now experiencing.

Additionally, air pollution, cigarette smoke, smog, car exhaust, toxic waste pesticides, herbicides, ultraviolet light, and drugs can all generate disease-causing free radicals in the body. Free radicals induce inflammatory reactions that cause life-shortening chronic diseases. Think about this, too: The average household carpet outgases over a dozen chemicals. Also in our homes, the place where we spend the most time, are paints, solvents, insecticides, greases, oils, lawn mower gas cans, a heated car engine, furnace, gas dryer, gas water heater, and washing machines—all possible pollutants, and we never give them a thought!

The chemicals given off in our environment can remain in the body for years, putting an enormous strain on our vital organs and glands. In fact, more than four hundred toxic chemicals have been detected in human tissue. This increased toxic burden on our bodies results in illness and disease: decreased immune function, arthritis, rheumatism, hormonal dysfunction, neurotoxicity, leukemia, obesity, chronic fatigue, depression, physiological disturbances, ADD (attention deficit disorder), and, of course, cancer.

Now, I realize that many of the things you have at home, at work, and around you are everyday luxuries. You're not about to get rid of most of them. However, there are some you can do without, especially now that you know their dangers, their impact on your body, and why you have chronic conditions you can't seem to shake. The purpose of this section is not to scare you. I just want to make you more aware so that you can lessen the effects on you and your family by eliminating some of them, buying the highest-quality food you can afford, and getting to the proper doctor if you feel you have been adversely affected by unwanted chemical poisoning.

TAKE CHARGE OF YOUR ENVIRONMENT

Buy high-quality air and water purification systems for your home.

Purchase natural-fiber clothing, bed coverings, and furnishings of cotton and wool whenever possible.

Use natural floorings or ceramic tile rather than carpets. But if you opt for carpet, choose natural fiber wool rugs and carpets.

Buy safe, natural, nontoxic paints and household cleaners to eliminate synthetic toxins.

Microwave your foods in glass; don't use plastic wrap.

Try to find ways to eliminate the use of plastics in your life: Drink water from glass bottles, heat baby's milk in glass bottles, and use fabric shower curtains instead of plastic.

Find ways to eliminate pests and rodents from your house without using chemicals. A helpful book is **1001 All-Natural Secrets to a Pest-Free Property** by Dr. Myles H. Bader.

Although we can limit our exposure to them, the chemicals in the air and water and soil are largely out of our control. Air pollution, cigarette smoke, smog, car exhaust, toxic waste pesticides, herbicides, ultraviolet light, and drugs can all generate free radicals in the body. We do have control over our diet and lifestyle, however. The choices we make also affect our organs, tissues, and glands. Of all the vital organs in the body, the ones that suffer the most abuse from our modern dietary and lifestyle habits are the colon and the liver. The liver is groaning from the effort of breaking down the massive intake of drugs and poisons. The colon was intended by nature to function as a smoothly flowing system that promptly and efficiently flushes digestive wastes from the body. Instead, it has become a stagnant wasteland. It's not pretty to think about, but I believe if we could see what we have lurking in our digestive systems, we would all change our eating habits overnight. Choosing real food, healthy food, is a part of the environmental assault over which we have control.

In this day and age, we now have the opportunity to do something about the environment that is aging us. The simple, pollutant-free life we inherited from our ancestors no longer exists. As I have said, we are experiencing an environmental assault unlike anything the human species has ever before endured. This is not hocus-pocus. Think about it: how different life is today relative to chemicals and preservatives, fake food, and bad oils. Think about the cooking oil used in fast-food chains. Think of all the processed food we ingest. All this bad food and all these chemicals and poisons have a negative effect on the state of our health.

These new-thinking doctors can help you reverse the damage. It's not too late. Take charge of your health and your personal environment. If you have been going from doctor to doctor and can't get to the bottom of your problems or are on too much medication, a good antiaging doctor might hold the answer.

INFLAMMATION

Hardly a week goes by without the publication of a new study uncovering another way that "inflammation" does harm to the body. The word **inflammation** is so overused that hardly any of us have ever really stopped to ask ourselves what exactly is inflammation.

Inflammation holds good news and bad news. When we cut our finger, an inflammatory response is triggered. It swells up and reddens. Sometimes it gets worse and becomes infected. Then, because of inflammation, it gets better. Another example: Inflammation is what turns the tissue around a splinter red or causes swelling in an injured toe. Inflammation is the body's natural healing mechanism. It activates a defensive attack the instant a deadly microbe slips into the body. Once this process subsides, healing begins. This is good inflammation, the body working at optimum.

Here's where we go wrong: The moment we experience recognizable inflammation, we run to the doctor and demand to be given something to stop it. Inflammation hurts, after all; it is painful. Swelling is uncomfortable, redness is sore, infection oozes and is not only sore but also disagreeable to view on our bodies.

What we fail to recognize is that, again, inflammation is our body's way of healing itself. When we stop the process with a drug or ointment, we leave our bodies confused. Now medicine takes over what the body is designed to do naturally; as a result, it takes longer to heal. The inflammation is driven deeper into the body, and it doesn't go away. Now it becomes harmful. That's bad inflammation.

Inflammation is not always as evident as the redness and swelling around a splinter. Inflammation can also be silent, lurking inside unbeknownst to us. Sometimes the problem is a genetic disposition (something we have inherited), and other times it is environmental (like smoking or eating fatty foods made from fake fats), that keeps the inflammatory process going, since habits like these contribute to the development of underlying plaques in our arteries and other problems. In these cases, inflammation becomes chronic rather than transitory, sticking around a lot longer than it is needed. When this occurs, the body turns on itself, with inflammation launching an attack on normal cells. Within this scenario lies a wide variety of diseases.

Chronic inflammation does harm to the body. In fact, chronic inflammation may be the engine that drives many of the most feared illnesses of middle and old age. Our Western lifestyle with diets high in sugar and saturated fats, accompanied by little or no exercise, makes it easier for the body to become inflamed.

C-REACTIVE PROTEIN AND INFLAMMATION

The top three killers today are heart attack, cancer, and stroke. Chronic inflammation plays a significant role in the development of each of these lethal diseases. If you have chronic inflammation in your body, it can be measured. One of the best and simplest ways to measure inflammation in your body is with a C-reactive protein (CRP) blood test. It detects a protein in the blood—C-reactive protein—that is a sign of inflammation within the artery walls. High levels of C-reactive protein indicate an increased risk for destabilized atherosclerotic plaque. When arterial plaque becomes destabilized, it can burst open and block the flow of blood through a coronary artery, resulting in an acute heart attack.

If you have this test—and you should—you want your levels to be below 0.5. Anything higher than that is an indicator that all is not well. Also, ask your doctor to order you a "high-sensitivity" CRP test. The standard test used by many labs does not measure the minute levels of CRP necessary to adequately determine cardiovascular risk. **Life Extension** magazine recommends ordering a low-cost high-sensitivity CRP blood test by mail by calling 1-800-

208-3444. I have nothing to do with this service, but I feel it will benefit you to know that it can be done at home and then have the results sent to your doctor to interpret. An antiaging doctor would be the best person to read the results for you.

Catch chronic inflammation now before it catches you later in life; don't wait until it is too late. Inflammation experts have determined that a CRP reading of 3.0 mg/L or higher can triple your risk of heart disease. Men with high CRP levels are three times as likely to suffer a heart attack in the next six years as those with lower CRP levels. The danger is even higher in women. By contrast, people with extremely low levels of CRP (less than 0.5 mg/L) rarely have heart attacks.

Those with elevated C-reactive protein have not only increased risk of heart attack, but also a two to three times greater risk of stroke. In people who have already suffered a stroke, higher levels of C-reactive protein predict the likelihood of another stroke or heart attack or dying within the next year.

What many doctors do not know is that people with high levels of C-reactive protein in their blood also have an increased risk of certain cancers. Chronic inflammation facilitates the transformation of normal cells into cancer and also increases the proliferation of existing cancers. People with the highest blood levels of C-reactive protein are three times as likely to get colon cancer.

Sometimes the reason for the initial inflammatory

cycle is obvious, as with chronic heartburn, which continuously bathes the lining of the esophagus with stomach acid, predisposing the person to esophageal cancer.

In addition to cancer and heart disease, chronic inflammation is involved in diseases as diverse as heart valve dysfunction, obesity, diabetes, congestive heart failure, digestive system diseases, and Alzheimer's disease—all "diseases of aging."

According to the book **Disease Prevention and Treatment** (fourth edition) published by the Life Extension Foundation, "Aging results in an increase of inflammatory cytokines (destructive cell-signaling chemicals) that contribute to the progression of many degenerative diseases."

Inflammatory cytokines can cause allergies by inducing autoimmune reactions; anemia, by attacking erythropoietins (hormones that stimulate the production of red blood cells by stem cells in bone); aortic valve stenosis (a narrowing of the aortic valve) by chronic inflammation that damages heart valves; and arthritis by destroying joint cartilage. Inflammatory cytokines do other dirty work. They are involved in congestive heart failure due to chronic inflammation that contributes to heart muscle wasting; fibromyalgia due to elevated inflammatory cytokines; and lupus due to an autoimmune attack by inflammatory cytokines. Kidney failure is caused by inflammatory cytokines that restrict circulation and damage nephrons, filtering units in the kidneys that remove waste products from the blood.

The beat goes on. Inflammation also destroys brain cells. People with CRP levels in the upper three quartiles are three times more likely to contract Alzheimer's disease.

In the last decade of her life, my mother became 98 percent blind with macular degeneration, a chronic eye disease that causes damage to the macula (central retina) of the eye. Affecting more than 10 million Americans, macular degeneration is the leading cause of blindness in people over fifty-five. The American Medical Association has published a new study indicating that systemic inflammation increases the risk of macular degeneration. This study evaluated 930 participants and found that people with high CRP levels were significantly more likely to develop advanced macular degeneration. The study concluded that "elevated C-reactive protein level is an independent risk factor for age-related macular degeneration and may implicate the role of inflammation in the pathogenesis of age-related macular degeneration."

I agonized as I watched my mother stumble around, trying to feel her way to different parts of her home. If we had known then about the C-reactive protein test, maybe we could have steered this disease off its course before it reached such a debilitating stage. Macular degeneration struck my mother with no warning. One morning in her seventh decade, she woke up and the lights were out. She could see nothing but about a 2 percent peripheral blur. It was pretty devastating, although she handled it well. I don't know what I would have done had it been me. My heart ached for her. I wanted her to see again all that she once saw, but there was nothing any of us could do for her.

Like a fire burning out of control, systemic inflammation is sometimes difficult to control. This is especially true in the elderly and the obese. Fortunately, there are ways to lower elevated C-reactive protein. The best way is to find a doctor who specializes in antiaging medicine, since elevated C-reactive protein is a result of aging. Other ways to guard against an outbreak of uncontrolled systemic inflammation and lower C-reactive protein is by managing stress, eating right, and taking the proper inflammation-suppressing supplements. The Life Extension Foundation recommends the following supplements and other agents to lower CRP:

- vitamin E
- borage oil
- fish oil (very important)
- DHEA replacement
- vitamin K
- nettle leaf extract
- ibuprofen, aspirin, or one of the statins (to be tried if diet and supplements fail)

As for lifestyle, here is where sleep is again a factor. If you skipped the section titled "The Importance of Sleep" (page 345), please read it now. Lack of sleep markedly increases inflammatory cytokines, which helps explain why pain flare-ups occur in response to sleep deprivation in various disorders. Menopausal women are at risk for high levels of CRP because hormonal imbalances make sleep impossible. It's like dominoes: hormones are off, can't sleep, disease has a chance to take hold, elevated CRP results, and so on.

Even modest sleep restriction adversely affects inflammatory cytokine levels. In reporting the results, a carefully controlled study by the Life Extension Foundation noted that sleep deprivation caused a 40 to 60 percent average increase in the inflammatory marker IL-6 in men and women, while men showed a 20 to 30 percent increase in TNF-a. Both TNF-a and IL-6 are potent proinflammatory cytokines that induce systemic inflammation. Here is another instance where the importance of restoring hormone levels to balance comes into play. Balanced hormones allow you to sleep!

INFLAMMATORY CYTOKINES: A PRIMER

As a health-conscious person, you should familiarize yourself with these terms, because excess levels of these cytokines cause or contribute to many disease states. Here are the acronyms that represent the most dangerous proinflammatory cytokines:

TNF-a = tumor necrosis factor–alpha

IL-6 = interleukin-6

IL-1b = interleukin–1 beta

IL-8 = interleukin-8

I urge you to take inflammation seriously. If you have a chronic cough, if you have chronic stomach discomfort, if you can't sleep, if you have leg pain, if you have chronic fatigue, if you are constantly clearing your throat, if you have a choking problem, if you feel nauseated frequently—these are all symptoms of inflammation. Most important, have a C-reactive protein blood test.

Remember this: As we age and become hormonally imbalanced (women and men), we lose the ability to "turn off" inflammatory reactions. This problem also occurs in younger people as a result of genetics, bad diet, and poor lifestyle habits. If you continue to smoke and eat badly, you are challenging your body to become chronically inflamed. Your body's immune system will end up attacking the arteries, brain cells, joint cartilage, and every organ system.

The symptoms we put off as "nothing," such as a chronic cough or hoarseness, is your body talking to you and warning you of what may come. Listen and make changes. A simple blood test can set you on a path of good health and change the course of your life. We are not necessarily genetically disposed to the ailments of our predecessors unless we take on their unhealthy diet and lifestyle habits. You have the opportunity to change the course of your family history by making a few simple changes.

CHAPTER 21

DR. MICHAEL GALITZER: ANTIAGING MEDICINE

Dr. Galitzer is my personal antiaging endocrinologist. His approach to medicine is to increase energy in the body. The question we all have to ask ourselves is not how old you are, but how young is your energy? It was Dr. Galitzer who introduced me to this concept. He practices energy medicine in Los Angeles and Santa Barbara, California. He is on the cutting-edge curve of the latest and greatest medical breakthroughs. It is a privilege to be taken care of by this kind, interested, and motivational doctor. Be sure to read the interview with "Wendy" to see the kind of work Dr. Galitzer is doing.

SS: Thank you for your time. You always have so much to say because you are naturally curious. I think curiosity is a great plus for a doctor because you keep up with all the latest information. But I have noticed that in the media, antiaging medicine gets a bad rap. They dismiss antiaging medicine as though it's not really medicine.

MG: Antiaging medicine is very real. It attempts to increase the energy of the body. Because lack of energy is associated with the aging process, I look to regenerate the body by restoring the ideal physiology and the optimum functioning of the cells, organs, and metabolism. The difficult thing is as we get older, we have less and less energy. The challenge as an antiaging physician is, how do you increase the energy with older people? How do you get them to have more energy? I use a lot of intravenous therapies, such as intravenous vitamin C or intravenous glutathione. These are great ways to increase energy.

SS: I know after my regular glutathione and vitamin C drips, I do feel energized, as well as strong and vibrant.

MG: It does have that effect. I also use herbs or other methods such as detoxification to remove toxins from the body. Bioidentical hormones are also effective for increasing energy.

To help people with energy, traditional medicine uses thyroid hormones, growth hormone, cortisol, and prednisone. In antiaging medicine, we use bioidentical estrogen and progesterone for restoring energy. Growth hormones also seem to help. Once we are able to increase energy in a person, we can then start the process of regenerating their body.

SS: Why do we lose energy as we age? Where does it go?

MG: It is spiritual and physical. Physically, we are exposed to far too many toxins from the environment, including heavy metals such as lead and mercury, and these exposures represent a major problem. As an example, I saw a guy two years after the fact who actually swallowed a mercury filling, and about a year later he started having rectal bleeding. His doctors didn't know what was wrong with him. They finally had to take him to the operating room, and after they opened him up, there was this huge cancer in the small intestine and inside the cancer was the mercury filling.

Mercury is the worst toxin in the environment, more dangerous than arsenic and lead. As a society, we are inundated with heavy metals like these, and they are making us sick. In antiaging medicine, we work to detoxify the body of these heavy metals.

SS: I have a friend, a famous clarinetist, who eats only sushi and raw fish. He lives a healthy lifestyle, but his doctors have found so much mercury in his system that he has been advised never to eat fish again. Why are fish so loaded with mercury?

MG: It has to be from the environmental toxins. It's a huge problem and is affecting the health of everyone on the planet.

SS: You mean from dumping or from sewage?

MG: Absolutely. Dumping and environmental toxins. The two big offenders are tuna and swordfish. Both are loaded with mercury. Your musician friend should take chlorella before he eats the fish;

the chlorella will help find the mercury in the gut to help move it out of the system.

In doing this work, I have found that certain people are mercury excreters. For some reason that no one understands, these people can be exposed to mercury, but it's not a problem. But there is a whole other group who are nonexcreters, and they are the ones who complain of chronic illnesses. With these people, taking out the mercury fillings from their teeth is important. After these fillings are removed, we must use a chelation sulfur compound called mercurialentis.

SS: Explain chelation.

MG: Chelation refers to the binding of a toxin, usually to a heavy metal. Mercury binds with sulfur; lead binds with EDTA. So in mercury chelation, we use sulfur compounds that bind to mercury. Chelation draws heavy metals out of the body and cleans out the system. We then do a urine test to look at how much mercury came out. Routinely, we find uranium and arsenic in the urine. Both are part of the contamination of the water supply. If a person has cancer and mercury toxicity, I wouldn't try to get the mercury fillings out. Instead, I would try to neutralize mercury within the body using selenium supplementation, 200 to 400 mcg a day.

SS: I have been putting that amount in my morning smoothie for years. Should people take selenium every day? I've read that selenium has anticancer and antiviral effects.

MG: Supplementation with selenium is a very good idea, as long as you don't go too high. Taking 200 mcg once a day is good.

SS: It's my understanding that when taking a bath with bath salts and oils and whatever, we take in 80 percent of that water transdermally. But what are we supposed to do, bathe in Evian?

MG: Of course, it is not realistic to bathe in bottled water. What you can do is put EDTA into the bath to pull lead out of the body. So you can actually do chelation therapy while taking a bath.

SS: What is EDTA, and where do you get it?

MG: EDTA is sold only to doctors. EDTA is ethylene diamine tetra-acetic acid. Technically, it is used as a food preservative to keep packaged food on the shelves longer. EDTA is a synthetic, or man-made, amino acid that was initially developed for intravenous use. First used in the 1940s for the treatment of heavy metals poisoning, EDTA chelation removes heavy metals and minerals from the body such as lead, iron, copper, and calcium and is approved by the U.S. Food and Drug Administration (FDA) for use in treating lead poisoning and toxicity from other heavy metals. Other ways of taking EDTA include EDTA chewing gum, swallowing it as a capsule or powder, or inserting it rectally as a suppository. Any way that we can draw these heavy metals out of the system is a major plus. You can do infrared saunas, which seem to help pull toxins out of the body, or colon hydrotherapy to help the colon detoxify. There are herbs and homeopathic remedies that neutralize pesticides and the chemicals in the body.

SS: So when a person comes to you who is healthy and proactive about their health, what do you do for them?

MG: We run a battery of various assessments, all very comprehensive. We measure body fat and body water, for example. There is a one-minute test using electrodes on the wrist and feet that measures body fat. We also want to know their basic metabolic rate and the number of calories they need to eat in order to lose weight. We want to know if there is water inside their cells; healthy people have 60 percent of their water inside their cells and 40 percent outside their cells. This helps us determine the health of their cell membranes. With this information, I can determine the level of their vitality and their ability to regenerate and create these cells.

Next, we conduct a heart rate variability test and look at the nervous system. We monitor their heart rate and stand them up for seven minutes. This gives me an idea about how strong their adrenals are.

After that, we run a test called blood/urine/saliva, or BTA (biological terrain assessment). The BTA has to do with where the patient lives and is based upon a test that originated in France in the 1950s. Back then, the French government studied clusters of cancer in various geographic regions. One area had a lot of cancer, and another area had very little, so they hired this hydrologist, Louis-Claude Vincent, to look into the differences. He concluded that where the soil and water were the healthiest, there was no cancer; where the soil and water were unhealthy, there were large levels of cancer.

The saliva test tells us what is in the lymph and digestive system. Blood tells us what is coming out of the cells. And urine tells us how well the patient excretes toxins.

From running these tests, we find that people often have too many acids in their bodies and that their blood pH is too high. What this means is that the liver, whose job is to detoxify the blood, is not filtering well. A healthy liver, on the other hand, is able to filter and clean the blood. With a healthy liver, people are able to sleep through the night. By contrast, people who have a malfunctioning liver frequently wake up about 1:00, 2:00, or 3:00 in the morning.

SS: You give me liver drops to detoxify; is there another way?

MG: Yes. Take a lemon and squeeze the juice out of both halves in eight ounces of water every morning. Other natural ways to detoxify the liver include consuming carrots, beets, zucchini, squash, watercress, and artichokes.

SS: I believe very strongly in a good diet for anti-aging. From your point of view, how important is eating right?

MG: Think of your body like a Ferrari. You've

got to use high-octane fuel in your Ferrari. Likewise, your physical body requires superb fuel. Balanced eating that includes real food, such as fruits and vegetables, is critical. Organic is best; this includes meat, free-range chicken, and fish—proteins raised without antibiotics and hormones.

SS: What else is important?

MG: The biggest obstacle in people's health is stress. It seems to me that every patient I see tells me about how stressed they are. Learning to destress is a challenge. Everybody has taken on more than they can handle, and consequently, they are driven by what they have taken on. Sure, you can detoxify, eat right, and exercise, but getting your emotional and mental state under control is the most important measure you can take.

Focus on what makes you feel good. Then use that feel-good energy to solve your problems. Express love to people or someone or something. Love your wife, your kids, your dog, your patients. Love the Lakers. If you ever need a refresher course, listen to the Beatles' "All You Need Is Love." Then do what kids do all the time . . . imagine. Imagine being absolutely healthy, every day of your life. Imagine living to a hundred with energy. See yourself as ambassador of longevity to the world.

Have fun in your life, whatever it is you are doing, your work, your family, your friends. Do what kids do . . . have fun. Some people say there is no fun in their lives because there's no one to have fun with. I advise them to make a list of all the fun things they can do on their own.

Be grateful for your life and for your family. Concentrate on the energy of the universe moving through you. If you can do these things in life, then you can get your head and your emotions together. Longevity will have a way of following.

SS: If someone has run themselves into the ground, eaten badly, smoked, consumed a lot of alcohol, stayed up late, overworked all their lives, and then they come to you, are you able to reverse the health of that person if they're willing to make changes?

MG: Definitely. There is never a lost cause. I believe everybody out there can get better. A lot of people ask, "What is more important, the patient's belief in the doctor or the doctor's belief in the patient?" I think it's the doctor's belief in the patient. That's because when the doctor believes in the patient, the patient gets it immediately. Once the patient gets it, all things are possible.

The art in this form of medicine is to meet patients at their level and move them up slowly, or sometimes quickly, depending upon where they are. With some of my patients, I have to get very basic with them. If they are addicted to junk food, for example, I show them how the Highway Patrol uses cola to remove bloodstains from the highway.

Everybody progresses at his or her own pace. I go over a plan for them. I tell them that I don't expect them to stop the colas and junk food tomorrow. It's a gradual process in which they start doing little things and then find themselves feeling better. Later, if they revert to their old ways and realize how bad they feel, they get back on the right path.

It is also important to recognize that different people age differently. One person who is eighty years old may have ninety-year-old bones but a fifty-year-old mind. Katharine Graham, the late owner of **The Washington Post,** comes to mind, sharp as a tack upstairs. But she was injured in a fall and died a few weeks later. After a fall, many elderly people just don't make it. They get immobilized, and their minds can't handle the immobilization. They get pneumonia from the immobilization; once that happens on top of the fracture, survival is difficult.

But the real key is that different organs age differently. My job is to find out which of your organs are aging the quickest. So something that improves protein regeneration, like growth hormone, will find its way to that organ.

SS: By the time a patient comes to you, they've all been around the block with traditional medicine. Aren't they desperate for help?

MG: Yes, and they are open to new things. The majority of my patients are women because of your book **The Sexy Years.** However, when I first started, I treated more men, especially men with prostate issues. I can do a lot to help men get their vitality back. Women are desperate to find a solution to their hormone issues. And we both know bioidentical hormone replacement is the only way, and it works.

SS: Yes, but I don't believe that people truly realize the major impact of blowing out their major hormones. I'm talking about the adrenals, cortisol, insulin, and thyroid. Women know about the minor hormones—estrogen, progesterone, testosterone, DHEA, and others. It seems to me that in antiaging medicine, you deal with the major hormones first.

MG: It's like a basketball game. Six of the players are women coming to see me; the other six are testosterone, estrogen, progesterone, insulin, thyroid, and cortisol. My job is getting these players to play well together.

One of the ways I do that is through "metabolic typing," a measurement of the body's response to sugar. Your metabolic type describes your hormonal area of weakness—the area you most need to build up. Fifty percent of my patients, for example, are "adrenal types"; 15 percent are "pancreas types"; another 5 percent might be "growth hormone types." By identifying the area of hormonal weakness, I home in on what hormones need to be elevated and strengthened.

SS: Antiaging medicine is preventive in its nature. The patient is part of the process by becoming aware of his or her symptoms, much as women need to do regarding their hormone imbalances.

So if a patient who was a "thyroid type" called you and complained of constipation and/or had cold hands and feet, you would see that as a symptom that his or her thyroid was low and needed building up, right?

MG: Yes. A patient must keep me informed about even the smallest symptoms. Symptoms are your body talking. I am not able to "hear" unless the patient keeps me filled in. When we work together like this, I am able to make them feel well quickly, and it is very exciting.

SS: So antiaging medicine is an art form because there are no rules. It's the intuitiveness of the doctor, who, in turn, must be able to identify the different metabolic types.

MG: That is where I have taken it. Everyone looks at it differently. Many doctors want to use blood tests, look at the hormones, and figure out which is low and high and make corrections.

But I feel that you also must figure out where the star player is. Half the time it's the adrenals that are burned out from everyone's stressful lifestyle. Once I strengthen the adrenals, balancing someone's hormones becomes much easier. Adrenals are the orchestra leader. When they are off, the whole body is out of tune. The adrenals are the body's response to stress, affecting the sex hormones (estrogen, testosterone, progesterone, DHEA, pregnenolone, and so forth). So when the body is under stress and the adrenals are tired, the body will convert estrogen to DHEA, testosterone to DHEA, and progesterone to cortisol.

SS: To survive?

MG: To survive at any cost, while the sex hormones go down to maintain the survival.

SS: Because now—when the body is stressed—is not the time to make a baby.

MG: Absolutely. Once we've identified the star player and strengthened it, we have one last component, and that's the coach. The coach is the leader. He's got to make the players play well together. In most cases, the coach is the liver. When the "team" is in a successful place and you keep the "coach" happy, that's when people show great results.

SS: So when a woman comes in and she's all out of whack because her minor hormones are gone, you first deal with the major hormones. That makes sense because I know from my own research that if one hormone is off, the entire hormonal system is off. If the adrenals are the orchestra leader, trying to balance the sex hormones of estrogen and progesterone would be futile until you get the adrenals straightened out.

MG: Yes, or any of the other major hormones.

SS: What I am starting to see is that these different metabolic types seem to dictate our reactions to how you are going to give progesterone or estrogen. What form of transport do you prefer, creams, drops, or capsules?

MG: As a rule, I prefer to use the cream, because with every pulse of the blood, it moves through the fat base. Most of us have such toxic livers that by the time a capsule moves through all the toxic sludge in the liver, it loses a lot of its effect.

SS: Do you feel that men need testosterone replacement as they age?

MG: I believe they do. When I measure men's testosterone levels, there is a huge range, anywhere from 200 to 900. But when I measure free testosterone, I almost always find it low. I also find it important to treat the prostate at the same time. I give them herbs, including saw palmetto and the extract of giant redwoods. Redwood trees live forever, and redwood extract seems to be a male tonic that helps the prostate. I also recommend other nutrients for the prostate, including vitamin E, selenium, fish oils, and zinc.

We know that testosterone gets converted to estrogen by an enzyme called aromatase, especially in men who are overweight. We try to block aromatase with chrysin in a cream form and also with zinc and vitamin C. By doing so, we are maximizing testosterone, preventing its conversion to estrogen, and at the same time treating the prostate.

SS: What does the future hold for antiaging medicine?

MG: The big hope is stem cell therapy, in which stem cells (cells that are capable of becoming all or many of the different kinds of tissues in the human body) can be injected into the brain, the heart cells, or other parts of the body in order to get them to repair damaged cells.

As far as patients are concerned, I believe we can

all live to be a hundred. When I ask my patients if they want that, they all say yes, but not if they are in a wheelchair or nursing home. People are now starting to realize that they are going to live longer. They are not going to be able to retire at sixty-five anymore. All insurance, including life insurance, is going to have to change drastically. In addition, there will be greater use of growth hormone in the future. Growth hormone enhances body proteins. It uses up fat storage, and it conserves carbohydrates. Growth hormone scares people, because they think it might fuel cancer growth, but it is really a metabolic hormone.

SS: But shouldn't you take growth hormone if it is low or missing?

MG: Yes, but you should have a fasting blood test first. Growth hormone tapers off naturally with age, so most people's growth hormones are low. When in range, it is at 130 to 350.

SS: What else do growth hormones do for you? My son, Bruce, injects HGH every day because his blood tests showed that his levels were very low. He loves the way he feels on it, and he also has a six-pack abdomen since he's been injecting.

MG: Growth hormone has many benefits. It promotes wound healing, improves vitality and energy, reduces body fat, increases lean body mass, strengthens muscles, and improves skin elasticity.

SS: Isn't it in a state of hormonal imbalance that disease can take hold?

MG: Yes, definitely, and also, if you look at the progression of disease as you grow older, you're exposed to more toxins. Your liver, kidneys, and lymph system no longer have the strength to pull out the toxins. Consequently, toxins start to accumulate in your body. Then your liver, kidneys, and lymph system call out to the glands for reinforcement. And they say to the glands, Come on, secrete more hormones and make us a little stronger.

Then the glands acquiesce and start secreting more adrenal hormones and thyroid hormones, but eventually the glands get tired. Ultimately, what happens is that you get a toxic body with very weak hormonal glands. And that's your setup for chronic illness.

SS: So it goes all the way back to where we started. By detoxifying the body of heavy metals, lead, mercury, and others, by strengthening the weakest major hormones and organs, whether they be adrenal, thyroid, the kidneys, or the pancreas, by replacing lost minor hormones, we can cut off at the pass the inevitable chronic illnesses that we were destined to have. That's how antiaging medicine works. We don't have to be sick just because we are old.

MG: Correct. It takes effort and a knowledgeable doctor, but the results are fantastic. But you have to start as soon as you recognize the validity of all of this. We want to feel good. We want to have energy. We want to jump out of bed in the morning. We want to see our kids and our grandkids. This kind of medicine can give you what you really want. Just stay open and find a physician who can really help you.

SS: I agree. Thank you.

DR. GALITZER'S TOP FIVE ANTIAGING RECOMMENDATIONS

1. Effective ways to increase energy are through intravenous vitamin C or intravenous glutathione.

2. One of the ways we ingest mercury (a harmful toxin) is by eating tuna and swordfish. You can help move mercury out of your system by eating chlorella prior to eating fish. Chlorella is a type of algae that is the world's richest natural source of chlorophyll and is sold as a food supplement. Another way to neutralize mercury in the body is to supplement with selenium, 200 to 400 mcg a day.

3. An easy way to detoxify your liver is to take a lemon and squeeze the juice out of both halves in eight ounces of water every morning. Other natural ways to detoxify the liver include consuming carrots, beets, zucchini, squash, watercress, and artichokes.

4. Choose organic foods for your diet. These includes meat, free-range chicken, and fish— proteins raised without antibiotics and hormones.

5. Prostate problems can be treated with herbs, including saw palmetto and the extract of giant redwoods. Redwood trees live forever, and redwood extract seems to be a male tonic that helps the prostate. Other nutrients also recommended for the prostate include vitamin E, selenium, fish oils, and zinc.

CHAPTER 22

DR. ROBERT GREENE:
THE ENVIRONMENT AND
BIOIDENTICAL HORMONE
REPLACEMENT THERAPY

Dr. Greene is one of the country's leading hormone specialists and founder of the medical clinic Specialty Care for Women in Redding, California, which caters to the unique needs of women with hormonal imbalance. His research has been published in prestigious medical journals, including Fertility and Sterility, The Female Patient, OB/GYN Clinics of North America, **and** The Aging Male. **He wrote the foreword to my book** The Sexy Years **and is the author of** Perfect Balance, **a book on hormone health. He is assistant professor at the University of California, Davis, School of Medicine and a genuinely nice guy. Dr. Greene's website is www.specialtycare4women.com.**

SS: You are always on the forefront of cutting-edge medical information. What's new?

RG: One issue that is new is the rise in breast cancer in China: A 40 percent increase has been reported. This amazes me because in this country everyone points to synthetic hormones as the cause of breast cancer. In China, they don't use those things.

SS: But to what do they attribute this rise in breast cancer? Pollution?

RG: Exactly. They have a big pollution problem. Their air is foul, and they are not conscious about chemicals and their effects on the body. Nor do these countries want to accept responsibility.

I don't think we have made it clear that all pesticides, preservatives, and fake food (I call these "bio-mutagens") are hormone-disrupting agents. They get into our bodies and do damage. Do you realize that in this country we actually consume about ten to twelve pounds of preservatives a year?

SS: How can a body tolerate that?

RG: The reality, Suzanne, is that we don't. That's why we have so many of the health problems that we have. It's also an issue with the cosmetics we are using. A lot of chemicals and preservatives have slipped into these products when there are much safer and healthier cosmetics available.

SS: I agree with you. I have started a line of organic cosmetics under my name. The skin is transdermal, it just makes sense; if we care about what we put into our bodies, we should be equally vigilant about what we put on our skin.

RG: That's wonderful. In my next book, I make the same point for my pregnant women, trying to impress upon them the effects of what they consume not only internally, but what they are putting on their skin.

When something is presented to the FDA as a new chemical or preservative to be added to food or to a cosmetic, the average time it takes to get that approval is three months. They accept these things under a category called GRAS (generally recognized as safe), meaning that it is safe until it is proven to be unsafe. That is scary.

Look at cigarettes, for example. They contain fifty-five different toxins, yet they are legal to sell. Did you know that when we consume a significant amount of nicotine, our bodies convert a lot of our estrogen into an antiestrogen? Called catechol estrogen, it has been shown to damage DNA and promote cancer. When I treat a smoker, even thin smokers typically, I need to give them a higher dosage of a bioidentical estrogen to relieve their symptoms, because their habit is converting into an antiestrogen.

SS: Does this apply to marijuana? Let's not kid ourselves; a lot of the baby boomers are potheads. They are of menopausal age when sleep is all but impossible, and marijuana is putting a lot of people to sleep.

RG: The biggest problem with marijuana is that

because it is not regulated, there is no incentive to grow organic marijuana. So what are these people ingesting? In Mexico, where a lot of it comes from, it is sprayed with paraquat, a highly toxic chemical.

And then there is the smoking aspect. Smoking anything is not good for you because smoking is an irritant.

SS: So let's get specific about hormone therapy. We know that stress, chemicals, fake food, preservatives, and the environment are wreaking havoc on our hormonal systems. What was once simply the domain of menopausal women is now affecting everyone from their thirties on. How are you treating your patients these days?

RG: I use a lot of estrogen gels because they are absorbed very quickly. I encourage my patients to not increase their dose the first month, and I always have them track their symptoms using a calendar. After the first month, if they show symptoms, I have them dose up a little bit according to an amount I give them. Then I schedule them to return in three months. That way, they have a record from their calendar of their symptoms. I can tell by their symptoms and what day on the calendar those symptoms occurred whether the problem is estrogen or progesterone. Realizing that we all have busy schedules and we have to charge for every visit, doing it this way cuts down on the number of office visits. It also empowers my patients to feel comfortable increasing or decreasing. Every man and woman has different needs. I am not worried about anyone taking too much because if they take too much, they won't feel well, and the same goes for too little. The object is "just right."

People often ask me: "Why are you such a big fan of bioidentical hormones?" It is because there is nothing our body makes in the way of a hormone that makes us feel better and at the same time does not harm us. There are a lot of drugs that can make you feel great, but all the while they are killing you. Bioidentical hormones are the safer route.

SS: You are also a fertility specialist?

RG: Yes, it is another of my hats. The doses you describe in this book on rhythmic cycling are comparable to the doses we give. When we are dealing with women who have lost their ovaries or are given hormones because they are using a donated embryo, we give them large doses of hormones. It's obviously safe enough to get pregnant, since pregnant women aren't dying and getting cancer. In fact, most cancer occurs in women who are in their seventies and eighties, not when they are pregnant.

SS: It is interesting that you mention this age group. I gave a talk in Wyoming to a group of older women, all of whom felt that hormone replacement was not for them—that they were too old. I tend to differ. I think replacing hormones in an older woman or man helps prevent them from getting sick. What do you think?

RG: Most older people say they don't have symptoms, but they don't realize that they do indeed have symptoms. They have accepted that they don't sleep well, that their bones ache, and that their memory fails them. They feel that these conditions are normal because all their friends are in the same boat. With an older patient, I always try to consider replacement unless they have symptoms they don't want treated. That is different. Then I must respect their wishes.

But certainly hormone replacement can be protective. Take Alzheimer's disease, for example. Several studies done on both men and women show if someone has an estradiol level of less than 20 pg/mL (picograms per milliliter), they are at highest risk of developing Alzheimer's disease and cognitive disturbances. Even if one of my patients feels good with an estradiol level of 10 or 15 pg/mL, I am concerned. Studies have been done on a variety of populations, and it always seems that less than a level of 20 pg/mL is definitely a problem. The brain functions better at higher levels of estradiol.

SS: If this issue came up in a man or woman's blood testing, regardless of their age, would you strongly urge him or her to go on bioidentical hormone replacement therapy?

RG: Absolutely. So many people have learned to settle and live with their symptoms. A blood test provides proof and often gives them a reason to try BHRT. Something else I have encountered—particularly among people in their sixties and seventies—is a vitamin D deficiency. Vitamin D is the only vitamin that is a hormone. It regulates calcium and bone metabolism. It has been nicknamed the "sunshine vitamin," because it is made in the body from exposure to sunlight. When a cholesterol derivative in your skin is exposed to sunlight, a chemical change occurs; it is converted into vitamin D, absorbed into the bloodstream, and taken into cells like a hormone through vitamin D receptors located throughout the body. Enough sunlight a day— around fifteen minutes—is sufficient for vitamin D production. However, when people have a low vitamin D level, not only do they lose bones, but they also lose strength and stability. Consequently, they are at risk for falls and dizziness if their vitamin D levels are low. Vitamin D deficiency in the elderly is more prevalent than we once believed. One reason is that vitamin D production declines in the elderly, usually because they stay indoors more and have less sun exposure. Older people also tend to eat fewer vitamin D–rich foods, such as dairy products. Research indicates that nearly half the women in this country who are being treated for osteoporosis are deficient in vitamin D.

We now know that people with vitamin D deficiencies have higher risks of cancer, such as breast cancer, pancreatic cancer, and colon cancer, because immune cells in the body also have vitamin D receptors. The current daily recommendation for 400 IU of vitamin D per day is about the minimum amount to prevent rickets, a bone disease widespread in children about a hundred years ago. However, we are really not worried about that disease in aging people. People require more vitamin D than the minimum amount.

SS: What should a person take daily?

RG: First of all, they should supplement with a version known as vitamin D3, which is more effective than another type known as D2. As they get older, people need a higher dose—at least 1,000 IU daily. This level not only strengthens bones, but makes people feel they have more energy, are less fatigued and less dizzy. Replenishing vitamin D also improves overall health by reducing cancer risk.

SS: In addition to treating your elderly patients, what do you do about your overweight patients?

RG: The average person in the United States is very insulin-resistant. These people need more human growth hormone. The main function of HGH is to offset the action of insulin, making it easier to manage blood sugar.

There is more to it than lowering sugar intake, however. An article in the **Journal of Urology** (volume 174) shows that testosterone has tremendous potential to treat insulin resistance. Physicians used to think testosterone aggravated insulin resistance; this new information proves otherwise. Testosterone doesn't make it worse; it makes it a whole lot better.

SS: Medicine is changing so rapidly. Those doctors who don't keep up are doing a disservice to their patients. Do you see hope?

RG: If doctors pay attention. But look at the way we now report health. The World Health Organization no longer talks about life expectancy; it talks about "disability-adjusted life expectancy," meaning how many years you will continue to breathe on the planet or, rather, how many years you will be awake and vibrant on the planet. What's scary is that in this country the disability life expectancy for the average woman is about eight years of disability before she dies. What we are trying to do with our new approach to medicine is to keep people healthier right up to their last day on the planet.

SS: Give me Dr. Greene's protocol for being healthy up to the last day.

RG: Most important, it requires being tuned in to your body and your body's senses. As a brain-related scientist, I always tell people, "Symptoms matter." To ignore symptoms is like ignoring a fire alarm.

Then make good choices, from eating organic foods to exercising. When people say to me, "I don't have time to exercise," my answer is, "You don't have time not to." Once you realize that you are so much less effective if you are not fit, the excuse dies away very, very quickly. Also, keep a journal, which is another form of meditation. Studies have shown that journal writing lowers cortisol by destressing your body. Anything that eliminates stress and slows us down in this high-stress environment will keep us healthier and happier. When you manage stress, eat properly, get proper rest, do yoga or exercise in some form, and still have symptoms, then I know it's time to fill in the gap with bioidentical hormones and supplements.

SS: Thank you, Dr. Greene.

DR. GREENE'S TOP FIVE ANTIAGING RECOMMENDATIONS

1. There is nothing our body makes in the way of a hormone that makes us feel better and at the same time does not harm us. There are a lot of drugs that can make you feel great, but all the while they are killing you. Bioidentical hormones are the safer route. Plus, they can be protective against cognitive diseases such as Alzheimer's. The brain functions better at higher levels of estradiol.

2. As we age, we need more vitamin D than the minimum amount—at least 1,000 IU daily of D3.

3. The average person in the United States is very insulin-resistant. These people need more human growth hormone. The main function of HGH is to offset the action of insulin, making it easier to manage blood sugar.

4. Make good choices, from eating organic foods to exercising. When people say to me, "I don't have time to exercise," my answer is, "You don't have time not to."

5. Get stress under control. Keep a journal, which is another form of meditation, for example. Studies have shown that journal writing lowers cortisol by destressing your body. Anything that eliminates stress and slows us down in this high-stress environment will keep us healthier and happier.

CHAPTER 23

DR. LARRY WEBSTER:
INFLAMMATION AND
THE ENVIRONMENT

I first met Dr. Webster on a medical radio show in
North Carolina and was impressed and moved by
his dedication and compassion. His mind is brilliant, and at times I have to slow him down so I
can comprehend. His passion for healing and his
ability to move forward in understanding the environmental assault on our health as a nation is
mind-boggling. Dr. Webster practices in Greensboro, North Carolina. He has been practicing
medicine for thirty years, attended Stanford University as an undergraduate, and interned in Oakland, California, at Oakland Alameda Hospital.
He spent twenty-five years working in emergency
medicine, which prepared him to handle just
about anything put before him. He has a lot to
teach to all of us.

SS: When we first met on the radio, you were so passionate and savvy about bioidentical hormone replacement, and I was thinking: Emergency room to bioidenticals is a circuitous route. How did you make this leap?

LW: It goes back to my time in the emergency room when I started observing that treating patients with drugs was working short-term, because we were saving lives. But for chronic patients, the methods we were using didn't seem to be effective. These patients kept coming back again and again, so I started looking into the cause of illness. Why are people sick? rather than, What drug would treat this symptom? What can I really do to help this person? That's how I got started into natural medicine.

Then I moved into the treatment of heart disease by eliminating heavy metals from the system. From there, I moved into the allergy realm, using homeopathic medicine. That is when I really started seeing changes in people's health. Because of these experiences, I started to analyze the body from a metabolic standpoint. I looked at: What does the body need in terms of nutrients? What is causing toxicity? Can the body be detoxified?

All of this led me naturally into the hormone realm. I knew that pharmaceutical drugs altered hormones. There were side effects, too, and I believed there had to be a better way, so I started using the natural approach to hormones. So it **was** a circuitous path.

Because I treat the whole person, hormones are an important aspect of my healing. But I also treat everything from fibromyalgia to chronic fatigue to heart disease, and I use different modalities to do this. It is clear that the environment is having a dramatic effect on people's health. Even the American Cancer Society says that 90 percent of all cancer is environmental because there are so many aspects of the environment affecting all of our different bodily processes.

SS: There has been much talk about inflammation, drugs, and disease. The issue seems to be that using drugs to prevent inflammation is counterproductive. It keeps inflammation from doing its normal work of healing and, thus, pushes inflammation deeper into the body. Inflammation then becomes chronic.

LW: You bring up a valid point. People suffer from so many chronic illnesses, including chronic fatigue, fibromyalgia, heart disease, hormone problems, polycystic ovarian disease (a health problem in which the body may make too much insulin, thus affecting numerous bodily systems), and breast cancer, all of which may result from treating misunderstood conditions with drugs that only masquerade as Band-Aids. **Time** magazine once had a cover story calling inflammation "the secret killer," meaning that it underlies all disease processes from Alzheimer's to heart disease to cancer. The problems at the cellular level in these conditions or diseases are related to inflammatory processes, which are coming from the environment, whether it be pesticides, herbicides, heavy metal toxins, stress, or electromagnetic fields. We're being bombarded at the cellular level, and our cells are inflamed with the production of proteins called cytokines, which inhibit the growth and activity of various immune cells. As a result, our cellular mechanisms just don't work as well.

If you look at the country of Gambia, Africa, the incidence of breast cancer is three in one hundred thousand, whereas in the United States it's one in six. In that country people are not overweight, and polycystic ovarian disease is not a factor. These people live longer than any other population on earth. I spoke with the minister of education for that country about the differences in the health of the people of our two countries. He told me, "We've got 80 percent unemployment, so we can't afford your chemicals."

SS: That's quite a statement!

LW: They don't eat processed food like we do, either. They may not have as much, but they eat better food. In developing countries, menopause is a much softer process than in this country. One reason is that these countries don't have the estrogen stimulation from the environment that we do. We have thirty times the incidence of breast cancer in this country. You can't ignore that fact.

SS: Clearly, something is not working with the

way we are being treated medically in this country. What do you think it is?

LW: Let me tell you a story: In North Carolina, a young doctor was verbally attacked by the Medical Board for using vitamin B_{12} and other natural modalities. At the time, I was treating one of the state legislators who was quite ill and diagnosed with Parkinson's disease. I discovered that he had large red blood cells, which is very significant for early pernicious anemia—in other words, a B_{12} deficiency.

After giving him regular vitamin B_{12} injections for a short time, this legislator was up and jogging. Prior to that treatment, he was falling on his face. As a lobbying move, we produced a testimonial videotape in which the legislator said, "Leave these natural doctors alone." We sent that video to every legislator in the state of North Carolina in both the Senate and the House, and the bill that would allow physicians to practice natural medicine without being regulated by the state passed 116–8 in both houses. The passage of that bill allows me to treat people naturally in the way I want without being evaluated by outside parties who have no understanding for what I'm doing.

SS: But there is a fear in general about alternative medicine, that somehow it's harmful. Yet look at the problems people are experiencing from mainstream medicine and prescription drug dependency and their side effects.

LW: As I said, I no longer wanted to treat the symptom of a patient's problem; I wanted to treat the **cause.** If that's considered "alternative," I'm sorry. I just want to do what is best for my patients, and a prescription for a symptom is not always the best way to go.

SS: Do men have fewer health problems, or is it hard for men to wrap their arms around antiaging and testosterone replacement?

LW: Men look at these issues as though they are all about erections, and most men have an ego to protect. But they need to understand that there are more testosterone receptors in the heart than anyplace else in the body. Testosterone protects the heart. For that reason alone, testosterone levels are important to check. But testosterone is about vitality and clear thinking. It also builds bone and muscle, so for a man who wants to get great results from his workout, replacement would help tremendously.

SS: If you were treating former president Clinton for his heart condition, would testosterone be a part of his treatment?

LW: Absolutely. He might not have a deficiency, but with his stressful life, it would make sense that he would. Just living in a polluted planet with tremendous amounts of pesticides and herbicides that have a major estrogenic effect—that alone will reduce a man's testosterone levels, and that has been proven. For example, some children are being born "hermaphroditic," meaning they have both sexual organs. This is environmental in origin. The environmental effect makes men's estrogen rise, thus telling the pituitary not to produce as much testosterone, so men are being adversely affected.

I have many men who come to me with much higher estrogen levels than women. This is not a good place for a man to be, because it makes balancing hormones very tricky. Environmentally, the major problem here is that we are swimming in a sea of abnormal estrogens that are confusing the body. This abnormal estrogen is coming from plastic drinking bottles, Styrofoam trays in which we buy our meats, and other sources of plastics.

SS: With regard to balancing hormones and heart disease, why are heart doctors not suggesting testosterone as therapy for a heart patient?

LW: All physicians seem to care about is cholesterol, which is really an indicator of low thyroid more than anything else. Generally, they don't look at cardioprotective compounds such as CoQ10 or L-carnitine. But men are being given Lipitor, Mevacor, and other statin drugs, which basically displaces CoQ10 from the body. CoQ10 provides energy and increases cardiac efficiency. So what happens when you take statins is that the body can run out of energy, and ironically, the heart may be affected. So instead of treating high cholesterol with a statin, a doctor should be looking at the thyroid levels first. In fact, this connection is well accepted in the textbook of endocrinology, where it explains hypercholesterolemia is related to hypothyroidism (underactive thyroid). So when a man comes in with high cholesterol, I first check thyroid TSH, T4, and T3. But more than blood results, you have to go on symptoms such as cold hands and feet, tiredness, high cholesterol, hair loss, weight gain, all symptoms you see in both men and women with underactive thyroid.

SS: What about women and PMS problems?

LW: PMS, irregular menstrual periods, heavy bleeding, miscarriages—these can be corrected most of the time by putting women on bioidentical progesterone and thyroid. One female patient of mine had had five miscarriages, and after thyroid therapy, she had a successful pregnancy and gave birth to a little boy last year.

SS: What about bloating? So many women complain about this problem.

LW: I think it has much to do with the estrogen– **Candida albicans** (yeast infection) connection. This is usually a problem when the progesterone is dropping down, creating estrogen dominance. Some studies have made a connection with an increase in interleukin-6, a protein inside cells that is often considered a "bad actor" of the immune system because of its association with inflammation injuries and malignant diseases. In this case, the inflammation is estrogen yeast, or **Candida albicans** overgrowth. One of the first things I would do for a woman with this condition is knock the yeast out of the body.

ss: Does everybody have yeast?

LW: Absolutely. Most men think yeast is only about vaginal yeast and, therefore, doesn't affect them. Not true. Take a look at the number of cancer and AIDS patients who are male and dying of yeast. Eighty percent of people with these diseases are dying of **Candida albicans** and other associated fungi.

ss: How do you get rid of yeast?

LW: Most important, as you have said in your books, Suzanne, eliminate sugar. With too much sugar, you develop insulin resistance. Not only does that throw off progesterone and estrogen ratios, it can also feed fungi and bacteria. In addition, insulin resistance can adversely affect a woman's ability to get pregnant. Not only that, too much insulin shunts fat into the peripheral tissues of the body, where it accumulates around the waist—a situation that produces excess estrogen.

In addition, there is a strong association between mercury toxicity and yeast. They feed each other. When I see a woman who has been treated with a strong antifungal like Nystatin and she continues to get fungal infections the minute she eats anything with sugar, even a white potato, I start wondering about mercury. Fungus and mercury have a pathological association; more than 95 percent of my patients have tested positive for toxic mercury levels.

ss: Is this happening as a result of the fish we eat?

LW: Yes. Fish and pesticide runoff, which has basically destroyed everything, including the ocean.

Seven years ago, when I was working out with a strength coach, I was in great shape and eating a fair amount of fish. Even though I was working out regularly, my heart was beating quite heavily. Then I noticed that my blood pressure had soared from 140/90 up to 160/110 in just a few months. I used kinesiology (muscle testing), which basically said that electromagnetically, my body had dangerously high levels of metal toxicity. So I did a chelation treatment on myself. This involved infusing the body with an amino acid that actually grabs onto the mercury and removes it in the urine so that it can be measured. The results showed that I had forty times the accepted levels of mercury in my body. I had been eating only orange roughy, which is supposed to be a safe fish. So that shows you that even the safe fish can be contaminated.

I was able to reduce the levels in my body through chelation and amino acids. With this treatment, my blood pressure came down, too. Now, do you think this approach would have been applied in traditional medicine?

Mercury is a killer because it is an inflammatory and a free radical. It will block all the energy at the cellular level and in the mitochondria, which are the little packets in the center of your cells that generate most of your energy.

SS: As you were talking, I was thinking that we all eat out so often—I know I do—and it's hard to find healthy food you can count on in restaurants.

LW: Yes. Restaurant food is rarely organic, so we are ingesting tremendous amounts of pesticides, herbicides, and chemicals—not to mention the lack of nutrients in our foods. All of these toxins are beginning to interfere with our metabolism at the cellular level. When you have inflammation, your cortisol is going to knock out your thyroid production or interfere with its efficiency. You will have a problem with the conversion of T4 to T3 thyroid. Also, estrogen dominance can occur. Everything is tied together hormonally. Overwhelmed by all the pollutants you've ingested, your liver has to detoxify your body.

Most people are not digesting their food properly, either. Much of poor digestion is a result of the food we're eating. Take chickens, for example. A report broadcast on ABC's **20/20** found that a number of different brands of chickens contain salmonella and **Helicobacter pylori,** a bacteria that has been implicated in ulcers. When people ingest this bacteria, it disrupts the GI tract. It also kills the cells in the gut that produce digestive acids. Inflammation in the gut is the result. I believe the major cause of acid reflux disease is related to **Helicobacter pylori.** When we take people off chicken and treat them with an herb called mastic, their acid reflux gets better.

SS: So they don't have to take Nexium or whatever?

LW: No. Knocking out the acid of the stomach with a drug like Nexium creates another set of problems. For one thing, it interferes with the production of a normal stomach substance called intrinsic factor, which facilitates absorption of vitamin B_{12} in the small intestine.

SS: So as a society, would you say we're generally in a state of **dis-ease**?

LW: Right. We're not getting the nutrients in our body that we need. We have inflamed guts because of all the pesticides, herbicides, and adverse chemicals that we are ingesting, along with all the bacteria and the fungus. Due to these problems, the gut is suffering. We're developing something called hyperpermeable gut, which refers to a gut that allows substances to pass into the bloodstream that shouldn't be there, from yeast to large undigested protein molecules. These are producing many of the allergic responses that we are now seeing in patients.

SS: What can do we do about this condition?

LW: Number one, give your body adequate nutrients to support your hormonal system. To get nutrients into the body, I use intravenous therapies; these bypass the gut so it starts to function better. This is why I have been able to heal people who cannot take anything by mouth because their gastrointestinal tract is so inflamed and defective.

Second, go organic, if you can. Organic food is the best defense, because it contains virtually no pesticides. What's more, organic meat is not injected with hormones like conventional meat. Did you know that the United States can't even sell nonorganic meat to Europe? It's sad when a whole continent won't accept our meat, yet we're eating it.

Third, digestives enzymes are crucial. So is L-glutamine, an amino acid that cuts down the inflammation of the gut wall. I recommend psyllium, a natural bulk-forming product, to patients with constipation, often a symptom of low thyroid. Once I can regenerate the thyroid, the GI function improves. Everything interrelates. I have to be careful, however, and not overtreat the thyroid, because doing so can overstimulate the adrenals. Overstimulated adrenals can put a person into a hyperthyroid, or overactive thyroid, condition. A patient with hyperthyroidism can't sleep, and his or her heart will be pounding like crazy.

I also have to be careful with vitamin B_{12} supplementation. If vitamin B_{12} is given prior to clearing out the yeast in the gut, the vitamin will overstimulate the growth of yeast. Again, everything is connected.

SS: Luckily, there are quite a few of you doing this work. Medicine is changing out of necessity.

LW: Sometimes my patients say to me, "Well, I'm gonna die anyway, so why do I want to go to all this effort?" I always answer: "It's about quality of life. And don't you want to participate in the next generation? Don't you want to see your kids and grandchildren grow up?"

As a doctor, it is so uplifting to see somebody who

says to me, "You know, I had no life before, and now I can enjoy life for the first time." I see thousands of patients, so when people have an interest in their health and a commitment to it, I will do anything for them to obtain their goal. Everyone deserves a worthwhile life in a very meaningful sense—in mind, body, and spirit. Each one of my patients is significant, and it is on them that I put my focus. Although it does not get written about in the newspaper, my work is my contribution to the world. Each and every one of us can do the same with our talents and gift.

SS: You are a beautiful person. Thank you.

DR. WEBSTER'S TOP FIVE ANTIAGING RECOMMENDATIONS

1. Men should definitely consider testosterone replacement. There are more testosterone receptors in the heart than anyplace else in the body. Testosterone protects the heart. For that reason alone, testosterone levels are important to check. But testosterone is about vitality and clear thinking. It also builds bone and muscle, so for a man who wants to get great results from his workout, replacement would help tremendously.

2. PMS, irregular menstrual periods, heavy bleeding, and miscarriages can be corrected most of the time by putting women on bioidentical progesterone and thyroid.

3. Eliminate sugar. With too much sugar, you develop insulin resistance. Not only does that throw off progesterone and estrogen ratios, but it can also feed fungi and bacteria. In addition, insulin resistance can adversely affect a woman's ability to get pregnant. Not only that, too much insulin shunts fat into the peripheral tissues of the body, where it accumulates around the waist—a situation that produces excess estrogen. Plus, there is a strong association between mercury toxicity and yeast. They feed each other.

4. Go organic, if you can. Organic food is the best defense, because it contains virtually no pesticides. What's more, organic meat is not injected with hormones like conventional meat.

5. Digestive enzymes are crucial to a healthy gut. So is L-glutamine, an amino acid that cuts down the inflammation of the gut wall. Another good supplement is psyllium, a natural bulk-forming product, for patients with constipation, often a symptom of low thyroid. Acid reflux gets better with an herb called mastic.

PART FIVE

AGELESS LIVING

Just before the funeral services, the

undertaker came up to the very

elderly widow and asked,

"How old was your husband?

"Ninety-eight," she replied.

"Two years older than me."

"So you're ninety-six,"

the undertaker commented.

She responded,

"Hardly worth going home, is it?"

CHAPTER 24

DIET AND SUPPLEMENTS

Good nutrition is essential to health. I have written extensively about the positive effects of eating real food in all of my Somersize books. But the moment you mention the words **healthy eating** to people, you can almost hear the inward groans. It conjures up diets of haylike food that is dry and tasteless. Not so! Healthy eating is simply eating **real** food. Real food is the food we grew up with: meat, chicken, and fish, **not** loaded with synthetic hormones and antibiotics; I'm talking about real fats like butter, cream, full-fat cream cheese, and olive oil, **not** man-made fats; fresh fruits and vegetables, but **not** sprayed to death with pesticides and chemicals to make them grow larger and more beautiful. By the way, have you noticed that since we've made our vegetables more beautiful and more colorful, they have also lost their taste? If you have ever visited Europe, did you notice the difference in the way their food tastes? It's not that they are better cooks; they just have cleaner, fresher, less-tampered-with, and therefore better-tasting food.

How did we get so far off track? How is it that we now have as many overweight people as we have underfed people? The answer is processed foods. We have gotten far away from real food, and we are paying the price. It's the sugars and the refined carbohydrates that are making us fat and affecting our health. We fill ourselves and our families with foods that are processed and refined with all the nutrition sucked out. Bad food is cheap, heavily promoted, and loaded with chemicals that make it taste really good. Healthy food is harder to get (you have to drive to the market, shop, and cook), and it is not promoted, plus it's more expensive. We have soft drinks and vending machines at schools and offices. Our portions are too large. We eat out more and cook less at home. Mom has stripped off her apron and grabbed her car keys to get to the closest, fastest, and most inexpensive restaurant to grab a quick bite to eat. Even our soil has been leached of its nutrients, rendering our fruits and vegetables less nutritious than ever before, even though they look "more beautiful." Add to all these things the overabundance of fast food in this country, TV, video games, and an intensive marketing campaign to get kids and adults to buy chemically sweetened products, and you have a perfect recipe for an epidemic.

Do sugar and processed foods really take enough of a toll on our bodies to have created the mess in which we now find our country? The answer is a resounding yes!

You must understand that eating badly negatively affects your hormones. You can't expect bioidentical hormones to do their job if you're eating junk and processed foods. Sugary foods and trans fats disrupt your hormones, so they can no longer keep your body on an even keel to give you the youthful energy and health that you want.

One of the major hormones in the body is insulin. Too much insulin throws off your body's hormonal balance. If one hormone is off, they are all off. It's like dominoes. All hormones work in concert and speak to one another. So if you are eating a diet loaded with sugar, chemicals, and fake food, your insulin will rise. The internal concert is off. Weight gain is the result, along with increased cholesterol and diabetes, which has reached epidemic proportions. Diabetes raises cortisol, and among many other destructive effects, it makes sleeping difficult. If you can't sleep, your insulin has no chance of going down, and the effect is continued high cortisol, which can eventually lead to heart attack and/or stroke—that is, if diabetes doesn't get you first.

Remember that insulin and cortisol are major hormones. When they are not working in concert, your minor hormones (estrogen, progesterone, testosterone, and others) don't have a chance. With obesity as the number one problem in this country, it's no wonder diminished health accelerates when hormonal decline begins. The body is already in bad shape!

Giving up sugar is a good start. By doing so, you can prevent your pancreas from oversecreting insulin, which will keep your blood sugar and hormones balanced. With balance comes weight loss, lowered cholesterol levels, a decreased risk of heart disease and cancer, and longevity. In healing insulin resistance, the body will unload the stored sugar in the cells, and your body fat will melt away. After the body releases the stored sugar, it then turns to your fat reserves to break down and use as an energy source. The result? You get thinner while your body is being fed a constant source of energy.

Here's something else: You can balance your hormones with good dietary habits. We go into hormonal decline very early in this country because of the poor choices we make when it comes to eating. Food is the building block of all cells in our body. Every cell requires protein, fat, and carbohydrates to reproduce. But with all the chemicals, trans fats, hydrogenated oils, fake food, and junk food that are a major part of the American diet, cellular reproduction becomes difficult, which is why we now have an epidemic of obesity not only in adults, but in children as well. Children are now getting fat because they eat very little real food.

It is a sad fact that in the poorer segments of this country people do not have access to real food. The bulk of their food comes from convenience markets, and there is very little real food available in these stores. Consequently, the fattest people in the country are also the poorest and in the worst health. This is a tragedy. Sadly, this is the first generation not expected to live as long as the present one, because of lifetime exposure to harmful chemicals and food additives.

Eating real food helps your body rebuild your biochemicals. Yet fake food, junk food, excessive sugar, excessive alcohol, and nutrient-empty foods like white-flour buns are doing just the opposite; they are a road map to bad health and premature aging down the road. We are youth obsessed in this country, but we can stay younger looking and have a more youthful interior if we eat real food and avoid sugar and chemicals. It's difficult to make young people understand this because they feel invincible. "Down the road" seems so far away from a young person's perspective. It's not until you reach middle age that you realize the harm done to yourself, but now the road ahead seems daunting. The good news is that it's not impossible to reverse the bad effects and poor choices we made earlier in life.

A good example of someone who did this is Dr. Paul Savage, whose wonderful story you'll read in chapter 26. Yes, even a smart doctor can get off track when it comes to eating. His dietary and lifestyle habits made him hormonally imbalanced at an early age. Yet he was able to reverse the damage and restore his body to youthful levels of hormones and energy.

What's more, he lost a tremendous amount of weight. His story is inspirational, and he now passes on what he has learned to his patients.

SUPPLEMENTATION

Unfortunately, today's foods are not as rich as they once were in vitamins and minerals. This is why supplementation is an important component of your daily diet. Vitamins are crucial in maximizing the number of years you can continue to enjoy good health.

The dietary reference intakes (DRIs) are values established by the Institute of Medicine for recommended daily nutrient intake.

The United States government has published recommended dietary allowances (RDAs) for nutrients, vitamins, and minerals—but these are based upon amounts needed to prevent deficiencies and are hardly enough to keep you alive. The recommended daily allowances are not enough to prevent the degenerative changes associated with aging. At least we now have the DRIs for nutrients. These include levels that may reduce the risk of heart disease, osteoporosis, certain cancers, and other diseases that have to do with diet. But these levels usually aren't enough to counteract the environment and its negative effects.

There seems to be a resistance to taking supplements, even though the published medical data on the benefits of vitamins are overwhelming. According to Dr. Ron Rothenberg, "We do not understand why the government and the media appear to be so opposed to supporting and promoting the benefits of vitamins. We do know, however, that vitamins, like many other supplements, are natural and therefore cannot be patented by the pharmaceutical companies. The pharmaceutical companies cannot make the types of profits they are accustomed to making with drugs for which they hold the patent. Drugs are big business!"

Both my husband, Alan, and I believe in supplementation. We originally started by recommendation from our internist, Dr. Soram Khalsa in Beverly Hills. At the time, I had not realized the extent of the damage to our food supply and that supplementation was necessary to achieve proper nutrition. Within a few weeks of taking vitamins and supplements, I noticed a profound increase in my energy and vitality. It's a lot to ingest twenty or thirty vitamins a day, and at times it can get pretty "gaggy." At one point, Alan got discouraged and stopped taking his supplements about six months into the program. He hadn't mentioned it to me; I simply noticed that he was dragging. He wanted to take a lot of naps. One day I asked, "Are you taking your vitamins?" This was when we realized the profound difference between his energy and mine. That was enough to make him a believer. With the environment in such a fragile state, it is crucial to augment your diet nutritionally. Until things change, this is the way it has got to be.

As for my regimen, I am sure to include

> calcium, to keep my bones strong
> vitamin C, 1,000 mg daily
> Saint-John's-wort for its calming effect
> vitamin E
> glucosamine for joints and cartilage
> selenium
> CoQ10 for heart health
> phosphatidylcholine
> zinc
> rhodiola
> Zyflamend
> white tea extract
> LycoPom, a combination of lycopene and
>   pomegranate (from New Chapter)
> Smoke Shield, to protect against environmen-
>   tal pollution (from New Chapter)
> reishi mushroom
> cinnamon
> multivitamin

These supplements change according to my stresses and traveling. But this should give you an idea of the way I augment my daily diet. I try to buy most of my supplements from my friend Paul Schulick at New

Chapter (website in Resources section), because I know him and know how deeply he cares about the purity and wholesomeness of his products. But many other companies offer fine products. Another good place to purchase supplements is through **Life Extension** magazine. They tend to do an article on the latest supplement, explaining its features and benefits, and then it is possible to order through the form in the magazine.

A good, qualified antiaging doctor is your best bet to finding the right fit for your personal needs. Unfortunately, acid rain and pollution are a part of the environment we can't avoid until our behaviors and habits change drastically. The best defense for each of us is supplementation. Many people pass off supplementation as "expensive urine," but I have seen and felt the results since my husband and I embraced this regimen. For us it's working; I believe it's worth looking into.

In addition to supplements, Dr. Galitzer, my antiaging doctor, gives me tinctures and drops to stimulate my major hormones along with my minor hormones. He also gives me formulas to regenerate my weakest organs.

He explains that when a patient comes in with numerous physical complaints, he realizes that many of the important organs are toxic and sluggish. He uses herbal drainage formulas to cleanse the body by stimulating the excretion systems of the liver, kidney, and lymph glands to rid the body of toxins that have accumulated over time.

The process of drainage reduces toxicity in the body, but organ function may still remain sluggish and susceptible to future physical, emotional, and nutritional stressors. These organs now need to be toned and strengthened in the same way you would build muscles at the gym. These formulas are homeopathic, derived from the plant (herb), mineral, and animal kingdoms. According to Dr. Galitzer, each organ is a unique bioenergy system. An imbalance in the organs frequently slows the process of doing what it knows to do naturally—that is, regenerate and renew itself. Several regeneration formulas can be taken together and used to complement bioidentical hormone therapy. These regenerative formulas support thyroid, adrenal, pancreas, and liver function. When used in combination with bioidentical hormones, they create an optimal result.

I never would have known this type of medicine and treatment was available had I not searched for it on my own. The effects are startling. For instance, if I drink a couple of glasses of wine the night before, the next day my liver tinctures do their daily work and let me know that my body does not tolerate alcohol well. For a few hours, I feel bloated and uncomfortable. That is my liver ridding itself of toxins. It makes me feel good knowing that the discomfort is short-lived and mildly unpleasant, that my body is detoxing itself of substances it does not want or need for function. This is how this new medicine works, and it is fantastic. It allows me to believe that a healthy life is available even under the negative environmental assault, if I am willing to put in the effort.

CHAPTER 25

WENDY: A VEGETARIAN
NO LONGER

Wendy was a vegetarian for many years, and to her surprise, that was a large part of her health problems. I met Wendy at a party at a friend's house and was impressed with her knowledge of hormones and how the body works. After spending ten years in great pain and ten years of medical doctors and the "standard of care" with no results, Wendy decided to take charge of her own health. Had she not done this, I fear she would have suffered the inevitable course that so many women endure: antidepressants, painkillers, weight gain, osteoporosis. She was on that path, but because she put forth the effort, she is now enjoying a quality of life she thought had passed her by. This is a woman who cares deeply about her health and the quality of her life. Today she is living a life she once only dreamed of.

SS: Your story fascinates me. What has been going on with you?

WF: For ten years, I had seen every doctor known to man, from New York to California. I was complaining of back pain and just overall body pain, and it was exhausting me. Basically, these doctors took lots of tests, and it didn't matter who I saw, their answers were always the same: "You're in great health. You just need to slow down a little bit. You need to relax and not be so type A."

SS: Did they offer you any kind of relief, such as prescription drugs?

WF: Yes, and I was told that if it got really bad, I could just take some anti-inflammatories to help get me through the really bad times. But it was bad every day.

SS: When you say "anti-inflammatory," do you mean Advil or ibuprofen?

WF: No. Vioxx—heavy-duty prescription. You know, the one they took off the market. These doctors were not prescribing Tylenol or anything over the counter. In the beginning, I took Vioxx, figuring if that's all that's wrong with me, that's what I'll do. I'm a good little girl.

SS: Did anyone suggest bone density tests?

WF: In the very beginning, my doctors would have me touch my toes, lay me on a table, and take my leg and bring it over my head. They told me that I was incredibly flexible, that I couldn't possibly be in that much pain if I was that flexible. I would look at them, not knowing what to say.

SS: Describe the pain.

WF: It was all lower back pain, with a burning in my upper back, shoulders, and neck. Just burning, burning constantly.

SS: Did it make sleeping difficult?

WF: It made everything difficult. It made life difficult. I would toss and turn. My husband and I bought different beds. I went through three different beds because we thought I must be sleeping on the wrong bed. My poor husband was beside himself. "How could you be in this much pain?" he would ask. "What's wrong with you?" I had no clue. My uncle was head of internal medicine at Montefiore Medical Center in New York City. He sent me to high-end Fifth Avenue doctors, but they all kept telling me that because I had so much mobility, it must be in my head. This all started at age forty. Well, come to find out ten years later, it was more than a back issue. Along the way, though, I kept saying to my husband that I have to keep trying, that there must be something seriously wrong with me, and that they just don't know what it is.

Then I decided to go holistic. I started massage and acupuncture, which actually helped me tremendously, but only for a short while. Then I became convinced that it was my posture. I've worn high heels my whole life. I probably have not developed certain muscles, and maybe if I go and take the Alexander Technique (which dancers do), it will help my posture and I will get better.

The woman who taught the class recommended

craniosacral therapy. I was open to anything. She put me on the table and told me that this type of therapy is the transfer of energy. "I'm going to relax all the muscles in your body," she said, "and I'm not even going to touch you." I thought to myself, Voodoo, but I was ready to try anything. Within ten minutes, I was drenched. She continued, "You have all this tension and stress in your head and shoulders, but it's calming you now. It's leaving." I walked out of there like a gazelle. I felt like a million bucks.

So I thought it was great. I'm a high-stress person, so I just need to calm down. At eighty bucks a pop, I couldn't afford that therapy every week.

SS: Along the way, with all this pain, were there any other symptoms of menopause such as depression or irritability?

WF: I was incredibly irritable and angry, although I'm a very happy person by nature. My husband, unfortunately, was the one who took the brunt. All day long, I would hold it in, but then at night I would take it out on him. But he kept saying, "We're going to find a solution." He knows me so well, and he knows that I am not a person who complains. I decided that I would live with this, and at this point, it was only two years. But I was now approaching fifty, and this had been going on for almost ten years.

Then we moved to the California desert, and I saw a building that said "Sports Medicine." I went in, after being in so much pain and not sleeping for so long. The doctor told me that my body was so inflamed. "If I don't give you some type of injection to get the inflammation down," he said, "I can't even work with you." I couldn't sit, I couldn't stand, I couldn't lie down—nothing. I was just a mess. I got epidurals and cortisone injections and then every kind of injection known to man.

SS: Are you talking about steroids?

WF: Definitely steroids. I was scared to death. This doctor wanted to inject my neck and lower back. I let him because I didn't know what else to do.

SS: What was your diet like at this time?

WF: At this point, I had been a vegetarian for ten years. I thought my diet was stellar. I thought I was never putting any chemicals in my body because I did read labels. I had sweets, but never as a daily occurrence. I drank a little bit of wine. I didn't smoke. I didn't drink sodas. I had coffee, but very little.

When it came to diet and exercise, I was in the zone, doing everything right. The doctors would confirm this, telling me, "You are so healthy. Your blood work is healthy. You eat right. There's nothing wrong with you, so it must all be in your head."

I'm not just saying this, but the first time I ever heard about hormones was four years ago. Prior to meeting you at a party, a friend of mine recommended a more forward-thinking doctor to me. I went for a physical, and she was the one who said, "Your blood work shows that you are nutritionally starving yourself. This is part of your fatigue problem. I don't know if you're a vegetarian for animal rights, for religious reasons, or whatever, but if these are not your reasons, I really recommend that you eat more protein." I countered by telling her that I ate a lot of soy, but she said it wasn't good for me.

That very night, my husband and I changed our diets (he was a vegetarian only because of me). We hadn't eaten meat in fourteen years. The doctor said I might get sick at first when I introduced these things into my system, so do it slowly. She advised that we start with eggs and a little bit of butter and see what happens. I immediately got sick. My stomach was killing me. She told me to go to the health food store and take enzymes while introducing these foods into my system, very, very, slowly, and drink lots of water. In a few days, I was eating eggs. Next, I was eating chicken. Then the doctor told me to get off the pill, which I had been on for seventeen years. She explained how my diet, my lifestyle habits, and the pill could be contributing to my back pain.

She also asked me if I had ever heard of Dr. Diana Schwarzbein. I then read Dr. Schwarzbein's book **The Schwarzbein Principle** and changed my diet. At my chiropractor's office one day, I noticed a flyer saying that Dr. Schwarzbein was going to give a seminar here. So I went to the seminar. Dr. Schwarzbein talked about vegetarians, who think they are so healthy, but in reality they're wreaking havoc on their whole systems.

SS: Yes—their bodies can't make healthy cells because they are not giving them the building blocks through correct foods.

WF: Then I met you at a party. By then I was already eating the Schwarzbein way and started feeling a little better. I was thrilled to hear you talking about Diana, and that's when I moved closer to the group. You were talking about hormones, and I thought, Okay—now this is my next step to feeling even better! At that point, since I was getting little help from the medical community, I was trying to be my own doctor. You were also talking about the importance of sleep, but I still did not think this related at all to my problems.

Prior to going to Diana's seminar, I did saliva testing through the mail. Anyone at the seminar who was tested she met with individually. That's when she told me to get off the pill and how my diet and the pill could be contributing to my pain. At this point, I had still not made the connection that since birth control pills were synthetic hormones, they were putting my hormonal system out of balance! I did get an appointment to see Dr. Schwarzbein.

SS: Did you get the feeling you were in the presence of great wisdom when you were with her?

WF: I was blown away. At her seminar, I don't think I ever closed my mouth. If you have any sense of wanting to get healthy, you immediately click with her. She just makes sense. Lights went off in my head. Now I know why I'm hungry all the time.

Now I know why I crave sugar like a maniac and why I fight constantly to not eat it, although I was eating it without realizing it, because I was on such a high-carbohydrate diet. I didn't realize that it all was turning to sugar.

SS: What was your weight like during this time?

WF: I always battled ten pounds. I was always starving myself because I needed to fit into something, so I would agonize over every morsel of food. I would gain weight, but it was more like I was bloating up because my hormones were so out of whack. The doctor then told me to stay on this path of eating because it's going to take a long time for the pill to get out of my system and to counteract all the years I had been a vegetarian. She said that it would take a good year for my system to really start acting the way I wanted it to. She also said, "Now don't get crazy if you gain a few pounds. This is normal, but one day, you'll wake up and wonder where it went." I probably gained about seven pounds, but I kept with it. I was eating three meals a day and snacking. I was just eating and eating.

SS: And you were making sure that you got protein, fat, and carbohydrates at every meal?

WF: Yes. I was so used to starving myself to stay fit that I never realized that this was not going to keep me thin. Then I read your first diet book, **Eat Great, Lose Weight,** in which you said exactly what Dr. Schwarzbein was saying, plus you listed all this great food we could eat.

SS: What was your libido like during this time?

WF: You know, my husband and I always had a great sex life, but when I was sick, I just didn't want to make love. My body hurt too much to be touched; my skin was crawling and in pain.

Month after month, my period came like clockwork, and then eight months into the program, my period was late. I called Dr. Schwarzbein's office, and they told me that she was no longer taking patients, that she was now only training doctors. I thought, Oh no!

I went out and bought **The Sexy Years,** and it was the book that saved my life. It had been nine months since I had seen Dr. Schwarzbein, and suddenly my small pants fit me again. My back was still hurting, but I did have more energy. This was all so encouraging. I was losing the weight by eating all this food. Dr. Schwarzbein had already told me it was going to take a year for the pill to get out of my system and for me to heal my metabolism. All those years of eating incorrectly had put my hormones completely out of whack. But reading her book and then your books, I realized that the birth control pills were a big contributor to my being hormonally out of balance. Now with my late period, you were telling me that I needed to fix my hormonal system.

I pored over your book. My husband would walk into the room, and I would be crying. There are so many great doctors in your book, and I was thinking, Who do I turn to, what do I do?

Then I read the chapter on Dr. Galitzer. I don't know why, but I just gravitated to him. I think because you said a girlfriend of yours went to him for a chronic condition, and no one seemed to be able to help her but Dr. Galitzer.

SS: Yes, he is my doctor, and he is a beautiful, kind, and brilliant person.

WF: It was hard to get an appointment with him. But finally I did. I walked in with my whole history all typed out. He said, "Wendy, this is all great, but we're not going to dwell on the negatives. We're going to move forward."

SS: Dr. Galitzer is a very positive person. He is an endocrinologist who deals in energy medicine. He identifies the weakest elements in your body, strengthens it, and gives it energy. It's quite amazing. Rarely does he do this with drugs.

WF: The first thing he said to me was, "Wendy, you have a thyroid problem. What you're complaining of is chronic fatigue, fibromyalgia, and overall body pain. You have trouble sleeping. You have trouble focusing, and you have absolutely no libido." I said, "Yes, and all of this makes me very irritable, unhappy, and I just feel awful all the time." When I left his office that first time, I felt excited.

The next thing he explained to me was that everyone has a dominant hormone in their makeup. "You have one system that basically maximizes and processes all your energy. You happen to be an adrenal type, and your adrenals are not functioning well.

That's why you are not feeling so terrific, but we're going to take care of that. We're going to boost your adrenals, and bring your thyroid back to normal. You're going to feel great. Also, we're going to clean out your liver and detoxify." He gave me tinctures, vitamins, and drops to start detoxifying my liver. I felt so comfortable in his presence that I believed him and decided I would do what he advised. One month later, when I went back to him, I was a completely different person.

SS: The initial reaction to detoxification is a little uncomfortable, right?

WF: Yes, but I believed in it. He was detoxing my sluggish liver. I had an underactive thyroid. I had acidity in my cells, and my adrenals were not functioning. I explained to him that my body ached from head to toe, like I was disintegrating. He told me that I was just toxic, but that I'd be amazed at how quickly I would start feeling better.

He gave me Wobenzym enzymes for the inflammation in my body. He had me drinking Japanese water with lemon every morning before I did my tinctures. He gave me the hormones pregnenolone and DHEA, which were both to help my adrenal fatigue. I knew from your book that these were minor hormones and that they were going to improve my memory. He also had me using glutathione cream for my immune system. I started cross-referencing with what he was saying to the information in your book. I kept thinking, What do women do who don't have access to this kind of medicine? I finally realized that it is up to each of us to get this information and then read and reread it until we understand it.

SS: That's how I learned it. We are the first line of defense. We are the generation of women who have got to figure this out on our own. We have to find the doctors who understand, and sometimes that takes time. Not all doctors are like Dr. Galitzer, or Dr. Schwarzbein, or the others that I write about.

WF: My friends started noticing a huge difference in me. For the first three weeks, I was pretty uncomfortable, like there was a war going on inside me. But I could feel that something good was going on inside my body. By week four, the pain was leaving. My ankles and knees were not killing me. My back was still hurting, but all the other inflammation in my body had subsided. I was starting to feel more energy. I still am not ready to join the circus, but I am definitely feeling better.

Dr. Galitzer gave me adrenal shots, a vitamin C drip, more tinctures, and more vitamins. My acidity had gone down. He said there had definitely been a virus in my system, and that it was attacking my liver and my thyroid, and we needed to get it out.

SS: And all this without drugs?

WF: Nothing—absolutely nothing but vitamins, tinctures, eating right, and getting rest. The only foods he removed from my diet were peanuts, and corn and dairy for a while. Instead of yogurt in the morning, he told me to take goat's milk yogurt.

By the second month, it was like, Oh man! I don't know what's happening to me, but I'm feeling really, really good. I had so much more energy. I jumped out of bed in the morning and started getting things done, not even thinking about the fact that there was no pain and no fatigue.

SS: Now, where are you hormonally?

WF: After two months, Dr. Galitzer said it was time to do a hormonal panel. We hadn't yet dealt with estrogen, progesterone, and testosterone. My tests showed that I was low in all three hormones and definitely needed replacement. He put me on estrogen, progesterone, and testosterone cream. I cycle progesterone on days 14 through 28. I needed more testosterone than any of the others. I was so low in that hormone.

SS: So what is your life like today? It's been a year since you started all of this with Dr. Galitzer.

WF: Suzanne, let's put it this way: I came from feeling like I had one foot in the grave, and today I am like 95 percent superwoman. I still have days when my back gets weird, but we're still working on this. Dr. Galitzer is looking into Raynaud's disease, a disorder of the blood vessels that supply blood to your skin. But I know that whatever I have, Dr. Galitzer wants to lick it for me.

SS: He will. He's like that.

WF: My husband is the happiest person in the world. We have our life back. All I know is that I went to doctors for ten years, and in just three short years, from hearing you speak, and listening to Dr. Schwarzbein, then reading your book, and finding Dr. Galitzer, I have gotten rid of 95 percent of my pain. I have my libido back. I am happy again. I am eating meat, chicken, and fish. I got hormonally balanced and detoxified.

I now realize that diet is mandatory, first and foremost. If I hadn't already changed my eating by the time I walked into Dr. Galitzer's office, it would have taken a lot longer to fix me.

Diet matters. It is the easiest and most significant change that we can make in our lives. It was my first step to wellness. As I learned, not everyone can be a vegetarian. For me, it was literally making me sick.

Hormones matter. They are not understood immediately. But every woman needs to know that hormones rule and can wreak havoc on our lives. I am not just talking about the sex hormones and menopausal symptoms. I am talking about the major hormones that affect our overall health. Also, every woman needs to understand the side effects of birth control pills. This knowledge was my second step to wellness.

Women need to understand that when you lose your hormones, things go wrong in your body that you would never connect to hormones. I have so many friends who are on sleeping pills, antidepressants, and anti-inflammatories. These are all solutions for the doctor, but not for the patient.

People need to understand the importance of

lifestyle and nutrition and then to understand that their body is a temple. If you're good to your body, then find one of these doctors who is more forward-thinking, and you can get your life in perfect balance. It takes work and determination and a belief that there is a better way than drugs. Learn about chemical imbalance and what causes all the acidity and toxins in your body. Stress and sleep matter, too. Learn to balance your stress and get more sleep.

As I said, the first time I heard you talking to these women about hormones, I didn't make the connection to me. I had a stressful childhood, and it caught up with me as an adult. Stress is such a part of all of our lives, and it makes us sick. I hope a lot of people read this book. It helps to know that others have gone through these things because it gives hope.

SS: Yes, information is empowering. We have all gone through what we've gone through, and these problems, whether they be physical or emotional, are opportunities to learn a great deal. Look at what this journey has done to your life.

WF: What I have learned from my journey is that there was a thread of truth in what all the medical doctors were saying about my slowing down and not being so type A. What they were really saying is my adrenals were burning out, and it was leading me down the path of physical destruction. With this hormonal imbalance, my poor vegetarian diet, lack of stress management, and poor sleep compounded the problem, and it slowly began manifesting itself in physical pain until I could no longer bear it.

I can't get my forties back, but Dr. Schwarzbein, Dr. Galitzer, and you are my angels! In a relatively short period of time, I have regained my quality of life. I'm still young and can look forward to wonderful, physical years ahead. I can't say enough good things about Dr. Galitzer.

As we continue to heal my body on a cellular level, he has now added an additional component—a very advanced chiropractor. I say "advanced" because he is not only dealing with my structure, he is also dealing with my intestinal tract. He believes I have gluten intolerance and that my years of being a vegetarian wreaked havoc on my body, creating toxins that have greatly contributed to my chronic back pain.

All the medical doctors I had seen were saying that I should not be in pain because I do not have any major disk problems. Well, they were right! I have a structural problem that probably stems from an accident I had as a child. I also have this intestinal problem that I actually created! Although on my ten-year journey I had been to chiropractors, not one was able to help me. I now understand that my body was too toxic and my hormones too out of balance for the adjustments to take hold.

I have made some further changes to my diet that may be temporary or may be lifelong. I'll have to wait, and I am taking supplements to heal my stomach. But the bottom line is that I wake up every morning happy and grateful. I have my life back, and I will never return to the old one.

I will be forever grateful to you for all the work you do on behalf of women's health. Your books explain the importance of diet, exercise, sleep, stress management, and hormones in a language that we can understand. You are incredibly honest in sharing your life experiences, and it has been a generous gift to so many of us. Thank you from the bottom of my heart!

SS: Thank you. Yours is an important story with a beautiful ending.

CHAPTER 26

Dr. Paul Savage: Nutrition and Hormones

Dr. Paul Savage is the chief medical officer of BodyLogicMD in Chicago, Illinois. He founded BodyLogic to share what he has learned from his personal journey about health and to dispel misconceptions about hormone therapy. His website is www.bodylogicmd.com, and his phone number is 1-866-535-2563.

SS: I am so pleased to speak with you. Please tell me about your organization and what you are doing in Chicago. What brought you into this arena of medicine?

PS: Even though I am a physician, I came into this new area of medicine because I did not know much about preventive health. You see, as doctors we are not really taught to treat a patient holistically in a preventive manner.

In 1996, I was thirty-eight years old and weighed

264 pounds. I was depressed. I had no libido. I couldn't get the weight off, no matter how hard I tried. What bothered me the most was that I had trouble sleeping. I would wake up at 11:00, at 2:00, and then pace the floor for two hours. Finally, I would go back to bed and get a couple of hours of sleep, but I never really felt rested. I went to my doctor, and he told me to eat better and exercise.

After leaving my doctor's office, it dawned on me that I did not know what to eat, nor did I know how to exercise. Do you do cardio? Weight lifting? What was best for physiology and good health? So I started on a quest: nutrition, dietitians, personal trainers, and so forth. I reached out to anybody who could teach me about health. I spent two years reading about nutrition, funneling through the maze of information out there, and realized how confusing it is. Everybody has a public relations angle or a marketing angle. It seemed the point was to confuse the population about what is healthy and what is not.

In my opinion, there is no such thing as a diet, only a proper nutrition plan. Sometimes you have to go back to what your grandmother taught you decades ago: Eat breakfast, lunch, and dinner. Have a nap after breakfast; have a nap after lunch. Turn off the TV; go out and play. Have two tablespoons of cod liver oil, and eat all your vegetables. You know, just simple rules.

After two years, I had lost fifty pounds, weighed 210, and had 26 percent body fat. I felt better, but I did not feel well. I was doing an hour and a half of exercise a day with my personal trainer, doing cardio, martial arts, and weight lifting. I was eating five meals a day of very good nutrition, but I could not lose more weight. That experience is what put me on this search.

At the time, I knew nothing about hormones. I did not realize how seriously my bad lifestyle and nutrition all those years had affected my hormone levels. I did not understand the connection, so I sought a bioidentical hormone therapist. He diagnosed that I had hormone imbalance, specifically too much cortisol and low testosterone. After being on bioidentical hormone replacement for five months, I dropped down to 14 percent body fat, my energy returned, and finally I could sleep again. It was amazing.

SS: Hormones were the missing component.

PS: Yes. This convinced me how important it is that we not only maintain hormone levels, but also return them to the same levels we had when we were twenty-five and thirty years old. Those are the age ranges at which our bodies operated at their peak—our healthiest prime.

Having had this incredible experience, I decided to leave my position as director of an emergency and trauma center, where I was treating gang members and gunshots and pretty hysterical people all day long—it was very stressful—and change the direction of my career. That is when I embraced this whole concept of hormones and replacing them naturally. I wanted to learn everything I could about bioidentical hormones, health, and nutrition.

I went to Alabama, Florida, California, Michigan, and New York and studied with a number of various experts on bioidentical hormones until I completed the picture. Finally, I understood that this missing component in health care was why people were not improving and getting well.

ss: When did you start BodyLogic?

ps: In 2003. The mission of BodyLogic is to help physicians come into the field of preventive health and age management by teaching them the proper way to help patients through nutrition, exercise, and bioidentical hormone therapy.

ss: Did they come?

ps: Did they ever! We now have five clinics nationwide because so many doctors want to come into this field but do not know how to do it.

I got my brother involved in starting BodyLogic. He is my twin brother, who is a retired vice president of AT&T and was also out of shape. He was 240 pounds, still smoking, and still drinking. I taught him the premises of health, and he markedly changed his life. He no longer smokes or drinks, and he exercises five times a week. He is down to 180 pounds and looks great.

When I discovered what bioidentical hormones could do for me, I was convinced of their importance. Once I opened my practice, suddenly there were a few thousand patients who wanted this help, and I needed to be able to have other doctors where I could send them.

SS: Is there any one patient whose story stands out in your mind?

PS: Yes. One of the interesting things about hormones is that they are not just for menopausal females. A thirty-two-year-old woman came to my office, tears streaming down her face. She and her husband were getting a divorce. Terrified, she explained to me that she could not control her anger. Each month in the last two weeks around the time of her period, she became (in her words) "a raging lunatic." She had severe cramps, clotting, and out-of-control moods. She was afraid to be around her two little boys, and they were afraid to be around her. Her husband was in desperate need, and he sought us out, too.

We diagnosed this woman with severe PMS, which is a progesterone deficiency, in the second two weeks of her cycle. Once we placed her on progesterone therapy for the last two weeks of her cycle, she improved markedly within three months. One day, this woman, her husband, and her two little boys came by my office to say, "Thank you for saving our marriage."

I see this all the time—the way that hormones dramatically change people's lives on a daily basis. In traditional medicine, it is very rare for people to come back and say thank you. In the emergency room, I truly saved people's lives on a daily basis, and rarely did they ever say thank you, but in this field, women are thanking me every day. My patient retention is over 90 percent.

SS: I know one forty-three-year-old woman who is struggling with her weight. She exercises, goes to sleep early, and tries to watch her diet, but she has about thirty pounds that won't budge.

PS: It sounds like a hormone problem and could be estrogen dominance. There are certain things that indicate hormonal imbalance:

1. estrogen dominance, which brings about unexplained weight gain
2. cortisol dominance; if cortisol is too high, you will gain weight
3. inadequate thyroid, either hypothyroid (low) or hyperthyroid (high)
4. low growth hormone

If a woman has estrogen dominance, we would lab test first, to be sure. Numbers from labwork are for clinical diagnosis only. A doctor has to look at other aspects, such as her stress, her weight, and her mental outlook. These are all part of the diagnosis. With estrogen-dominant females, we find out what is blocking the progesterone because that is what balances the estrogen.

SS: How do you discover this?

PS: Through clinical history or through saliva testing. Although there are not many things that block progesterone production, it can be due to dietary deficiencies. For example, vegetarians don't get enough cholesterol, which is required to manufacture hormones. The other way we can remove the blocking action is by increasing fiber in the woman's diet. I frequently put estrogen-dominant females on a high-fiber diet, which would include any food that is green and leafy or crunchy when you bite into it, such as apples, pears, apricots, berries, spinach, kale, broccoli, or cauliflower. Increasing your fiber intake helps regulate estrogen levels.

Finally, we replace the estrogen-dominant female with progesterone to help balance the estrogen/progesterone ratio. This brings her back into balance, and she then is no longer estrogen-dominant.

SS: Does the weight dissipate as long as she continues to eat right and exercise?

PS: Right. When estrogen is in balance, your metabolism increases. Too much, however, can slow it down. Estrogen can put on fat; progesterone helps take it off. Progesterone is also a diuretic, so it helps you lose water weight. When women are bloating, it indicates that they have too much progesterone. It's all a fine balance.

SS: Many women have a difficult time on their progesterone cycle, because they feel bloated and can put on as much as five pounds.

PS: If you are putting on five pounds, bloating,

getting cramps, and feeling irritable, or experiencing any one of these symptoms alone, you are not on enough progesterone.

SS: It sounds like bioidentical progesterone replacement could be a better remedy for young women than taking over-the-counter pain medication and diuretics. Tell me, what is the average dose of progesterone you give a woman? I know it's different for everyone, but there must be some kind of "norm."

PS: Depending upon the female herself, if she is active, thin with a higher metabolism, she will need more progesterone. By contrast, if she is sedentary, older, and has a slow metabolism, she will need less. Every woman is different. Some need more, some need less.

SS: What about the person who has high cortisol?

PS: I diagnose this type very frequently; usually they are younger, active professional females.

SS: Because they are not sleeping enough?

PS: Poor sleep quality is definitely one of the things that can increase cortisol levels. But you have to ask yourself, why aren't you sleeping? Usually stress is the big offender, and it causes cortisol to go up. Cortisol has two functions, and let me explain this in terms of our ancient defense mechanisms. First, it is in your body to help you with the fight-or-flight response; in other words, it helps you mobilize energy to run away from a dinosaur chasing you. Second, it helps cool down your body and your joints after you flee in order to decrease inflammation in your body. Of course, back thirty-five thousand years ago, we didn't get chased by dinosaurs every moment of the day. But in today's world we are constantly under stress; we are constantly chased by what I tell patients are "dinosaurs"—family stress, work stress, relational stress, financial stress, and emotional stress. We are constantly pushing ourselves without letting ourselves rest. As a result, our adrenals are constantly pumping out cortisol. Chronically elevated cortisol shuts down your metabolism and says, "Okay, fat, give me all the food you've got because we are under attack and we need to store food." As a result, you start absorbing many more calories than you normally would with a regular working metabolism. All your extra energy is stored as fat because cortisol has actually turned down your metabolism.

SS: So what's the remedy?

PS: The remedy is to get the cortisol to come down by eliminating stress through stress management and life changes. Many people are under the false impression that because they are stressed and constantly on the go, one or two light meals a day is sufficient, instead of breaking down food into five or six different meals every day with sufficient amounts. Eating one or even two meals a day makes your body think that it is starving. This induces stress, and stress increases cortisol.

SS: I have written about this extensively in my

Somersize books, that by skipping meals, you actually **gain** weight because it raises cortisol, and that you must eat properly to lose weight.

PS: You need a constant influx of food throughout the day so your body understands that it is not starving and not stressed. Through nutrition, you can bring your cortisol down and thus lose weight.

You also need exercise, even though initially, exercise elevates your cortisol. But exercise also relieves stress, so long-term it will lower your cortisol. Find an activity that you like to do—yoga, tai chi, martial arts, weight lifting, or running—that will relieve your stress level. Vacations are important, too, but the bottom line is to find an activity you like to do to relieve your stress level.

SS: What about the person with underactive thyroid?

PS: Underactive thyroid is one of the most under-diagnosed diseases in the United States today. Some studies suggest that 75 percent of women have underactive thyroid and go untreated. For physicians, it is a very complicated issue because we have gotten to the point of using only lab tests to diagnose low thyroid, when other issues are involved. For example: weight gain, sluggishness, constipation, dry skin, depression, or missing the outer corner of the eyebrows. These are all symptoms of low thyroid that you have to stay attuned to, in addition to the blood test.

SS: So just because your blood test says you are

normal, it really is not the indicator. The diagnostic savvy of the doctor plays a role, too, correct?

PS: Yes. The doctor has to listen to physical symptoms of the patient. Five years ago, if a blood test indicated that the TSH was over 5, that indicated a problem. Now it's been lowered to 1 or 2 [pg/dL] so we are getting more and more broad on how we treat this disease.

SS: Let's talk about adrenal burnout. It's a difficult concept for people to understand.

PS: When the adrenals get fatigued, you have too much stress, and you have called on your adrenals too much. Once the adrenals tire out, they no longer produce enough cortisol. We see patients all the time with low cortisol levels, and you can tell by looking at them that they are completely fatigued. They have difficulty waking up in the morning, but feel a little better around noon. At around 4:00, they need a nap, and after dinner, they feel better than they do most of the day but quickly tire out and have a difficult time sleeping. They are more sensitive to the environment, and they have infections that last longer than is normal.

It is essential to try to reach this person by explaining the importance of nutrition, exercise, and lifestyle. You try to get them to stop doing the things that are stressing the adrenals, such as not eating properly, not exercising enough, and having too much stress.

After that, I talk to them about herbal agents, supplements, and vitamins that can help increase the production of the adrenals. If I still can't reach them and I realize they are not going to change, my last resort is to give them hydrocortisone. Cortisone is only for people at end-stage adrenal fatigue. It is not a jump start, and it should not be used frivolously. Its side effects include osteoporosis and psychosis.

SS: I know how burned-out adrenals feel because in my career, I have burned out my adrenals five times. I have vowed to myself that I will never do that again, but at the time I did not understand the effects of overwork on my body. I guess you learn from your mistakes. I now value my good health so much that I will go to bed before pulling an all-nighter and figure out tomorrow how to finish the job when I am well rested. Maybe it's called "maturity."

PS: Statistically, 83 percent of women and 80 percent of people under the age of forty have adrenal stress, meaning they are producing too much cortisol. You can tell an adrenal-fatigued person by how many cups of coffee they drink in a day.

SS: That's interesting, but isn't coffee in small amounts an antioxidant?

PS: A cup a day is fine, and there are theories about its antioxidant effects, but when you start putting too much caffeine into your system, it stimulates the adrenals in a negative way. Like everything else, it's about balance. Take wine, for example. A glass of red has positive effects on your blood pressure, but if you exceed two or three glasses daily, you can start having liver problems.

SS: Let's talk about men. Men seem to be reluctant to investigate antiaging medicine on their own.

PS: As a man myself, finding out what was at the root of my problems—weight gain, fatigue, stress, lifestyle, and hormonal imbalance—was astounding. Then I began to realize that other men were having the same problems. I consider it an honor that I have hundreds of men in my practice, and I do very well with them. I am treating them for adrenal, cortisol, thyroid, and their testosterone. But I have to say it's usually the women who come to me first, who get the biochemistry of it, and then sign up their husbands.

The thing about male menopause that is different from menopause is that women lose over 90 percent of their estrogen within about twenty months, while men lose their testosterone over two to three decades. It's so gradual for them that we don't have that sudden feeling of falling off a cliff. Instead, we just take this long stroll down this never-ending path, and then one day we turn right and go, "You know what? I don't feel the same. I don't feel energized, I don't feel vital, I don't feel mentally sharp, I don't feel as sexual, I don't feel as strong as I used to feel." One of the great misconceptions held by men is that they feel that testosterone causes prostate cancer. Unfortunately, this belief keeps men from entertaining the idea of replacing testosterone.

SS: It is an environment of balanced testosterone that prevents prostate cancer.

PS: When you read the literature on testosterone and prostate cancer, you find the predominance of this literature shows that, in fact, testosterone does not cause prostate cancer. Further, testosterone is beneficial for a man's mood, memory, mind, libido, heart health, strength, metabolism, and bone health. When you see an elderly man flopped over, thin skin, pale, no energy, poor vision, can't pee, irritable, grouchy, isolated—these are all symptoms of a testosterone deficiency. I try to prevent that from happening with my male patients, because once a man gets to that point, trying to bring him back is very difficult. I do not feel that testosterone, or any hormone for that matter, should diminish with age.

SS: You seem to have a great passion for your work. When you leave your office each day, how do you feel?

PS: Tired, but satisfied, extremely satisfied. The greatest thrill comes when I am outside of my office and someone will come up to me and say, "I saw you on television, and what you said makes sense." Or when other doctors come up to me and say, "How can I learn to do what you are doing?" It is absolutely wonderful to know that I can impact physicians' lives and work, because when you impact a physician, you are in turn impacting their patients.

SS: Thank you for your time, Dr. Savage, and continue doing your great work.

DR. SAVAGE'S TOP FIVE ANTIAGING RECOMMENDATIONS

1. Dietary deficiencies can compromise progesterone production. For example, vegetarians don't get enough cholesterol, which is required to manufacture hormones. The other way we can remove the blocking action is by increasing fiber in the woman's diet—adding any food that is green and leafy or crunchy, such as apples, pears, apricots, berries, spinach, kale, broccoli, or cauliflower. Increasing fiber intake helps regulate estrogen levels.

2. When estrogen is in balance, metabolism increases. Too much, however, can slow it down. Estrogen can put on fat; progesterone helps take it off if it is in the right ratio. Progesterone is also a diuretic, so it helps the body lose water weight. When women are bloating, it indicates that they have too much progesterone. It's all a fine balance.

3. Poor sleep quality is definitely one of the things that can increase cortisol levels. But you have to ask yourself, why aren't you sleeping? Usually stress is the big offender, and it causes cortisol to go up. Cortisol will come down by eliminating stress through stress management and life changes.

4. Many people are under the false impression that because they are stressed and constantly on the go, one or two light meals a day is sufficient, instead of breaking down food into five or six different meals every day with sufficient amounts. Eating one or even two meals a day makes the body think that it is starving. This induces stress, and stress increases cortisol.

5. Exercise also relieves stress, so long-term it will lower cortisol. Find an activity that you like to do—yoga, tai chi, martial arts, weight lifting, or running—that will relieve your stress level. Vacations are important, too, but the bottom line is to find an activity you like to do to relieve your stress level.

CHAPTER 27

PAUL SCHULICK:
HERBS AND ANTIAGING

Paul Schulick is founder and CEO of New Chapter and a Master Herbalist. He is so pure and honest in his search for the finest herbs on earth that when he could not find the quality of ginger he wanted, he started a ginger farm in the rain forest of Costa Rica to grow his own. If we all thought like Paul, there would be no war and we would all live to be 150 years old and happy. Paul Schulick has been my dear friend for many years.

SS: I am thrilled to bring your knowledge to the public. People don't understand herbs and supplementation. For years, you've told me about herbs such as turmeric, green tea, ginger, and curcumin, among others. What supplements do you most frequently recommend?

PS: There are literally hundreds of different supplements that could be recommended. Even when recommendations are made with the best of intentions, there are huge choices involved. If stranded on a desert island, I would want with me the following eight supplements:

- selenium
- rhodiola
- cinnamon
- coenzyme Q10
- omega-3 fats
- LycoPom, a new formulation of lycopene, pomegranate, and cinnamon
- Zyflamend, a formulation that is a combination of ginger, turmeric, green tea, and rosemary
- reishi mushroom

SS: So let's talk each one through, beginning with selenium.

PS: Successful aging involves how well you can protect yourself against life-shortening diseases such as cancer. Selenium is a mineral that helps guard against cancer. Published in the **Journal of the American Medical Association,** a large-scale study involving 1,312 people over an eight-year period pointed out the incredible value of selenium. With selenium supplementation, the researchers found there was a 46 percent reduction in lung cancer, a 58 percent reduction in colorectal cancer, and a 63 percent reduction in prostate cancer when people took 200 millionths of a gram of selenium. It's like nothing, a little speck of this trace mineral, but it elevates the body's detoxification capabilities. Selenium works by elevating certain enzyme systems in the body that help fight free radicals.

SS: In which kinds of foods would you find selenium?

PS: Almost every green vegetable is very high in selenium. However, the selenium content of food depends upon the soil in which the plant is grown, and many soils around the world are selenium-depleted. In some of the epidemiological research (population studies), investigators found that the soils with the lowest amounts of selenium were also (not surprisingly) the areas that have the highest incidences of multiforms of cancer. Selenium is a highly abbreviated answer to cancer protection, but it's really one of the most important nutrients and one of the simplest to take.

SS: If we eat adequate amounts of broccoli, kale, and dark green leafy vegetables, do we need to supplement with selenium?

PS: It all depends upon where the broccoli is grown.

SS: If we buy organically grown vegetables, are we getting those foods from selenium-rich soil?

PS: Not necessarily. That's why supplementation is important; it's insurance that we take in sufficient selenium. It's a relatively inexpensive supplement. You can take it in its yeast form, too.

SS: Does your company, New Chapter, sell selenium in yeast form?

PS: Yes. It's called Selenium Food Complex.

SS: Let's go to the next supplement on your list: rhodiola. I've been taking it for years because you gave it to me and I trust your instincts, but please explain why.

PS: Rhodiola is native to arctic eastern Siberia, Alaska, Lapland, and Scandinavia and has been used as a medicine for several centuries for increasing stamina, mental fortitude, and athletic performance. It has a pronounced antifatigue effect, too. If you are to age successfully, you need to have energy and a positive mood state so that you're motivated to exercise.

SS: So you are saying that with rhodiola you will feel in the mood to exercise because you will have the energy to do so?

PS: Yes. Many people who are depressed don't exercise. Why aren't they exercising? They don't have the energy, nor do they have the brain chemistry that gets them off the couch to move. So an herb like rhodiola gets people moving; in that regard, this herb may be helpful in treating obesity. It may also dampen food cravings.

The beautiful thing about rhodiola is that it was discovered in Russia as part of a process to help elevate the consciousness of athletes.

Rhodiola has a pronounced antifatigue affect. It improves exercise endurance. Also, it helps the general fatigue that people suffer from so much in our culture. If one is to age successfully, one needs to have his or her brain chemistry in good shape and needs to have the experience of having energy so one can exercise.

SS: Why are we all so lacking in energy and stamina? Why are we having such trouble sleeping? And why are we so fat?

PS: I have to go to a broader perspective to answer that. We lack a sense of deep connectiveness with the earth. When I'm in Costa Rica, or when I'm taking a walk in the woods, there are literally thousands of life forms all around me, chirping and singing. You feel such a oneness with the force of creation that it's almost impossible to be depressed or feel a lack of energy. But in today's world, we live in self-imposed cages. We don't get out enough. We don't experience the force of nature. As a result, I think we are like animals in a zoo. We lack our connectiveness with the earth, a void that saps our vitality.

SS: When my mother died, I had an uncontrollable urge to hike the mountains that I love so much in the desert. But it was more than that. I wanted to go to the highest part of the mountain that I could get to. Maybe it was to be close to her, or maybe it was just to get away from all things of the earth and just **be.** Sometimes I go back up to that spot, just to feel her. So I know what you mean about the oneness. I remember on that day, it was the only way I could heal my heart—through nature.

PS: Why does everybody go to the beach? What is it about the beach that attracts people? It's the primal force of creation. We just need more of that. It is in our natures.

I went to the movies the other day; it's rare for me to enjoy a movie these days (I have kind of gotten stranger and stranger, as I'm getting older). But what I noticed were all the previews for all the different movies that I didn't come to see. The assault on the senses was amazing. That people need this . . . but if you're not going to go to the ocean or you're not going to go to the top of a mountain or you're not going to go into the woods or into the rain forest, the only alternative is this assault on the senses. It's the end result. Just as you were saying at the beginning of this interview, our health care system is not working. It is failing, and it's failing miserably, because more and more people are feeling sicker at a younger age. It's a sign of our times.

ss: Let's talk about the third supplement, which is just so natural—cinnamon. Are you talking about cinnamon that we buy at the grocery store to put into our cookies or sprinkle on oatmeal?

PS: Yes, the same one. If it's added to our diets, people would be a lot healthier.

ss: Tell me why.

PS: Compounds in cinnamon have been shown in research to significantly lower blood levels of glucose, triglycerides, and cholesterol—and may represent a treatment for diabetes, which is now the fifth deadliest disease in the United States, one that kills 210,000 people annually. A study sponsored by the

U.S. government looked into how different foods affected elevations in blood sugar—and produced an unusual finding. When people ate apple pie, their blood sugar stayed relatively normal, as opposed to spiking upward as you might expect. After all, apple pie is high in sugar.

The researchers found that the apple pie contained cinnamon and that cinnamon enhanced the metabolism of sugar in fat cells by a factor of twenty times. It normalized blood sugar.

Research also shows that there are constituents in cinnamon depending upon the species of cinnamon. There are two major species of cinnamon. There's one called verum, which is a true cinnamon, and the other is called aromaticum, or cassia. This species has a number of constituents that if you consume a lot, it might not be healthy for you. But at the dosage or serving size of 1 gram, it was found to be highly effective.

SS: Do you sell cinnamon supplements?

PS: We sell it in a very small capsule in the form of an extract, so it's very concentrated. One dose is equivalent to 1 gram of cinnamon, which is about a quarter of a teaspoon of cinnamon.

SS: So I could either take your supplement, or I could make it a point to use a quarter of a teaspoon of cinnamon in my cooking a day?

PS: Exactly.

SS: Now, how about coenzyme Q10?

PS: Coenzyme Q10 is a vitaminlike nutrient naturally produced by the body but available as a supplement. It is responsible for converting food, oxygen, and water into energy. The heart muscle contains highly concentrated amounts of coenzyme Q10 due to the high energy requirements of cells located there. Given supplementally, coenzyme Q10 may help reduce high blood pressure, treat heart disease, prevent and treat cancer, and provide general antiaging benefits.

SS: Is there any difference between taking coenzyme Q10 in capsules or as chewables?

PS: With my company, our whole philosophy has been to deliver nutrients in the form of food, so we make coenzyme Q10 in a cultured food form, but packaged in a capsule.

SS: Next on your list are omega-3 fats.

PS: Now considered essential in the diet, omega-3 fats, found most abundantly in fish, have a wealth of antiaging benefits. They may help prevent heart disease, block inflammation, fight weight gain, and alleviate depression. Besides fish, you can obtain these healthful fats from omega-3-rich eggs, flax, and walnuts.

SS: What about omega-3 supplements like fish oil?

PS: Fish oil capsules are an excellent source, especially if you don't like eating fish. I take 4 grams every day.

SS: The next supplement on your list is LycoPom, which is a combination of lycopene and pomegranate. From writing my own books, I know that lycopene is a powerful antioxidant found in cooked tomatoes.

PS: That is correct. Lycopene is also found in a number of herbs, including saffron and rosehips. What I found to be quite remarkable is that of all the risk factors for prostate cancer, the number one risk factor (according to a Harvard study) was a lycopene deficit. Also, a shortfall of lycopene is a significant factor for cardiovascular disease among women, according to other research. So lycopene is one of these nutrients that I think is really, really important.

The other ingredient is pomegranate. It is a simple fruit. There is an antioxidant test gaining a lot of popularity called ORAC, which stands for oxygen radical absorbance capacity. The ORAC is being considered a model to evaluate the free radical scavenging capability of a food. Compared to wine, green tea, tomatoes, and all the foods that are considered to be potent antioxidative foods, pomegranate rated among the highest of all of them. More so, as I said, than wine or green tea. It has five times the ability of vitamin E to inhibit the oxidation of low-density lipoproteins. Pomegranate, again, is one of these kinds of wonderful foods. There are a number of companies that sell pomegranate juice. That could be very beneficial for cardiovascular health.

SS: How much pomegranate juice would you need to drink a day, a glass, two glasses, to get the benefits?

PS: One glass, or eight ounces. It is also available

in supplement form. In LycoPom, you get lycopene, plus a supplemental dosage of pomegranate that is equivalent to fifteen pomegranates, so you can get a fairly effective therapeutic amount in a relatively small capsule.

SS: Let's talk about Zyflamend.

PS: Zyflamend is a combination of herbs that include turmeric and curcumin. Curcumin is actually an extract of turmeric, which is the spice that gives curry its color and flavor. Both herbs are known primarily as anti-inflammatory herbs. But they have other well-researched properties. Research suggests that they are protective against heart disease, diabetes, even cancer.

Zyflamend also contains green tea, which is a powerful antioxidant. Studies show that populations that consume the largest amounts of green tea happen to also have the best overall health. We are now also doing research with Zyflamend at the Cleveland Clinic, at Columbia University, and at MD Anderson Cancer Center.

SS: So could you not get the same effects by cooking with it?

PS: No. When you're cooking with these herbs, all their oils are extracted and the biologically active compounds are lost.

SS: You've used the term **oxidation,** a word most people have heard but don't really understand. What does it mean, and why should we be concerned about oxidation?

PS: I was asked that same question when my daughter was in elementary school. To explain oxidation, I peeled an apple and asked the kids, "What's going to happen now that I've removed the skin from the apple?" All the kids chirped up, "It's going to turn brown."

Of course, they were right. The brown discoloration was a sign of oxidation—oxygen hitting a substance and spoiling it. The same thing happens in our bodies. I showed the kids that I could preserve what's inside the apple by keeping the order, the integrity, the synchrony, of those nutrients intact. So when you look at a food like ginger, or garlic, and you leave them out, they'll be good for a couple of months on your shelf because they have a certain organization, a certain intelligence, which is very profound.

When you take those things into your body, you're taking in organization and integrity, which then traps oxidation. We can only live without food for a couple of weeks at most. We can go without water for maybe a day or two, but it is oxygen that is our key nutrient. Proper management of oxygen is the key to longevity.

SS: Thus **oxygenation!**

PS: The beauty of the herbs that are in Zyflamend is that they are all very powerful free radical scavengers, all of them. Zyflamend delivers green tea also, which is a wonderful food, and virtually every research study that comes out indicates that populations that consume the largest amounts of green tea are the ones that have the best overall health. To me, the World Health Organization kind of said it all when they listed Japan as being the number one country in the world with healthy life expectancy.

One of the other herbs we included in the formulation is rosemary. A number of years ago, I was formulating a bar. To make the bar the most stable, the bar formulators told me I had to add one-tenth of 1 percent of a rosemary extract. I said, "My God, that's such a small amount! It will really have that kind of effect on a bar? It's going to give me an extra six months shelf life on the bar and it's not going to degrade?" Then it came to me: Shouldn't rosemary be able to do it for a human body as well?

I looked at Rutgers and other prestigious universities that were doing research on rosemary, and I found that it does have self-protective effects that are quite profound.

Again, the right chosen herbs can have profound antioxygen effects. And, Suzanne, the whole inflammation process is at the root of Alzheimer's disease, diabetes, cancer, heart disease, and autoimmune disorders. All of these diseases have at their root oxidative stress, which is poorly managed utilization of oxygen. The beauty of these herbs is that they help the body manage oxygen so it doesn't cause these premature aging processes.

SS: Fantastic.

PS: Columbia University is constantly doing research, and so is MD Anderson on cancer. They're finding dramatic effects at normalizing cell growth in terms of reminding cells what their missions are. A cell that loses its genetic integrity, by nature, should commit suicide in a process called apoptosis. However, when the body's systems lose some of their intelligence, cells lose this genetic programming to commit suicide. Instead, they undergo rapid and uncontrolled cellular growth, which we call cancer. The way to correct that is to infuse the cells and remind the cells of their innate intelligence.

The beauty of herbs like ginger, turmeric, green tea, and rosemary, which are in Zyflamend, is that they remind cells when they're not behaving themselves to undergo apoptosis.

Here is something amazing to hear: Keep in mind that MD Anderson is one of the leading facilities in the world in drug development for cancer treatment. The lead researcher there, Bob Newman, said that we pretty much are done with drug development. We've done everything that we can do. We've come up with the best chemicals that we can think of to kill cancer cells. We're done, it's over. The future of drug development is going to be in polypharmaceutical herbal development.

Newman says that we consider a drug for cancer to be effective if it can extend life by three months. Very few people talk about the quality of those three months. But people who are just flat-out brilliant say they have no doubt that herbs are the future. In the five thousand years that people have been using turmeric or ginger or green tea, how many fatalities have been reported from people taking too much turmeric? How sick do people get? So they get a little diarrhea or they have a little stomach upset. But their hair is not falling out, and they're not dying from the treatment. This is very exciting. The beauty of it is that you're seeing these very brilliant, different types of minds at work here, beginning to see the light of herbal medicine. It's just very, very promising.

SS: Which takes us to the reishi mushroom.

PS: Yes, it's almost mystical in nature. It is the number one medicine in traditional Chinese medical practice. This mushroom has been referred to as the mushroom of immortality. It contains constituents that lower cholesterol, regulate blood pressure, and boost the immune system by countering viruses and bacteria. There are hundreds of references on the immunologically active effects of the reishi mushroom. It works on virtually every system of the body.

SS: Is reishi mushroom something you buy in a capsule form?

PS: You can buy it in a capsule or in extract form. I was initially attracted to it because of its reputed effects on the nervous system. It strengthens memory and sharpens concentration. Interestingly, it was given to the Taoist monks of China to calm the mind and improve the value of meditation. To me, anything that I could use that could safely and effectively get me out of what is referred to as my "monkey mind" was very attractive to me.

SS: What's interesting to me about the supplements and herbs you've chosen if you were stranded on a desert island is that vitamin C isn't there. Nor are some of the newer ones like phosphatidylcholine. Where do you place those other supplements in terms of importance? Also, Alan and I take about thirty supplements a day. Do we take too many?

PS: Those are good questions. I try to apply common sense as much as I can. What I am enthusiastic about are herbal supplements because they're plants, foods that you should be able to get from your diet. If you were left with plant-based, herb-based supplements, you would probably be the healthiest.

Ultimately, I believe when our bodies come down with an infection, it's that the energy systems of the body just need a recalibration. I'm kind of a strange person with regard to coming down with flus or colds or whatever. I really believe they are a good thing, as long as they are happening not more than two or three times a year. I really do believe it's the way the body tunes itself up. One of the most important things the body can do to heal itself is to go through a periodic cleansing like that.

My dad was a physician and fifty-nine years old when he passed away. He used to be so excited that in ten years he'd never had an infection. I really believe he would have been better off had he had a number of infections. Infections can help fortify your immune system.

SS: Because of the inflammation?

PS: Yes. This issue reminds me of what Hippocrates used to say: "Give me a fever and I'll cure any disease." Once your body temperature gets raised, your immune system goes into a hyperactive wonderful mode. All those white blood cells start gobbling up anything that shouldn't be there. If you ever look at somebody after they go through a good fever, they look wonderful. Drinking fluids is very important when you're feverish. It helps you keep flushing.

SS: I was saying to my husband, Alan, the other day that he has a built-in health barometer in his head. He's an old soul, you know. He has always consumed enormous amounts of blueberries and enormous amounts of pomegranate juice and fruits. He eats lots of nuts, raw nuts, cashews, and almonds. He's always munching on things. It's interesting how he naturally gravitates to all that is proving to be so beneficial. When it's blueberry season, he'll just eat them by the case. So in a way, he listens to his body and what his body is asking for, and he goes and gets it.

PS: In some ways, Suzanne, I believe that people like yourself are facilitating, whether you're aware of this or not; you are part of a mission of humanity. You're part of a voice of consciousness for the better part of humanity. And you are . . .

SS: Using up energy.

PS: You are using up energy but you're also doing what you're called to do. You don't have to do this.

SS: Well, thank you. It's a privilege to deliver this information.

PS: When you're out in the world, your body is under enormous demand, and you have to breathe polluted air; more and more research is showing that polluted air ages you quite rapidly. Unless you use the appropriate measures, even though your mind is in wonderful shape, your body will show the wear and tear of the pollution.

SS: One last thing: I find what you're doing in your company so interesting. I find its values are in the right place. As someone who started this company, what was your mission? What were you trying to accomplish?

PS: Our company slogan at New Chapter is "Delivering the Wisdom of Nature." This is based upon our very deep belief that for every disease, there is a plant or a remedy that the divine force has offered.

SS: Thank you, Paul.

PAUL SCHULICK'S TOP FIVE ANTIAGING RECOMMENDATIONS

1. The eight best supplements to take for health and antiaging are selenium, rhodiola, cinnamon, coenzyme Q10, omega-3 fats, LycoPom (a formulation of lycopene, pomegranate, and cinnamon),

Zyflamend (a formulation that is a combination of ginger, turmeric, green tea, and rosemary) and reishi mushroom.

2. Omega-3 fats are important in the diet because they help prevent heart disease, block inflammation, fight weight gain, and alleviate depression. You can obtain these healthful fats from fish, fish oil supplements, omega-3-rich eggs, flax, and walnuts.

3. Pomegranate juice is among the best foods in terms of antioxidant content. A good practice is to drink one eight-ounce glass a day, or you can take supplements containing pomegranate extract.

4. Green tea is also high in antioxidants and beneficial compounds. Virtually every research study that comes out indicates that populations that consume the largest amounts of green tea are the ones that have the best overall health.

5. Herbs like ginger, turmeric, green tea, and rosemary help protect cells and make it possible to normalize cell growth to protect against cancer, which is characterized by uncontrolled cell growth.

CHAPTER 28

DR. RON ROTHENBERG: HUMAN GROWTH HORMONE, THYROID, AND MELATONIN

Dr. Ron Rothenberg is an antiaging specialist who has had several careers, from pediatrics to tropical medicine to emergency medicine and now full circle back to preventive medicine. Dr. Rothenberg was the tenth MD in the world to become fully board certified in antiaging medicine. He specializes in advanced preventive medicine, BHRT for men and women, and what has been called "the ultimate executive physical." Over one-third of his patients are physicians, and he has educated more than twenty thousand physicians in hormone optimization and antiaging, preventive, and integrative medicine. He is the founder of the California HealthSpan Institute in Encinitas, California, and director of the Menopause Institute in La Jolla, California. He is a full

clinical professor of family and preventive medicine at the University of California, San Diego, School of Medicine.

SS: How does a doctor go from the emergency room to antiaging medicine and the Menopause Institute?

RR: The emergency room is a great place for a doctor to get experience in the entire world of medicine. We deal with everything. We're not cardiothoracic surgeons, but if an emergency patient comes in with a knife in his heart and needs to have his chest cracked and heart sutured, we'll give it a try. It's all about saving lives. I was one of the first doctors in the country to be board certified as an emergency medicine specialist. It is interesting that like antiaging medicine and bioidentical hormone replacement today, years ago the prevailing idea in the medical community was that emergency medicine was not necessary. Well, thirty years later concepts change, and emergency medicine is definitely mainstream. But after a while you have to leave the emergency room or it will kill you. The hours are so long and the stress so intense that at some point you have to make a change.

It was my own journey. I'm sixty now, but at about fifty-two or so I was starting to feel my age—just a gradual decline. I was doing okay, still surfing and practicing medicine. But everything from memory to body composition to libido was a little bit off. So

I started looking into this on my own. At that time there were **Newsweek** articles on hormones and vitamins, but I still had the conventional doctor mind-set—oh, vitamins, expensive urine, ha-ha, what a big joke. Then I started reading the original medical literature to see what information there was that could make me healthier. I studied the benefits of limiting the high-glycemic-index carbohydrates and began a 40/30/30 Zone-type nutrition plan. I began to exercise regularly (surfing is great, but there are long spells with no waves) and combined resistance and aerobics. I began a regimen of vitamins and antioxidants. My hormone levels were measured, and when a deficiency was present, I began replacing my declining hormones with bioidentical ones. I began changing, mentally and physically. The other doctors in the hospital said, "What are you taking? We want some of that." But it's not just "taking a pill"—it's a whole lifestyle based upon nutrition, exercise, stress reduction, and supplements. From there, I developed an antiaging medical practice. It's interesting that now about a third of my patients are physicians. And if you count nurses, vets, and other health care people, it's about half.

SS: What is the mission of your institute and your menopause clinic?

RR: The mission of the California HealthSpan Institute is to provide ultimate state-of-the-art preventive and antiaging medicine. We spend almost all day with a new patient designing customized plans of nutrition, exercise, stress reduction, vitamins and neutraceuticals, and bioidentical hormone replacement when needed in men and women. We continually fine-tune the programs based upon our patients' needs and new medical research.

The mission of the Menopause Institute is to provide accessible, cost-effective bioidentical hormone replacement therapy for women. It is specifically priced so that anyone can afford it. At the moment, women who need bioidentical hormones are not usually covered by their insurance and certainly not by their HMOs. I didn't want to only have an "elite" practice that provided advanced quality health care. I realized that women who need hormone replacement have to have it, and I wanted to do something that would make it affordable, personal, and advanced.

Every week at least one or two people, unprompted, say, "This is the best I have felt in as long as I can remember." That's what I wanted to accomplish when I went into medicine.

SS: Let's talk about human growth hormone. There's been so much controversy.

RR: I've been studying this in depth for eight or nine years.

SS: Can you dispel the fear of HGH? We make human growth hormone until we're about twenty years old, and then it starts declining.

RR: Right. We do make some HGH all our lives. It peaks in the teenage years (fourteen to eighteen) or so. Then it stays stable from, say, twenty to thirty. Somewhere in the mid-forties, the curve takes a sharp dive south. That's called somatopause. Every hormone has a "pause" . . . menopause, andropause, and so forth, but HGH is at its highest level in our youth when we are healthiest and strongest, with the least disease risk and the least cancer risk.

SS: Who should take HGH?

RR: You would only want to take it to treat a deficiency disease, meaning, "Are you at present deficient, do you have adult growth hormone deficiency?" When we treat with HGH, we are treating adult growth hormone deficiency, which is a known disease entity. We never treat with HGH for sports performance, bodybuilding, aesthetics, or antiaging. Everyone is on his or her own curve, but the deficiency affects most of us sooner or later. An HGH deficiency affects brain functions, since HGH is brain food. HGH is a big molecule, with 191 amino acids, but there's an active mechanism that imports it into the brain through the blood-brain barrier. All brains cells need HGH and IGF-1. IGF-1 is produced by the liver as a response to HGH.

SS: Isn't it a measure in older people that the better the brain function, the higher the growth hormone level?

RR: Correct. The higher the HGH and IGF-1, the better the brain. We need it for our immune system. That is what guards us against the cruel world. Growth hormone is a constant stimulus to produce

T-cells and B-cells (lymphatic cells that filter out invading organisms) and make the immune system work. Then there's body composition—more bone and muscle, less fat; HGH plays a role there. Growth hormone is important for heart function. Growth hormone reverses atherosclerosis in the carotid arteries. Then there is quality of life, which is a general term and hard to measure scientifically, but surveys show that keeping growth hormone levels balanced would save lives and give a better quality of life. Adults with growth hormone deficiency are happier and healthier when treated. HGH replacement is a powerful tool to reverse the destructive course of growth hormone deficiency.

SS: There's a lot of controversy about HGH because there haven't been a lot of long-term studies on this hormone. Many researchers and doctors are worried that it promotes cancer growth.

RR: Try typing "growth hormone" into pubmed .com and you'll get around 52,709 articles. It is one of the most studied compounds in medicine. There have been children on growth hormone who have been followed for twenty years at this point, so there are very long-term studies. If you look at the endocrinology literature, I could pull more than thirty studies, and the conclusions are the same. The risk of cancer, either recurrent cancer or new cancer, is not greater with growth hormone replacement therapy.

SS: Do you think growth hormone is as essential to replace as all of the other hormones?

RR: Well, there's a hierarchy. I mean, growth hormone injections are expensive, so sometimes people have to draw the line. I would start with the basics first. Assess the need for and treat deficiency of estrogen, progesterone, and testosterone in women and testosterone in men. Assess the needs for thyroid and DHEA. Look for adrenal fatigue. Once again, not everyone needs growth hormone replacement therapy.

SS: Do you think in time the price will go down?

RR: I hope in the future it will cost the same as insulin injections, which are relatively inexpensive. This therapy can help people with HGH deficiency in so many ways. There is a study in Denmark, patients over seventy-five years of age given growth hormone on the day of a hip fracture, treated for a couple of months, and 95 percent return to their former lifestyle. It's incredible.

SS: Is there any age where it would be dangerous to take HGH?

RR: Again, growth hormone replacement therapy should be used only to treat either pediatric or adult growth hormone deficiency. It should not be prescribed if not needed. I've had Olympic athletes come to me asking for HGH before the last Olympics. This use is not appropriate on many levels. I wouldn't give it to someone who doesn't need it to treat a deficiency disease. Young adults would not be treated unless there was serious pituitary disease. No one is too old to treat with HGH for growth hormone deficiency. You could be diabetic and treat obesity-related diabetes with lifestyle coaching and growth hormone. It is an absolutely amazing way to treat diabetes in patients with growth hormone deficiency.

The theoretical concern of administering HGH is that it sounds as though growth hormone makes things grow, so if there is a cancer hiding somewhere, the thinking is that it might grow. But extensive years of study have shown that not to be the case, that this theoretical risk is nonexistent. Teenagers have sky-high growth hormone levels but have relatively low rates of cancer. You need growth hormone for cellular replication, so if you don't have any HGH left, you are not going to be in very good shape on a physiological level. As your growth hormone increases, your IGF-1 made by the liver increases. Then a hormone and a carrier protein called IGF binding protein 3 (IGFBP-3) increases. This IGFBP-3 is an anticancer hormone.

Now, HGH doesn't make you immortal. Could someone on growth hormone replacement therapy get cancer? Of course. Otherwise, it would be too good to be true. The medical literature discusses the theory of treating cancer patients with growth hormone in terms of immune system stimulation and better quality of life.

On the HGH package insert it says not to use it with an active malignancy. There's an extensive discussion of this issue by the Growth Hormone Research Society published in the **Journal of Clinical Endocrinology.** The Growth Hormone Research Society concludes that the statement about not using HGH in active malignancy is not based upon any data and should be removed.

SS: So this was just a presumption?

RR: Right. This was the theory like the old theories on testosterone. It was thought that because men have more heart attacks than premenopausal women, testosterone must be the cause. Turns out that it is just the opposite. Testosterone prevents heart attacks in men.

SS: Would HGH accelerate weight loss?

RR: Yes. Women in the studies done at Johns Hopkins lost 14 percent of their fat mass, and with men it's even more dramatic. You see, HGH is lipolytic, meaning it dissolves fat.

SS: It dissolves fat. That's enough right there to make people run out and get this stuff.

RR: Yes, but then you need the correct lifestyle—here's the other side of it. If you consume unlimited carbohydrates, things could get worse with HGH. You could become more insulin-resistant, store more fat, and get closer to diabetes. You've got to have the right lifestyle with it for it to work. And you need the deficiency in the first place as determined by a physician with experience in the field.

ss: But if you're willing to exercise, eat real food, good food, sleep, and then add HGH to this regimen, you're ahead of the game, wouldn't you say?

RR: Oh, very much so, but as I continue to stress, only if you need it, only if you have adult growth hormone deficiency.

ss: So, used properly, HGH is a wonderful addition to your hormone supplementation?

RR: Yes, this is a hormone that sets the background vibration of life. Some things about it are subtle. It's not like you get a shot of it and, wow, what a rush. After you have been taking HGH replacement for years, you just live your life. You don't even notice the feeling because you're living on a much higher level, mentally, physically, and emotionally.

ss: When a woman comes into your clinic for the basic sex hormones like estrogen, progesterone, or testosterone, would HGH would be a next step?

RR: It might be. Other basic hormones to evaluate include DHEA and thyroid. We should determine if HGH is needed on the basis of history, physical exam, and labwork.

ss: When you give someone HGH, do you give them a blood test first? Or do you just presume by their age and by looking at them that they are deficient?

RR: We always get blood tests and sometimes twenty-four-hour urine tests. Like so much in medicine, a diagnosis is on the basis of clinical medicine, history, and physical combined with lab. The older someone is and the lower the IGF-1 test is, the more likely it is that he or she has adult growth hormone deficiency. Also, the "phenotype," which is the physical appearance, can give you a clue. For example, someone whose skin is droopy and saggy, who has more body fat and less energy, is more likely to have HGH deficiency.

There are aesthetic effects to treating HGH deficiency. More collagen is grown under the skin, so it can eliminate fine lines and wrinkles improve. There is sometimes reversal of thinning hair and graying hair.

SS: There's a lot of discrepancy on how to administer HGH. Some doctors are very nervous about giving it more than once a week. That doesn't make sense to me.

RR: Would you treat diabetes one day a week? Of course not. People will not get the benefits injecting once a week. You administer it every day and as early in the morning as possible, or you can take it before you go to bed at night because your body normally produces HGH in your sleep.

HGH is used to treat a deficiency disease. You're replacing an absent hormone. If a person is to be healthy and you don't have enough at fifty, you're not going to start magically making more at sixty. Once the well runs dry, the well is dry. If you think you're treating a deficiency disease, then you do it every day. You don't give them a weekend off.

SS: What is the lowest dose you give of HGH?

RR: I keep it simple. I usually start treatment at 0.2 mg a day, and then after about a month, if there are no side effects, go up to 0.4 mg a day. Most men end up in that range. After another month in most women, I will increase to 0.6 mg a day. Women need more than men, and most women will end up at 0.6 mg a day. Some patients may have side effects on those doses, and I treat them with as little as 0.1 mg a day.

SS: What are the side effects of HGH?

RR: The four possible side effects of growth hormone replacement therapy are edema [ankle swelling], numb and tingly fingers, aching joints, and insulin resistance getting worse, not better. If a side effect develops, you decrease the dose or stop for a few days. If you stop the HGH replacement, the side effects disappear.

By the way, if a woman is on oral estrogen (which she shouldn't be on anyway because it's very inflammatory), it's not even worth trying growth hormone. Estrogens given as a skin cream or gel are fine.

SS: Why is that?

RR: Oral estrogens stop liver production of IGF-1, which is an important component of the growth hormone effect. Even with endogenous estrogens in a premenopausal woman, or transdermal estrogens in a woman receiving the right kind of bioidentical hormone replacement therapy, HGH works, but not as effectively as it does with men. I find with some patients I have to fine-tune the HGH dose because of the side effects I just mentioned.

SS: What is the dose that you take?

RR: I'm on 0.4 mg per day.

SS: And how do you feel?

RR: I feel great. I mean, I don't notice it anymore. At first, there was a dramatic change in energy and quality of life. I've been doing it for eight years. So it's not like, wow, here comes the growth hormone. I feel great, even though my lifestyle is not as good as it should be. I should exercise more, and my kids sometimes say, "What a hypocrite for a nutrition expert guy! You ate all the Ben and Jerry's."

SS: Well, we're all human. The messenger doesn't always live the message. I feel you have to give yourself a little wiggle room.

RR: Right. So I could do better, but I know I feel better. I'm operating on a healthier and a higher level mentally and physically than I was eight years ago.

SS: You do have great vitality and youth about you. How young would you start someone on HGH?

RR: It is very individual. We are assessing whether the patient has adult growth hormone deficiency. This would be extremely unlikely for someone in their thirties, possible in their forties, and more likely in their fifties and sixties. I would never prescribe it for bodybuilding, looking good, or athletic performance. But if there is a deficiency in patients who are in their forties or fifties, why wait for those patients to fall apart?

SS: So using IGF as a measurement, when the levels come back is there any level that is alarming?

RR: If someone has acromegaly, which is a condition of growth hormone excess from a tumor of the pituitary, the level could be alarming. That is the Andre the Giant look. Sometimes people who don't understand HGH fear that you could get acromegaly from growth hormone replacement for adult growth hormone deficiency. I have never seen that happen with proper treatment and monitoring. It is possible, however, when HGH is bought without a physician in the loop and used for bodybuilding or sports performance. Sometimes huge doses are taken in this abuse setting—ten times higher than the correct treatment dose. So abuse could be dangerous, but that is completely different from appropriate medical treatment.

SS: So is that what the controversy is about regarding HGH, because certain athletes abuse this hormone?

RR: Yes. HGH is not allowed to be used in professional or amateur sports, so use in that setting is cheating. Also, huge abusive doses are sometimes taken, and the athletes are usually young and do not have adult growth hormone deficiency. There is neither medical supervision nor testing.

SS: And what could that do to them?

RR: Anything bought illegally is dangerous. You don't know the effects because it's not regulated. You don't know what's in the bottle. I mentioned acromegaly before. There's too much skeletal growth signal. Jaws and hands get bigger. Teeth don't match anymore. It creates a weird look when abused, and that is not healthy. This condition will create a lot of medical problems, and with this kind of increased level, there might be a risk of certain cancers. Low growth hormone people (which is a pituitary insufficiency) have much higher cancer rates.

SS: Interesting. Why is that?

RR: My educated guess is because you need growth hormones for your immune system to get rid of cancer.

SS: Let's talk about thyroid.

RR: Great. I love to talk about thyroid because so many people can be helped by thyroid optimization, and in my opinion, so many people are not treated or are undertreated for hypothyroidism.

The TSH is a number that's traditionally used to look at thyroid. The pituitary gland tells the thyroid to make some thyroid by producing TSH. It's an indirect signal. Over the years that I've been in medicine, what has been considered normal has gone from 10 to 5 to 2.5 to 2.1 in conventional endocrinology. The optimal value is probably lower. But this wasn't looking at the right hormone. This is looking at the signal to make thyroid. There are two thyroid hormones to consider: T4 and T3. T3 is the active hormone, and T4 is the prohormone. Your body has to change T4 to T3. So ideally you have to measure T3, and usually that hasn't been done. If you don't do that, you really don't know their active hormone level. Traditionally, we were taught in medicine that all you need is T4 to treat hypothyroidism. This may be pharmaceutical company propaganda, since there are different brands that contain only T4, like Synthroid or Levoxyl. But that's not even the active hormone. Under times of stress, mental stress, physical stress, trying to lose weight with dieting, illnesses, and anxiety, you stop converting the T4 to T3. It's a method of us going into hibernation. When times get stressful, there is a mechanism for shutting off the thyroid. If there's no food, you'll survive until you get some. We are looking at the wrong lab test if we just look at TSH. We're treating with the wrong drug if we just use T4. A better way to treat patients is with a mixture of T4 and T3, like Armour thyroid or a compounded equivalent. Armour thyroid is a porcine (pig) product, but unlike horse estrogen (Premarin), porcine thyroid is bioidentical to human.

SS: What is thyroxine—where is that from?

RR: Thyroxine is T4. Thyroxine, Synthroid, and T4 are all the same thing. It is synthetically made, and that is okay. It is bioidentical, but you need the other thyroid hormone, T3, to go with it. So we can have the wrong tests, the wrong drug, even though sometimes the tests might look normal. You can tell by the patient's symptoms that they are screaming, I'm hypothyroid! Their hair is falling out, they can't lose weight with exercise, they're losing the outer third of their eyebrows, their hands and feet are freezing, they're constipated, there's no energy in the afternoon, they can't think. There's a terrific British book called **Your Thyroid and How to Keep It Healthy** [by Dr. Barry Durrant-Peatfield]. The scandal is that people aren't being treated properly. And hypothyroidism has been drastically increasing in society.

SS: Why?

RR: First, people are kept alive longer than ever before. At the turn of the century, if a baby was hypothyroid, it wouldn't have survived chicken pox or any of the diseases we no longer worry about because we now have infant vaccines and better ways to keep people healthy. Hypothyroid people died from infectious diseases such as tuberculosis.

Second, I think, as hypothyroidism increases, hypothyroid men and women are attracted to each other. They both have the same slow lifestyle, and guess what? They reproduce. So now we've got even more hypothyroidism.

SS: So if a woman's or a man's thyroid is low, what is the remedy for that?

RR: First you look at lifestyle. Then micronutrition. Is there adequate selenium and iodine in the diet and supplements? Sometimes just optimizing these minerals can improve thyroid function. Iodine deficiency is rare here in San Diego, where we eat a lot of fish. I am an avid surfer (not a great surfer), so it's hard for me sitting out there on the water, chewing on kelp, to remember that people in the goiter belt in Michigan don't get any iodine. Many people don't even get iodized salt since they are advised to follow a low-salt diet. But most people need iodine. When nutritional and functional treatments do not solve the problem, I treat the patient with a combination of T3 and T4. Most of the time, a patient goes to the doctor, and the doctor treats hypothyroidism with only T4, or thyroxine. As I mentioned earlier, patients feel better, think better, and have a better quality of life on the combination. We follow up with blood and urine lab tests. We make sure there are no side effects; we confirm there is no bone loss or irregular heartbeats. Then we ask the all-important question, "How do you feel?" The most important part of medicine is clinical, not high-tech.

SS: Let's talk about the hormone melatonin and using melatonin supplements.

RR: That's a good way to sleep.

SS: Because that's a natural, normal sleep?

RR: Yes. That's the signal to our brain that the sun has gone down. You see, the retina is an outgrowth of the brain. Light shines on the retina, which suppresses melatonin production. Lights off, and melatonin is produced. Melatonin is a very powerful antioxidant, anticancer hormone. So yes, this is a supplement that helps people sleep. And it's very safe; there's no such thing as an overdose on it.

SS: Well then, shouldn't that be a part of the

whole regimen for aging people? Because everyone I speak with has trouble sleeping from middle age on.

RR: Absolutely, as we age, melatonin production decreases dramatically.

SS: So shouldn't melatonin be automatically supplemented? And is some melatonin better than others?

RR: I think so, because almost everybody feels good on melatonin. Some of my patients tell me they have vivid dreams, which is cool, if you like that. But it can be scary to some people, for whatever reason, so not everyone feels right on it. But you can adjust the dose. Sometimes less is more. Just a tiny dose is all someone needs, say, 0.25 mg. Others need 3 or 6 mg in a time-release form.

SS: Is it dangerous to take too much?

RR: No. There are some studies relative to cancer treatment where they give 700 mg along with conventional chemo and radiation, and the patients have a better outcome.

SS: Can you get melatonin at a health food store?

RR: Yes, you can get it at a health food store, and it's probably the real thing. It's not exact milligrams as getting it from a compounding pharmacy, however.

SS: Is a prescription necessary?

RR: Hormones from a compounding pharmacy require a prescription. It's odd that only in the United States can you purchase melatonin over the counter. Same for DHEA, which is weird, because it's not a vitamin, it's a hormone. In Canada, you can't get DHEA and melatonin at all.

SS: I think melatonin has been the forgotten hormone.

RR: In the animal world, melatonin will increase animals' life span and health span. You give mice melatonin every day (because they're nocturnal), and they live 50 percent longer.

SS: Is that because they're sleeping well?

RR: Sleeping well and the antioxidant effect of quenching free radicals that can damage DNA.

SS: I was reading in **New York** magazine recently about Bill Clinton. In the last year since his heart problems, we've all noticed that he looks more fragile. Now, being president of the United States has got to be probably the most stressful job; and then there was the whole Monica thing. So we can assume this stress has blunted his hormone production. In this article, it mentions that he wears out his colleagues because they have to stay up playing cards with him until 3:00 and 4:00 in the morning. The guy never sleeps; he goes to bed at 4:00 a.m., and then he's back up again at 6:30 or 7:00. As a doctor, what do you think when you hear this?

RR: Bad for the former president in terms of premature aging. He apparently has cardiovascular disease, since he had a bypass operation. The major factor in cardiovascular disease and other diseases of aging appears to be inflammation. Lack of sleep and lack of healthy lifestyle can increase inflammation and cause premature aging.

SS: They make fun of President Bush going to bed so early, but whenever I hear this I think that's a good example. He goes to bed early, and he takes vacations. There is something to learn from that.

RR: And he rides his mountain bike around the ranch. When you look at him, he looks healthy.

SS: He really does. He doesn't drink, he doesn't smoke, he goes to bed early, he takes a vacation, and he gets mocked for that, but I feel it's a good example. In Europe vacations are considered as important as work. In this country, that seems weird.

What do you see in the future of antiaging medicine?

RR: The next generation of doctors is already hungry for this information. It's all right there in the regular medical research. This isn't some alternative medicine. This is out of the **New England Journal of Medicine,** in **Circulation,** in the **Journal of Clinical Endocrinology.** As physicians, we have got to find the articles that relate to what we're interested in and then read and absorb them.

SS: So you're hopeful?

RR: Yes, I'm more than hopeful. There has been a change happening in just the last nine or ten years. I realize this when other physicians are referring patients to me for hormone optimization. Or urologists are saying to me, "Well, okay, you can put the guy on testosterone, and I'll follow him with you." Men and women can live long, healthy lives if we take advantage of the newest information. I see it every day in my practice, and it's a great feeling as a physician to see these improvements in my patients. It makes all the hard work worth it.

SS: Thank you so much for your time.

RR: You're welcome. Thank you for allowing me to share my passion for this field of medicine with you.

DR. ROTHENBERG'S TOP FIVE ANTIAGING RECOMMENDATIONS

1. You would want to take HGH only to treat a deficiency disease, such as adult growth hormone deficiency, which is a known disease entity. I usually start treatment at 0.2 mg a day, and then after about a month, if there are no side effects, go up to 0.4 mg a day. Most men end up in that range. After another month in most women, I will increase to 0.6 mg a day.

2. Even though you might take HGH to help you control your weight, you must still follow a healthy diet and an exercise program. You've got to have the right lifestyle with it for HGH to work.

3. When someone has a low thyroid, I'll start him or her on Armour thyroid. If there's a philosophical or religious objection since Armour is derived from pigs, I'll have a compounding pharmacy make up an individually tailored mixture of T3 and T4. Then I wait to see how the patient feels.

4. Sleep is a huge component of antiaging. Sleep and growth go together, meaning you make growth hormones only in deep sleep. But if sleep is poor, people today take a sleeping pill, which is **not sleep.** It's simply a suspended state, and none of the healing hormones are doing their work.

5. Taking melatonin is a great way to help with sleep, plus it is a potent antioxidant. You can adjust your dose. Sometimes less is more; just a tiny dose is all someone needs, .25 mg. Others need 3 or 6 mg, perhaps in a time-release form.

CHAPTER 29

YOGA AND EXERCISE

For years, I have been getting the message "You should do yoga." It was said to me by my doctor, by my friends, by overhearing something on television, in magazine articles—I was even left a gift certificate on my front gate to "join them at the local yoga center for a complimentary free trial class." I was deaf and blind and resistant, probably because it was coming at me too hard and strong, and since I'm stubborn, probably because it wasn't my idea.

It wasn't until a year ago Thanksgiving that my son, Bruce, organized a yoga instructor to come to the family compound in the desert as a gift. That way all of us could take yoga classes together for the week. Well, I would never turn down Bruce for anything, and the chance to do any activity with the family is always a thrill.

To my surprise I took to it from the very first class. The breathing and stretching felt better than any form of exercise I had ever done before. There was a peacefulness, beauty, and elegance to it, and I loved the focus and concentration. I opened my eyes at one point, and the sky looked more blue; **vivid** is the word I'd use to describe it. The birds were singing more melodically, the bees were "bee-ing." I was one with nature, and something about it all felt so . . . right.

That experience alone was enough to convert me to this ancient form of exercise. After the family left to go back home to their own lives, I continued with our yoga teacher, and to my great surprise and delight, so did my husband, Alan. Now we had this great activity to do together three or four mornings a week.

Unlike other forms of exercise that I have tried over the years, yoga made me look forward to the alarm going off in the mornings. Instead of dreading the next hour, I found myself leaping out of bed to get up, go outside, breathe in the fresh air, and begin the luxurious stretching that is such a part of yoga.

I had always noticed that our cat, Chrissy Snow (I know, I know), a beautiful white Persian, woke up every day of her life and stretched and scratched and stretched some more. Nature knows. Now I was taking part in this ritual of nature, and my body loved it.

I have always exercised. I've had trainers come to my house for years. But there have always been pockets of fat here and there on my body that just wouldn't go away no matter how hard I worked out. It was as if a couple of pieces of pie had settled right on the back top of my hips, like two pie shelves. Twisting, crunching, and sit-ups did nothing for these shelves . . . and they were laughing at me. Then the skin on my back started to drape, like a curtain, starting just about at the bra line. I lifted weights and did push-ups and not much happened; the curtains remained, flapping and waving. But with yoga, in a few weeks I began to see results such as I had never experienced before. The breath (it is all about the breath) would seep down into those fatty areas with each stretch and inhale; as I exhaled the breath would melt the fat. Literally, in a few months these problem areas were tighter, smaller, and smoother. I have not seen my hips, thighs, and back look this good in years. The big surprise is that I so loved the art and form of yoga that I stopped thinking of it as a means to improve my figure outwardly. I did it because my body and soul were wanting it, needing it. It was natural and felt as though my body had been looking for this outlet all my life. I took to yoga because it made me feel centered and in touch with my "self" and nature; the exciting result was a long, lean, flexible body.

For the first time I feel that I have found a form of daily exercise that I will do my entire life. I can't see myself ever stopping. It is the one form of exercise that has no age barriers. It is not competitive; even my husband and I are not looking over our shoulders to check each other out. If you do that, you lose concentration, and concentration is required to hold these poses.

I am now two years into yoga. I consider myself a beginner, and that is the exciting part. Every time my body is able to move forward to another pose that in the beginning felt impossible, I feel a personal triumph. I am now doing back bends . . . imagine being so flexible that I can do a back bend at sixty! Who would have thought? Between hormone replacement, which has kept my bones intact, and yoga, I can only imagine (and look forward to) what my body will allow me to do by year three. I am getting close to doing a handstand without my instructor standing guard—that amazes me.

So now I am going to do for you what so many tried to do for me for many years while I remained deaf to it. Try yoga. Try it. Before long, you will be waxing poetic as I am.

Yoga is great for cardio as well. Last summer, I debuted my one-woman show on Broadway. It was highly energetic; I ran back and forth from one end of the stage to the other and leaped and danced and sang and talked for ninety minutes each night, and the only form of exercise I did to get in shape was yoga. I was never out of breath onstage. Truly remarkable. My singing was better than ever before because now I used my yoga breath to pull the oxygen from the lowest part of my diaphragm. Singing became effortless.

The primary aim of yoga is to restore the mind to simplicity and peace. Yoga frees you from confusion and stress. Other forms of exercise strain muscles and bones, but yoga rejuvenates the body. By restoring the body, yoga frees the mind from the negative feelings caused by the fast pace of our modern lives. We are all going a mile a minute. We have lists in our heads, we walk down the street with cell phones, multitasking. We are a generation of superwomen and supermen, and it is making us sick. We have to find something to counterbalance the insanity, and for me yoga is the answer.

"Yoga is a light which, once lit, will never dim. The better your practice, the brighter the flame," said B. K. S. Iyengar, a yoga master.

I agree. Once the light of yoga was lit within me, I knew I would do this forever. It is now a part of me. I feel better, lighter, calmer . . . thinner (now you're listening). After a yoga session, my mind becomes tranquil. Regular practice helps you face the turmoil of life. Our bodies are our temples. We need to care for them, and yoga keeps not only your body, but also your mind, healthy and active.

Yoga can heal parts of our bodies that have been injured, traumatized, or simply ignored and neglected. Western medicine can accelerate the healing process but all too often cannot tackle the source of the problem. Yoga is wonderful for ailments because it stimulates injured parts of the body by increasing the blood supply to those areas. The body is a complex piece of machinery, a finely connected network of muscles, joints, nerves, veins, arteries, and capillaries. The science of yoga classifies ailments that afflict the body and mind into three basic categories:

- self-inflicted ailments, caused by neglect or abuse of the body
- congenital ailments, present from birth
- ailments caused by the imbalance of any of the five elements of ether, air, fire, water, and earth in our system

Yoga can treat all three categories, but it requires a commitment to the treatment.

Yoga is good for people with cold extremities, which is caused by a slowdown in circulation when blood collects in the torso and fails to correctly reach the extremities. It gives rise to ailments of the chest and of the intestinal and abdominal organs. It is often the result of a sluggish thyroid, stress, or nervousness. Headstands and/or shoulder stands are great for the thyroid because the reverse position allows the blood to flow down and flush the thyroid with fresh blood.

Yoga is great for the heart and circulation, varicose veins, high blood pressure, low blood pressure, blocked arteries, angina, heart attack, colds, breathlessness, sinusitis, bronchitis, asthma, indigestion, acidity, and constipation.

I don't know anyone over the age of fifty who isn't troubled by constipation at some time or another.

For some it is chronic and ongoing. Yoga is magical in its alleviation of constipation. After a series of yoga twists and positions, relief is immediate. This alone makes yoga worthwhile.

Yoga is also great for diarrhea, irritable bowel syndrome, duodenal ulcers, gastric ulcers, ulcerative colitis, incontinence, obesity, diabetes, low immune system, physical fatigue, muscle cramps, lower, middle, and upper backache, osteoarthritis, skin conditions and skin health, the brain and nervous systems, the mind and emotions, women's health, men's health, and the balancing of the hormonal system. Need I say more? And you'll get thin and flexible.

In the next chapter, you'll read about what my yoga instructor, Julie Carmen, has to say about yoga.

CHAPTER 30
JULIE CARMEN: YOGA

Julie Carmen and I met filming a movie together in Tucson, Arizona. Several years later, we found ourselves virtually as neighbors living in Malibu, California. It seemed serendipitous that we would find each other again. I enjoy Julie's technique; she has studied with several of the great yogi masters, and her approach is gentle yet informative. She explains each position thoroughly and motivates us to want to do the positions perfectly. She is a natural teacher, and I think you will get turned on to yoga after reading her interview, even if you have never thought about it.

SS: Thank you for your time. Through you as my teacher, I have come to love my yoga practice, but for those who have no idea of what to expect, walk me through the reasons why one would want to do yoga.

JC: Yoga "tunes the instrument"—in other words, your body. I couldn't imagine if, for instance, I was in an orchestra and played the violin, that I would not tune my instrument before playing. Each day, whether we're going off to a stressful job, or being with children, or perhaps struggling with a personal illness, you can deal with your day more effectively if your body has been tuned.

SS: Yes, but most people are interested in an exercise program because they want to get their bodies in shape. Tuning the instrument comes afterward because (as I now know) you get turned on by what yoga does to your body. You see results like never before.

JC: Yes. Yoga has been practiced for more than five thousand years, so it's a time-honored system. Yoga aligns the joints into their natural, healthy posture, so that in a short period of time, muscle groups develop and maintain that alignment with a beautiful sculpting. With a balanced yoga practice, you'll notice that there is definition in your glutes. Your stomach becomes more scooped; there's more of a waistline, and your torso elongates so that your rib cage lifts out of your pelvis. Yoga helps you develop the muscle strength to be able to maintain that lift, so whether you're sitting in the car or at a desk or computer, your waist is still long.

There are a lot of spine stability exercises in yoga. It really depends upon what the teacher teaches, but those spine-stabilizing postures help keep length in the waistline, and this also increases digestion and respiration so that the lungs aren't sitting right on the stomach. There's some space in there, so you can actually take a deep breath and digest more efficiently.

Also, the neck is held long through yoga practice, and that gives a lifted feeling. A youthful look is about posture. A twenty-year-old who has been carrying a backpack and sitting over a Game Boy or video games can look older than his years just because his posture has collapsed.

SS: That's so true. Look at elderly people. My father-in-law had beautiful posture and walked erect and straight at the age of ninety-two. He always seemed so much younger than his years. Yet an elderly person who is hunched over looks frail and fragile.

JC: Absolutely. You see a sixty-year-old with magnificent posture and say, "Wow! What's their secret?" The secret is posture, and yoga is famous for developing magnificent posture.

SS: Frankly, Julie, I don't think sixty is "old" (laugh), seeing how that is my age!

JC: You are so right! Sorry! It's difficult to equate that age with you. It used to be deemed "old."

SS: But no more! I worked out for years with a trainer, and I always had fat deposits around the upper part of the back of my hips and waist, and then there was this extra "stuff" that popped out from under the back of my bra strap. No matter how hard I worked out, it wouldn't go away. With yoga it is **melting** away. Why is that?

JC: Yoga is thorough. There are thousands of postures. A teacher is able to look at a body without a lot of clothes on and see where there are fat deposits.

Usually the muscles in that area need more developing and strengthening. There's a balance between stretch and strength. So the answer to your question is twofold: Number one, the cardio system has kicked up, and a strong yoga practice can make the heart beat fast for an extended period of time so you're burning fat. And number two: You're strengthening the muscles underneath where there are fat deposits so you're toning that area. It's different from weight lifting in a targeted way. Also, it relates hormonally because hormones are affected by yoga postures. For instance, if we're upside down for five to seven minutes in different comfortable inversions, just being in that position affects the thyroid gland and stimulates thyroid action.

SS: And we know from this book that the thyroid is a major hormone. I love the visual you create when I'm upside down. Can you tell me what you say?

JC: Well, the blood flows in reverse and stimulates the thyroid. If you just have your legs up a wall, lying flat on your back relaxing, the blood will flow down and pool. I use poetic images such as "Imagine it's a waterfall, and the blood and all the liquid in your body is draining out of your feet, draining out of your legs, and pooling or landing into a beautiful lake into a pool, which is your thyroid." Those relaxing images also allow the brain to relax and not pump the stress hormones. Now if you have a hyperactive thyroid or high blood pressure, you should check with your doctor about having your head below your heart.

SS: The first time you did that image for me, I could feel this lake at my thyroid, which I loved. Now what about constipation? As we get older, it seems that everybody has trouble with constipation. Is yoga good for that?

JC: Yoga twists are good for constipation. You first want to warm up the body and then do gentle twists where you're compressing the digestive organs, twisting and putting pressure on the colon, on the liver, and on the kidneys in your back. Then you unwind the twist and release the pressure. That area then fills up with nutrients and oxygen and blood, and then you twist again. You create stimulation in that area. Being upside down also helps because gravity is pulling in an opposite way. If you're standing all day long, often blood pools in your feet or intestines, and there's a downward pull because of gravity. If you're upside down in a shoulder stand or a headstand, eventually gravity's pulling in a different direction.

SS: Everybody's stressed. Is yoga a destressor?

JC: Yoga is a calming form of exercise. It has a calming effect. I divide thoughts into past, present, future. If you are thinking about things that you need to do later on or tomorrow, that's future. If you are thinking about what was, that's past. In yoga, we concentrate on being in the present. You focus your mind on the simple path of inhale and exhale. The definition of yoga, which means "yoke," is the yoking together of the mind, body, and breath. There are moments in yoga even after practicing for a short while where all of a sudden you'll say to yourself, "Wow, that was it! I wasn't thinking about my shopping list or picking up the kids from school. My mind was really on the alignment or the breath or the flow, or the movement, and the noise in my head didn't bother me. Nothing distracted me in that moment." What we search to do in yoga is extend those moments of unity. Yoga is not merely exercise; it's a practice that we do as often as possible, hopefully on a daily basis. It unifies our mind with our breath.

SS: Yes, but the beauty to me is twofold: Yoga calms and focuses me while sculpting my body into a shape I've never had before, even when I was young. I have never had any exercise that I have enjoyed this much or seen better results physically. Initially, I found it difficult to focus and concentrate on each movement because of all the "noise" in my head. You know, all the "future" stuff.

JC: A sensitive teacher will make it just hard enough to quiet your mind, but not so hard that you add stress. It's in a range between being a couch potato and being a total overachiever. There is a delicate balance where you find the edge, and you have to focus enough that you won't be wiped out by the next wave. I treat yoga as an extreme sport in that way, because I like to find a person's edge, where there is no room for extraneous thought.

SS: How long can a person do yoga? Could an eighty-year-old do yoga?

JC: Yes: 103-, 106-year-olds do yoga, and pretty strenuous yoga at that. It's a matter of knowing your body. It's like anything; it's a process of getting to know "who you are." Your "self" is manifested in your body and in your strengths, weaknesses, and illnesses. Getting to know all that constitutes your "self," including your hormones, your injuries, and your stage of life, will allow you to adjust your yoga practice to fit your level of ability.

SS: Is there a danger for an older person? As we age (without BHRT), men's and women's bones get weaker. Could they hurt themselves?

JC: Everything should be done in the context of that person's overall health. I say it's better to exercise than to risk getting diabetes and cardiovascular disease from doing nothing. A sensible yoga practice in the context of that person's overall health is right for anyone at any age with any condition.

SS: What has yoga done for you?

JC: It has completely transformed me. It has made me a better mother and made me more present with my child and in my life. I am less anxious, and it has made me more joyful.

SS: When you're in the car, or temple, or at a school function, do you find yourself consciously breathing or adjusting your posture or sitting up straight as a result of yoga?

JC: Well, I try to be aware of my posture. Of

course, there are times I forget, but I do find I am more awake.

SS: I find that I am also constantly adjusting my posture to breathe more deeply to relax and bring up my energy.

JC: Yoga is an energy system. We're extending the life force; we're extending our breath. If we feel sluggish, we want to increase our energy. If we're feeling hyper and manic, then we want to slow down, and yoga will help. Throughout your whole practice, Suzanne, we use a practice called Ujjayi. That's a strong inhale, strong exhale, and even breath. When I say, "Empty all your air out, and then take in a breath into your lower lungs, hold it, then into your middle lungs, hold it, then into your upper lungs, hold it, hold it as long as you can, and then let it all out with control," you can feel the breath working.

SS: Yes. I swear, that is how I believe the fat that I couldn't get rid of literally melted off . . . through this kind of controlled breathing and stretching. To me it's miraculous. Women my age have joint pain, watery eyes, sinusitis, allergies, and other conditions from the drastic drop in estrogen and progesterone. I believe yoga is a perfect complement to bioidentical hormone replacement. Yoga keeps you limber at a time when your body wants to stiffen up. It stimulates the hormonal system to counteract these conditions brought about by hormonal decline.

JC: Well, hormones are your area of expertise. I am learning from you.

SS: That's how it works. We women help one another. What about men? Most men think yoga is for girls, that it's a sissy sport.

JC: Half of the people in my class are men. Things are changing. Some men come to me and say they want to do yoga because they are not flexible anymore.

SS: Look at Alan, my husband. When he started he was very stiff . . .

JC: And now he stands on his hands and does back bends in only two years of practice.

SS: He loves yoga, and his love handles have melted away. Yoga has reshaped his body with no significant change in his diet (which has always been good) and lifestyle. We still go out a couple of times a week and enjoy our life immensely.

JC: Love handles disappear because there is a lengthening of the waist and strengthening of the muscles that keep length there. When you stretch and elongate, this lengthens the spine, without congesting or compacting the area. A lot of men are dealing with heart disease, depression, high blood pressure, and stiffness of the joints. Yoga has helped people deal with those conditions. Did you know that yoga was done **only** by men until the 1930s? It was only meant as a practice for Brahman boys.

SS: There you go. Once again, we women have

had to struggle even for the right to do exercise. What do you say to the person who doesn't want to do any kind of exercise? What would you say to that person in order to turn them on to yoga?

JC: Eventually, everybody who has a consistent yoga practice looks and feels remarkably better, and it has a positive feedback loop. That's when people start saying, "Oh my God. You look so great, you look so much better. What have you been doing?" So the physical changes are stimulating and encouraging. But it's the change in energy that really gets people turned on. You don't realize how sluggish you can get until you take the steps to reverse it.

SS: Yes. I find on the days I do yoga there is a spring in my step. I feel lighter, more joyful, and of course I love that my body looks so youthful as a result.

JC: Yoga fills your brain with a thought of inhale/exhale, stretch, and contract. If you fill your brain with those thoughts but think about it as breathing in compassion, breathing out compassion, it leaves no room for negativity, worry, depression, anxiety, and stress.

SS: What a lovely way to end. Thank you.

CHAPTER 31

BEAUTY

I t's not easy to keep it all together these days. You've got to work at it, but at the same time there are so many wonderful benefits with new technology and advancements. This chapter will give you some of my personal recommendations for maintaining a youthful appearance. Today, we have available to us new techniques for youthfulness such as fillers like collagen and Botox. The face lifts of old look strange and outdated, and today's advantages used in moderation can help you maintain a youthful appearance without looking "strange." Even so, collagen and Botox injections are often grossly overdone, and the result can look grotesque: lips that resemble a duck's or faces that appear frozen from overuse of Botox. The object is to look natural.

If you choose to use fillers as a beauty advantage, remember that it's all about good taste. Anything overdone is not good taste. You have to go slowly, use less rather than more, and exercise good judgment. The outcome should look natural and refreshed. If it doesn't, you will attract attention, and not in a good way. An overdone woman or man can get mocked and ridiculed. This reaction from people is never the intent of the person who has had the procedures, since anyone who sees a doctor for face work desires to look better. An overdone face does not look better!

When you have these procedures, be sure to go to a reputable doctor and never to a beauty salon or nurse's office. Injectables and other cosmetic procedures can be dangerous stuff, so you want a doctor to oversee the procedure you're having, plus ensure the quality of the filler and the cleanliness of the environment. These things are a must.

That said, here are my tips on how you can have ageless beauty:

First and foremost, get a good haircut. This is what makes middle-aged women stand out. With a fresh, hip haircut, you can dress conservatively but still have a youthfulness about you. Nothing ages a woman more than an "old-lady haircut." Color your hair or put in highlights to freshen your look. You don't have to do anything drastic like punk red with blue streaks—that would be "desperate"—but highlights or a lighter color can do wonders for any woman.

Second, update your makeup to appear ageless. So many of us tend to keep doing the same makeup we did when we were younger. It was great then, but as your face ages, a different look and different colors are essential. Smudge shades of brown across your lids and in the creases to give a smoky effect and depth. Line your eyes with a brown/black pencil and then smudge it so it is not a rigid line. Add mascara, eyebrow pencil, and a light touch of blush either at the tops of your cheeks or to add depth at the bottom of the cheekbone. Experiment. See what looks best on you. You be the judge.

Third, have regular facials if you can afford them. It is dreamy to spend an hour every week or two having soft hands massage your face and neck, clean your face properly, tighten with masks, and moisturize. It's an hour just for you to relax and relieve stress. This has a positive effect on your hormones. If you can't afford to go to a facialist, then give yourself regular masks. They really do work. Also, use a daytime moisturizer with sunblock. At night, use night cream on your face and throat and décolletage.

Fourth, have your brows professionally shaped and tinted. This is a major beauty tip and one that all women in Hollywood know is a must. In fact, they stand in line waiting for Anastasia in Beverly Hills, who is known as "the definitive brow expert" because of the way she shapes and grooms brows. I go to Faith Valentine in Malibu. She does a great job, and I never have to stand in line. Great-shaped brows can change your face, making you look fresh and awake. By contrast, the wrong shape is a detriment to your face. A professional can shape brows that are perfect for you. Shaping gets rid of the gray that has started to infiltrate your brows and promotes a natural look. If you need to add a little pencil to fill in the shape, match the color to your tinted eyebrows. Using too much eyebrow pencil will make you look old.

Fifth, have your eyelashes dyed dark brown or black. That way, you won't have to wear mascara every day, nor will you look washed out without your makeup. Brush a little bronzing powder over your chin, cheeks, the sides of your forehead, and the tip of your nose—just enough to look as though you spent the weekend in the sun.

Sixth, to keep yourself ageless, lose weight. Your hormones are fighting you, yet it is a war you can win. The war starts with understanding good nutrition. I always say if it comes in a bag or a box, it is probably fattening. In other words, eat fresh delicious real foods, including lots of vegetables, and cut out the breads and desserts.

Most people go on a diet and immediately cut out taste by eliminating all the things that make food intriguing: salad dressings, olive oil, and butter. Your food can be great-tasting with butter sauces and wine-reduction sauces, and they will not make you fat. Chicken piccata, for example, is one of my favorite meals, dripping in lemon-butter sauce. Instead of a big plate of potatoes, pasta, or bread, I load up on the sauce, and this method has kept the weight off me for over a decade.

My next beauty tip for appearing ageless is to dress in clothes that accentuate your positives and cover up your negatives. A bare midriff, for example, is not going to serve you well, even if you are thin. You'll never be as thin and as tight as the twenty-year-olds, so why put yourself in that position? I always tell my ladies to dress hip and sexy, but not desperate. You don't want to look as though you're wearing your daughter's clothes. Don't show skin that is no longer looking great. It is better to cover up and show off your shape. Solid colors work well, and unless you have a perfect figure, don't chop yourself in half with one color on top and another on the bottom. This shortens you, whereas if you wear all one color, you'll look thinner and longer. Overweight women often make the mistake of wearing two-piece print outfits, which makes them appear larger. Prints are difficult if you are carrying around any weight, so stick with solids.

Finally, the beauty tip that has served me so well over the last fourteen years is the FaceMaster, which is a nonsurgical face-lift. I will tell you right now that this is a machine that I manufacture, and I am reluctant even to mention it because it will sound self-serving. But honest to God, I have used this device almost every day for fourteen years, and I truly feel it has arrested the aging process on my face. The Face-Master uses a microcurrent that pumps up the muscles under the skin to hold up the structure and, thus, keep the skin from sagging. My partner in this venture, Dr. Peter Hanson, likens aging skin to an old barn with a sagging roof. If you were just to replace the shingles, the roof would still be sagging. What you need to do is build up the supports of the barn to strengthen and hold it up; then your new shingles will look like a brand-new roof. Using the FaceMaster several times a week works your face the same way free weights work out your biceps. It takes only about fifteen minutes a day. I do it lying in bed in the morning while having my daily cup of perfect coffee made by my husband.

The result of daily use is quite remarkable: natural, fresh-looking skin. The first time you use the FaceMaster, try doing only one side of your face. Then look in the mirror, and you will see that the FaceMastered side is higher and more lifted. Your eyebrows are higher, your cheekbones more pronounced, and your jawline stronger.

Women have been using this technology for decades in Europe, where I first encountered it. A friend of mine flew from Saint-Tropez to Geneva for her treatment. It was that important to her, to leave her vacation to be sure she didn't miss her appointment. When she returned, I was stunned at the difference in her face. This treatment—called a "microcurrent nonsurgical face-lift"—is also given in fancy salons from Los Angeles to New York City. The Tracie Martyn Salon in Manhattan gives these facials, for example. Go there and try it out; you'll see the difference it can make, and then you can buy a machine of your own for under $100. (By the way, the salon price for one treatment runs from $200 to $300.) I interviewed Dr. Hanson so you can learn for yourself the efficacy and safety of these treatments.

CHAPTER 32

DR. PETER HANSON: NONSURGICAL FACE-LIFT WITH THE FACEMASTER

Dr. Peter Hanson is a Western-trained medical doctor, acupuncturist, and author. He runs the Hanson Peak Performance Clinic for pain management, and he is the author of The Joy of Stress, which has sold over 1 million copies. I first met Dr. Hanson several years ago when we got together working on the FaceMaster. The FaceMaster is an ingenious little machine that gives a nonsurgical face-lift. In his clinic, Dr. Hanson was using a similar device for pain management. It works on the theory that electricity is your friend in small doses and has great healing properties. Dr. Hanson and my team worked together using the same technology for the face to bring this device to the public. It gives the appearance of a face-lift without surgery, and the results are fantastic. This interview is going to sound like an infomercial, but I am always asked about my

beauty regimen, and this truly is my primary beauty secret, and I use it almost every day. It is small enough to fit in my purse, and on the rare day I don't use it, people ask me if I am tired. Let me put it this way: If my house were on fire, I would grab my FaceMaster.

SS: Good morning, Dr. Hanson. Let me first ask you to describe what kind of doctor you are.

PH: I am first a medical doctor specializing in family practice and emergency medicine. But I also specialize in alternative medicine, and my expertise is in medical acupuncture and alternative treatments for pain and for stress.

SS: How does medicine interact with something like the FaceMaster?

PH: I first started working with medical acupuncture for Bell's palsy in 1980 and started to see the effects that electrical stimulation deep into the tissues had on the face. The effects were dramatic. We were able to see that we could stimulate all twenty-two muscles of the face with electrical stimulation using an acupuncture needle placed correctly at the beginning and end of the muscles and that it had an immediate impact. And then, of course, everyone who had this done said, "Gee, what about for me, who has no Bell's palsy? What about just using it for cosmetic purposes?" We weren't changing the outer structure of the skin—you need a skin product to do that—but we could see that the tone of the skin had improved dramatically and that it had a tremendous effect on changing the appearance of the skin.

SS: Is it the skin that ages, or is it the muscular structure under the skin that ages?

PH: Obviously, we know that skin ages on the surface, and for treating that, you can use moisturizers or a host of other treatments to smooth the outer layer of the skin. But in terms of the deep layers of the skin, there is an underlying sagging of the muscles that occurs with aging. Rubbing a product on your skin will do nothing to help the sagging muscles. Those muscles have to be tightened in the same way that you might go to the gym to tighten your biceps and other muscles.

SS: Yes, but can't we just do facial exercises to get the same results?

PH: Ah, that would be so easy. You can do facial exercises day and night, and all you are going to get is increased wrinkling. There is no way to exercise the muscles in the face. That is why the FaceMaster is so awesome. The FaceMaster affords us a chance to get right up close to the muscles. We don't need to place deep electrodes because the facial muscles are very close to the surface. In fact, there is hardly any distance between the skin and the bone, so the muscles are in between. With the FaceMaster, we can reach these muscles with probes dipped in conductive solution rather than using needles. For home use, this became a logical vehicle for transporting the electrical microcurrent. You can't really use probes to affect the biceps because they are too deeply seated. On the face, however, everything is handy, very easy to get to, and it works really well.

SS: But isn't electricity dangerous?

PH: Well, sticking your finger into a light socket is probably not a good idea. But the electrical current used for medical purposes is very, very, small and much less powerful. In fact, the current we use is called microcurrent, which is millionths of an amp. This current is actually a very healing current.

SS: Do you think if a woman used a FaceMater regularly, she wouldn't need to have a face-lift?

PH: So much depends upon the individual. It is important to remember that there are cases in which we will see people with severe drooping eyelids, like your one eye, Suzanne, which has been corrected with the FaceMaster. If you are considering a face-lift because your facial muscle tone is poor, you can be assured that using the FaceMaster should at least put off the need for a face-lift.

SS: I have been using my FaceMaster for fourteen years now, and I truly believe it has helped tremendously in arresting the sagging process. When I have a facial, the aesthetician always remarks that I have such good facial tone. I know that that tightness is from using the FaceMaster so religiously. I love the results of using this machine. It makes my eyes appear clearer, whiter, more alive, and less tired. Over the years, I have been able to sculpt my cheekbones in much the same way using free weights in a gym would tone and sculpt the biceps or any of the other muscles.

PH: It is nice to be able to use the full menu of possibilities and realize that before you leap into surgery, or even after you have surgery, you can still do something about your muscle tone. Keep in mind that muscle tone is never addressed by surgery. There is no operation to pump up muscles.

SS: If you had surgery, would this speed up the healing process and help with the scarring?

PH: We use it routinely on people who have had surgery, and they are thrilled with the results. It tones the muscles as it runs a current through the scar tissue. The technology is known to speed healing. Postoperatively, surgeons routinely implant electrodes above and below a scar level, and the scars heal better as a result. Moreover, the patients usually don't need pain pills.

SS: Do muscles have a memory?

PH: Absolutely. Let's say a bodybuilder like Arnold Schwarzenegger took one year off and then went back to the gym. It would take no time at all for his muscles to bounce back because he has had a whole lifetime of using them.

SS: How often should a man or a woman use this device?

PH: It works if you use it once or twice a week, but for a full face, you could use it every other day and touch up areas as needed.

SS: Well, that's good because I do use mine almost every day.

PH: And that's okay. We just want to make sure that it is used as instructed. We don't want people using it for eleven hours at a time and ending up with their muscles in spasm.

SS: Is this a machine that works on a man's face as well?

PH: Oh yes, because muscles know no bounds. A man's face responds beautifully. Look at Alan's face when we only did half of it as a demonstration. The half that had been FaceMastered was visibly higher, firmer, and the eye was more open. In general, the one side of the face that had been done looked much better than the one that hadn't had a treatment.

We are specialists in the muscle area. Ninety percent of the appearance problems that people have as they age are directly related to muscle tone, and the other 10 percent concerns inherited bad bone structure or sun damage, which clearly does need to have some dermatology treatments.

SS: Do you think microcurrent is the future?

PH: Absolutely. Microcurrent has several other applications. We use it in our office as an alternative to drugs. It seems odd for a physician to be in the business of taking people off drugs, since most medical doctors believe that every symptom in the human body has to be caused by the lack of a brand-name drug. Clearly, there is more to pain than just a Vicodin deficiency. If you find a new, nondrug way of treating pain, such as using a microcurrent, the patients are very grateful.

SS: Then why is the medical community behind relative to understanding the healing properties of microcurrent and electricity?

PH: Rather than use the word **brainwashing,** I'll explain this using the word **paradigm,** meaning pattern or model. In the history of medicine, the paradigm is interesting. First of all, doctors think in terms of traditional Western medicine. Right off the bat, that phrase is an oxymoron. In 1941, there was a doctor in England who worked in a venereal disease clinic. He spent all day, every day, injecting arsenic into the veins of anybody who had venereal disease, because they did not have antibiotics then. So Western medicine only goes back to 1941. Prior to that time, we were very, very dangerous. We were a bunch of loose cannons. So we have some nerve applying the term **traditional** for Western medicine because it is really not that old at all.

Doctors have been using electrical stimulation since 1856, dating back to Italy, where they had the first acupuncture needles left over from Marco Polo and the galvanic batteries. So, basically, we know that electric current has been tried for more than a century, and it has been tried safely in the post–World War II years in China, where medical practitioners routinely used electricity to stimulate their acupuncture needles.

We have also found that with the electrical stimulation of acupuncture needles, we increased the patient's levels of endorphins and ACTH [adrenocorticotropic hormone], which are the precursors of cortisone. And acupuncture restores the body to normal balance.

Electricity can even be tested by blood samples to make sure that it does work. We have found that it restores normal hormone and chemical levels, namely endorphins and cortisone, in chronic pain patients, for example, and thus improves their inflammation. Even so, doctors still think you need a drug every time you have a symptom.

SS: Why is it that I fly all night and when I arrive my eyes are red, scratchy, and tired? Then I use my FaceMaster, and they go clear and fresh.

PH: It has to do with restoring the balance of the normal blood supply to the area.

SS: So it's about circulation?

PH: Yes, it restores proper circulation and eases inflammation. The eyes go red because of inflammation, often caused by dry eye or dust in the area. Stimulating with electricity gets the body back to normal, restoring its levels of cortisone, and that is probably the mechanism by which the red goes out of the eyes.

SS: Well, this is my little beauty secret. And to think it's good for me, too! Thanks, Dr. Hanson.

DR. HANSON'S TOP FIVE
ANTIAGING RECOMMENDATIONS

1. Ninety percent of the appearance problems that people have as they age are directly related to muscle tone, and the other 10 percent concerns inherited bad bone structure or sun damage, which would require dermatology treatments. Rubbing a product on your skin will do nothing to help the sagging muscles. Those muscles have to be tightened through an electro-microcurrent, or nonsurgical face-lift, or the Face-Master. This addresses the underlying muscle tone rather than being limited to just the superficial skin, sanding off the skin or moisturizing the skin.

2. The nonsurgical face-lift restores proper circulation and eases inflammation in areas of redness, such as the eyes. Stimulating with electricity gets the body back to normal, restoring its levels of cortisone, and that is probably the mechanism by which the red goes out of the eyes.

3. If you are considering a face-lift because your facial muscle tone is poor, you can be assured that using the FaceMaster should at least put off the need for one.

4. If you do facial exercises day and night, all you are going to get is increased wrinkling. If you were to spend your whole life scrunching up your face to exercise the muscles, your facial skin might fold all the skin lines into permanent positions.

5. Sun-damaged skin needs to be treated by a dermatologist. In addition, creams and lotions are the best bet for sun-damaged skin.

CHAPTER 33

THE WRAP-UP

Now you know what I know. After reading about the advances being made relative to our health, I hope you will take advantage of the opportunities presented here. The changes you need to make are not drastic, not really. They simply involve choices.

Now that you know how great you can feel with balanced hormones and the major health benefits of replacement, I'm sure you have already chosen to make an appointment with the doctor nearest you. Using natural hormones is as easy as rubbing cream into your arms or thighs each day.

For those of you who want to go further, you can add supplements, vitamin B injections, and/or HGH injections. I'm sure after reading Dr. Ron Rothenberg's interview and the section on HGH, you are at least interested. If lack of energy is plaguing you, you were probably turned on by the possibilities that Dr. Michael Galitzer and Dr. Larry Webster are offering to restore energy. Now that you have read how the environment is harming us, you will want to meet with an antiaging doctor to see about ridding your body of these dangerous pollutants.

Soon you will be like me, passing the word to anyone who will listen about the glorious effects of real hormone replacement and the abilities of new doctors to restore energy and reverse aging. This is the way medicine will change—through a grassroots effort. We of this generation are once again leading the way. We don't want to accept inferior health care. We don't want to accept anything less than superb quality of life. We don't want to accept sickness with aging.

As for nutrition, it's clear that eating real food and choosing organic food, if you can afford it, is the way to go. Real food tastes better and offers greater nutrition. You can still enjoy all your favorite dishes; it's not as though you are being asked to eat plates full of hay.

Yes, it is harder and harder to eat in restaurants these days because the quality of food is compromised for financial reasons. As consumers, it is important to question your butcher and to ask your favorite restaurant to start serving organic meat, chicken, and fish. Be vocal; it brings results. If you are willing to pay a little more for the sake of your health, the owners will comply. After all, they are in business and do not want to compromise their profits.

Once you get your health in balance, you can finish off any emotional work you still need to do to let go of old angers and resentments, because they cause stress. Find yourself a good therapist to help you accomplish this one. All therapists are not created equal. Sometimes you have to try a couple until you find one with whom you feel comfortable.

By now you realize the dangers of stress. Had I not been able to do the work and find true forgiveness for my alcoholic father, I believe my stress would have made me a very sick woman. I believe my breast cancer had a lot to do not only with the chemicals I was given for birth control, but also the pain and anger of my childhood had to be a factor. I believe I "entombed" that anger in my body until I reached a place in my life where I could handle it. My "tumor" changed my life. It was the wake-up call for just about everything. It put my life into perspective, not only regarding a new approach to my health, but also in terms of giving me a better emotional perspective. I realized that by not forgiving my father's alcoholism, I was letting the disease win. A brutal childhood takes so much from your life; by not getting to the bottom of that sadness, hurt, and anger with the help of a good therapist, you allow it to continue to take from your life; it negates happiness, and the stress can make you sick. My brutal, violent childhood has turned out to be my gift. I have done the emotional "work" to undo the pain, anger, and resentment I harbored for so long. Doing this work has enhanced my life more than I can describe, and it led me to understanding and true forgiveness. I have come to be grateful for this childhood because it forced me to confront myself and transform my life into a life I love living. If what I project professionally and personally as a public person is something that appeals to you, then everything in this book is what I have done to get to this place.

By looking deeply into who you really are, you will realize that the key to all of this is doing the work to love yourself. Taking care of **yourself** requires self-love. Without that, you are never going to care if your liver is cleansed or not. People do destructive things to themselves and their bodies when they have no self-love. I know this sounds very 1960s, but think about it. If you really cared for yourself and valued the life you are living, you would not treat your body with such disregard. This could be the key to why you are gaining weight or why you are in such poor health. You can change your attitude, and you can reverse your poor health. But it is going to take some soul-searching to find out why you have never bothered up to this point. The fact that you have read this book means that you are ready. Take it from someone who has done the work. Yes, it is agitating at times to stir up the past, but we have to know where we came from to understand where we are today. That understanding unlocks the answers that you have been hiding from. When you feel clear about the past, the future holds nothing but excitement and joy. As I said in the beginning, good health brings joy, balanced hormones bring joy, and a well-running body brings joy. Emotional health brings joy.

So do the work. Listen to what these doctors are telling you. They have explained the medical answers to fight the damage that has been done to our planet that is affecting each one of us personally. They have given you the key to unlock the answers to the ravages of aging that we are seeing all around us.

This information and these tools are your hope and your chance. We all want to live a long, healthy life and die healthy. Now you know how.

Thank you for taking the time to read what I have to say.

GLOSSARY

16 alpha-hydroxyestrone: A metabolic estrogen that has the capacity to damage cellular tissue and is safely metabolized and excreted from the body using vitamin B_{12} and folic acid.

Acromegaly: A disorder that is caused by chronic overproduction of growth hormone by the pituitary gland and is characterized by a gradual and permanent enlargement of the flat bones (as the lower jaw) and the bones of the hands and feet, abdominal organs, nose, lips, and tongue, and that develops after puberty is complete.

Adenomyosis: Endometriosis, especially when the endometrial tissue invades the myometrium (the muscular layer of the wall of the uterus).

Adipose tissue: Connective tissue in which fat is stored and that has the cells distended by droplets of fat from excess stimulation of insulin. Adipose tissue is metabolically active and can contribute to inflammation and cause further deposition of fat.

Adrenals: A pair of small glands, one located on top of each kidney. The adrenal glands produce hormones that help control heart rate, blood pressure, the way the body metabolizes food, and other metabolic functions.

Adrenarche: An increase in the production of adrenal hormones by the adrenal cortex that usually occurs just prior to and during puberty.

Adrenocorticotropic hormone (ACTH): Stimulates the adrenal cortex; more specifically, stimulates the secretion of glucocorticoids such as cortisol.

Anabolism: The building and support of cellular tissue in the body.

Androgenic: A male sex hormone (such as testosterone) effect.

Andropause: A gradual and highly variable decline in the production of androgenic hormones, especially testosterone, in the human male, together with its associated effects. Symptoms include erectile dysfunction, fatigue, muscle wasting along with increased body fat, diminished mental function, and others that define a condition described as male menopause.

Angiogenesis: The stimulation of blood vessel formation.

Anthroposophic: Medicine that is not FDA-approved but must be prescribed by a doctor, such as Iscador, an immune system builder made from mistletoe extract.

Antioxidant: A natural or synthetic agent that helps protect cells from the damaging effects of free radicals by providing neutralizing electrons.

Apoptosis: A process that programs the death of cells and is effective in limiting the growth of tumors.

Armour thyroid: Thyroid tissue derived from pork thyroid glandular tissue that provides the body with both T3 and T4 thyroid hormones.

Aromatase: An enzyme or complex of enzymes that promotes the conversion of an androgen (such as testosterone) into estrogens (such as estradiol).

Atherosclerosis: Degenerative vascular inflammation characterized by fatty deposits and fibrosis of the inner layer of the arteries.

Autoimmune: Of, relating to, or caused by antibodies or T cells that attack molecules, cells, or tissues of the organism producing them. The production of antibodies against tissues of the same body producing the antibodies, which results in tissue destruction and loss of self-immune recognition.

Bilateral oophorectomy: Surgical removal of both ovaries, with marked reduction in the body's production of natural hormones.

Candida: A normally occurring fungus in the body that becomes pathologic with overstimulation through excess intake of sugar or depression of the body's immune system by metabolic and psychological stressors.

Catechol estrogens: Estrogens metabolized in the liver and kidney, some forms of which can contribute to increased cancer risk.

Chelation: The removal of heavy metals by amino acids that attach to metals and remove them through the kidneys. Effective in the treatment of heart disease, hypertension, and other conditions.

Choline: A substance found in animal and plant tissues that is essential to normal fat and carbohydrate metabolism and necessary for brain and nervous function.

Chronic: Marked by long duration, by frequent recurrence over a long time, and often by slowly progressing seriousness. A condition denoting a long-term disease presence in the body that often will increase in severity over time.

Chrysin: A substance that is used to help reduce the conversion of testosterone to estrogen and reduce estrogen levels.

Circadian: Being, having, characterized by, or occurring in approximately twenty-four-hour periods or cycles (as of biological activity or function). The rhythmic release of hormones over the course of a twenty-four-hour period.

Cortisol: The primary stress hormone. Cortisol is the major natural glucocorticoid in humans. A hormone (adrenal) released in response to metabolic or emotional stress that stabilizes blood sugar, blood pressure, and so on but in excess causes a deterioration of metabolic bodily processes.

Craniosacral therapy: A therapy used to balance the electromagnetic status of the body and support bodily healing.

C-reactive protein: A protein produced by the liver that is normally present in trace amounts in the blood serum but is elevated during episodes of acute inflammation (such as those associated with neoplastic disease, chronic infection, or coronary artery disease).

Curcumin: An Ayurvedic herb used to reduce inflammation, improve circulation, and boost the immune system.

Cytokines: More than one hundred proteins produced by white blood cells that regulate immune aspect or cell growth and function associated with cellular inflammation.

Dioxin: Any of several persistent toxic heterocyclic hydrocarbons that occur, especially as by-products of

various industrial processes (such as pesticide manufacture and paper milling) and waste incinerations.

Dopamine: A protein-derived neuroreceptor substance that regulates nerve transmission in the brain
and muscles.

Ductal carcinoma: A cancer of the breast involving
the ductal breast tissue. A benign form of breast cancer unless invasive in a minority of cases.

Endocrinology: A science dealing with the endocrine glands (a gland, such as the thyroid or the pituitary, that produces an endocrine secretion).

Endometrial ablation: Removal of the endometrial
lining of the uterus to remove tissue proliferation, reduce excess bleeding, and reduce uterine cancer risk.

Endometriosis: The presence and growth of functioning endometrial tissue in places other than the
uterus that often results in severe pain and infertility.

Endometrium: Cellular lining of the uterus.

Endorphins: Proteins produced in the brain that act
as a narcotic by binding to narcotic opiate receptors
that reduce pain perception.

Epidemiology: The study of disease patterns in
populations to help regulate disease patterns.

Erythropoietin: A hormonal substance that is
formed especially in the kidney and stimulates red
blood cell formation.

Estradiol: The most hormonally active estrogen, which is converted to both estriol and estrone.

Fibromyalgia: A chronic disorder characterized by widespread pain, tenderness, and stiffness of muscles and associated connective tissue structures that is typically accompanied by fatigue, headache, and sleep disturbances.

Fluoride: A compound of fluorine, in part derived as a by-product of aluminum production, used to help prevent dental cavities. Toxicity is a possibility, and dosage is important.

Follicle-stimulating hormone (FSH): A hormone from the anterior lobe of the pituitary gland that stimulates the growth of the ovum-containing follicles in the ovary and activates sperm-forming cells.

Gamma-aminobutyric acid (GABA): A nonexcitatory amino acid that raises the central nervous system. Excitator threshold reducing susceptibility to convulsions and CNS (central nervous system).

Genomics: A branch of biotechnology concerned with applying the techniques of genetics and molecular biology to the genetic mapping and DNA sequencing of sets of genes to help predict the incidence and outcomes of clinical disease patterns.

Glutathione: An antioxidant peptide useful for the detoxification of chemicals and heavy metals and reducing cellular inflammation.

Helicobacter: Gram-negative bacteria proven to cause ulcers and gastritis and ultimately gastroesophageal cancer found primarily in chicken and other poultry.

HER2-neu: Herpes II virus found in genital viral lesions.

Hypercholesterolemia: The presence of excess cholesterol in the blood.

Hyperinsulinemia: The presence of excess insulin in the blood.

Hyperpermeable: Describing a membrane such as the lining of the gut that allows excess diffusions of substances through it.

Hyperplasia: An abnormal or unusual increase in the elements composing a part (as cells composing a tissue).

Hypertrophy: Excessive development of an organ or part—specifically, increase in bulk (as by thickening of muscle fibers) without multiplication of parts.

Hypogonadism: Functional incompetence of the gonads, especially in the male, with subnormal or impaired production of hormones and germ cells.

Hypothalamus: A structure in the brain that releases hormones to stimulate the pituitary to in turn release hormone regulators affecting bodily hormonal systems (thyroid, adrenals, and so on).

Hypothyroid: Of, relating to, or affected with hypothyroidism (deficient activity of the thyroid gland).

Immunologic: Relating to the immune system function of the body.

Inflammation: A bodily condition indicating inflamed cellular energy production, contributing to many disease processes in the body.

Interleukin: Any of various compounds of low molecular weight that are produced by lymphocyte macrophages and monocytes and that function especially in regulation of the immune system and especially cell-mediated immunity.

Kinesiology: The study of the principles of mechanics and anatomy in relation to human movement. Also used in applied kinesiology to read the electromagnetic balance of a body.

L-glutamine: An amino acid used for muscle function, gastrointestinal repair, and detoxification.

Lipid system: System of the body that involves the use and metabolism of fat-related compounds.

Lipoprotein: Any of a large class of conjugated proteins composed of a complex of protein and lipid that carry lipids in the bloodstream.

Lupus: Lupus erythematosus, an autoimmune disease adversely affecting the lungs, heart, skin, joints, and the like.

Luteinizing hormone: A glycoprotein produced in the pituitary that stimulates progesterone secretion from the corpus luteum in the ovaries of females and testosterone production from the testes in males.

Macular degeneration: Progressive deterioration of the macula lutea in the retina, resulting in a gradual loss of the central part of the field of vision.

Melatonin: A hormone that is derived from serotonin and secreted by the pineal gland especially in response to darkness. It has been linked to the regulation of circadian hormonal rhythms and has strong antioxidant function in the prevention of cancer.

Menarche: The age at which a young female begins menstruation.

Metabolism: The whole range of biochemical processes that occur within us (or any living organism). Metabolism consists both of anabolism and catabolism (the buildup and breakdown of substances, respectively).

Metastasis: The spread of cancer from one part of the body to another. Cells that have metastasized are like those in the original (primary) tumor.

Mitochondria: Structures in the cell in which energy is produced in the Krebs cycle.

Modality: A form of application or employment of a therapeutic agent or regimen.

Mucosa: Mucous membrane or moist tissue layer that lines the hollow organs and cavities of the body.

Necrosis: Death of living tissue—specifically, the death of a portion of tissue differentially affected by local injury (as loss of blood supply, corrosion, burning, or the local lesion of a disease).

Neuromuscular: Of or relating to nerves and muscles especially jointly involving nervous and muscular elements.

Neurotoxicity: Any toxic element adversely influencing nervous function.

Norepinephrine: An adrenal medullary hormone that is the chemical means of transmission across synapses in postganglionic neurons of the sympathetic nervous system and that helps to maintain blood pressure.

Oncogene: A gene having the potential to cause a normal cell to become cancerous.

Osteoblasts: Bone-forming cells stimulated by progesterone and testosterone.

Osteoclast: Any of the large multinucleated (having more than two nuclei) cells closely associated with areas of bone resorption necessary in the proper remodeling of bone.

Osteoporosis: A condition that affects especially older women and is characterized by decrease in bone mass with decreased density and enlargement of bone spaces producing porosity and brittleness.

Paraquat: An herbicide that is used especially as a weed killer and is extremely toxic to the liver, kidneys, and lungs if ingested.

Pathogenesis: The origination and development of a disease.

Perimenopause: The period around the onset of menopause that is often marked by various physical signs (such as hot flashes and menstrual irregularity).

Permutation: A complete transformation or change.

Pernicious anemia: An anemia with severe neurological deterioration secondary to impaired vitamin B_{12} absorption.

Peroxidase: An enzyme that hastens the transfer of oxygen from peroxide to a tissue that requires oxygen. This process is essential to cellular energy production.

Phosphatidylcholine: A phospholipid that helps the brain manufacture neurotransmitter function, enhancing memory.

Phosphatidylserine: A phospholipid that maintains brain cell membranes that helps with dementia and depression.

Phthalate: A stabilizer used in plastics that is toxic to the liver and other tissues.

Pituitary: The main endocrine gland; produces hormones that control other glands and many body functions, especially growth.

Polycystic ovaries: A condition of multiple cysts associated with infertility, weight gain, and other symptoms.

Prolactin: A protein hormone of the pituitary gland that induces and maintains lactation in the postpartum mammalian female and can disrupt the function of other hormones.

Pylori: The openings from the stomach into the duodenum of the small intestine.

Quartile: A fourth of a whole.

Recolonize: To reinstitute bacterial growth especially in the gastrointestinal tract to improve digestion and absorption.

Rectus abdominis: A long, flat muscle on either side of the linea alba extending along the whole length of the front of the abdomen, arising from the pubic crest and symphysis, inserted into the cartilages of the fifth, sixth, and seventh ribs, and acting to flex the spinal column, tense the anterior wall of the abdomen, and assist in compressing the contents of the abdomen.

Selenium: An element that is used as a component of thyroid hormone activation and heavy metal chemical detoxification.

Serotonin: A chemical in the brain involved in the transmission of nerve impulses. Serotonin can trigger the release of substances in the blood vessels of the brain that in turn cause the pain of the migraine owing to its vasoconstrictive effect. Used for weight control, sugar craving, depression, muscle aches, and pains.

Sleep apnea: Brief periods of recurrent cessation of breathing during sleep that is caused especially by obstruction of the airway or a disturbance in the brain's respiratory center and is associated especially with excessive daytime sleeping.

Statin: Any of a group of drugs that inhibit the synthesis of cholesterol and promote the production of LDL-binding receptors in the liver, resulting in a marked decrease in the level of LDL and a modest increase in the level of HDL circulating in blood plasma. Side effects include liver damage, reduction of coenzyme Q10, and memory problems.

Stenosis: A narrowing or constriction of the diameter of a bodily passage or orifice.

Thyroxine: One of the principal hormones secreted by the thyroid gland consisting of the amino acid tyrosine with four attached iodines (T4). T4 is deiodinized to the more active T3, which promotes metabolism in all tissues of the body.

Transdermal: Relating to, being, or supplying a medication in a form for absorption through the skin into the bloodstream.

Troche: Lozenge.

Tumor necrosis factor-alpha: A protein that is produced chiefly by monocytes and macrophages in response especially to endotoxins, that mediates inflammation, and that induces the destruction of some tumor cells in the activation of white blood cells.

RESOURCES

ANTIAGING DOCTORS, SPECIALISTS, CLINICS, AND INSTITUTES

CALIFORNIA

Dr. David Allen
2211 Corinth Avenue
Suite 204
Santa Monica, CA 90064
310-966-9194

American College for
    Advancement in
    Medicine
23121 Verdugo Dr.,
    Suite 204
Laguna Hills, CA 92653
800-532-3688

American Health
    Institute
Dr. Michael Galitzer
12381 Wilshire Blvd.,
    Suite 102
Los Angeles, CA 90025

800-392-2623
www.ahealth.com

Dr. Catherine Arvantely
1151 Dove St., Suite 110
Newport Beach, CA 92660
949-660-1399
www.drarvantely.com
wellness@drarvantely.com
    (E-mail)

Dr. Jennifer Berman
421 N. Rodeo Dr.
Penthouse 1
Beverly Hills, CA 90210
310-432-6644
www.bermansexualhealth
    .com

THE CENTER FOR
ANTIAGING MEDICINE
1270 Coast Village Circle,
Suite 2
Montecito, CA 93108
800-392-2623

DR. YUN-CHING CHEN
720-A Capitola Ave.
Capitola, CA 95010
831-462-6013
831-462-4494 (fax)
www.emotrics.com

DR. MARC DARROW
Assistant Professor
UCLA School of Medicine
11645 Wilshire Blvd.,
Suite 120
Los Angeles, CA 90025
800-REHAB10
310-231-7000
www.1800rehab10.com

DR. JOE FILBECK
8929 University Center
Lane, Suite 202
San Diego, CA 92122
858-457-5700
www.palmlajolla.com

DR. DAVID L. GREENE
459 W. Line St.
Bishop, CA 93514
760-873-8982

DR. ROBERT GREENE
1255 East St., Suite 201
Redding, CA 96001
530-244-9052
www.specialtycare4women
.com

DR. HANS GRUENN
Longevity Medical Center
2211 Corinth Ave.,
Suite 204
Los Angeles, CA 90064
310-966-9194
www.drgruenn.com
www.i4sh.com
ceo@drgruenn.com (E-mail)

DR. PRUDENCE HALL
1148 4th St.
Santa Monica, CA 90403
310-458-7979

DR. CATHIE LIPPMAN
Lippman Center for
Optimal Wellness
291 S. La Cienega Blvd.,
Suite 207
Beverly Hills, CA 90211
310-289-8430
310-289-8165 (fax)
www.CathieLippmanMD
.com

Dr. Gary London
9201 Sunset Blvd.,
   Suite 401
Beverly Hills, CA 90069
310-207-4500
www.garylondonmd.com

Dr. Robert Mathis
9 E. Mission St.
Santa Barbara, CA 93101
805-569-7100
www.BaselineHealth.net

**MENOPAUSE
   INSTITUTE**
877-5 MENOPAUSE
www.menopauseinstitute
   .com

This is a one-stop shop that
has outstanding BHRT pro-
grams and a highly skilled
medical staff to assist with
menopause, andropause,
and PMS. They have loca-
tions all around the country
and the cost is affordable for
every woman, man,
and girl.

Dr. Philip Lee Miller
Los Gatos Longevity Institute
15215 National Ave.,
   Suite 103
Los Gatos, CA 95032

408-358-8855
www.antiaging.com

Dr. Wendy Miller
   Rashidi
Women's View Medical
   Group
299 West Foothill Blvd.
Upland, CA 91786
909-982-4000
www.womensviewmedical
   .com

Dr. Uzzi Reiss
414 North Camden Dr.,
   Suite 750
Beverly Hills, CA 90210
www.uzzireissmd.com

Dr. Ron Rothenberg
California HealthSpan
   Institute
320 Santa Fe Dr., Suite 301
Encinitas, CA 92024
760-635-1996
800-943-3331
www.eHealthSpan.com
Located on the campus of
   Scripps Memorial
   Hospital, Encinitas, CA

DR. GARY RUELAS
Integrative Medical Institute
  of Orange County
707 East Chapman Ave.
Orange, CA 92866
714-771-2880
www.integrative-med.org

DR. JOSEPH SCIABBARRASI
2001 S. Barrington Ave.,
  Suite 208
Los Angeles, CA 90025
310-268-8466
310-268-8122 (fax)
www.DrJosephMD.com

DR. JULIE TAGUCHI
317 West Pueblo St.
Santa Barbara, CA 93105
805-681-7500
drtaguchi@thewileyprotocol
  .com (E-mail)

DR. DUNCAN TURNER
219 Nogales Ave., Suite A
Santa Barbara, CA 93105
805-682-6340
www.duncanturner.com

DR. RONALD WEMPEN
Health and Energy Medical
  Clinic, Inc.
14795 Jeffrey Rd., Suite 101
Irvine, CA 92618
949-551-8751

949-551-1272 (fax)
lifenergy@cox.net (E-mail)

T. S. WILEY
Wiley Systems
P.O. Box 50734
Santa Barbara, CA 93150

For lists of certified doctors
and registered pharmacies in
your area providing the au-
thentic Wiley Protocol, go
to www.thewileyproto
col.com for links and information.

COLORADO

DR. PETER HANSON
Cherry Creek Center for
  Healing
3300 East First Ave. #600
Denver, CO 80206
303-733-2521
www.peterhansonmd.com

FLORIDA

DR. ROBERT CARLSON
1762 Hawthorne St.,
  Suite 4
Sarasota, FL 34239
941-955-1815
800-815-7443
www.hghtest.com

www.4pbr.com

www.preventaging.org

DR. HERBERT SLAVIN
7200 W. Commercial Blvd.,
  Suite 210
Lauderhill, FL 33319
954-748-4991
www.Drslavin.com

GEORGIA

DR. DANIELA PAUNESKY
3400 Old Milton Pkwy.
Bldg. C, Suite 380
Alpharetta, GA 30005
770-777-7707

IDAHO

DR. PAUL BRILLHART
1110 E. Polston Ave.
Post Falls, ID 83854
208-773-1311
www.drpaulbrillhart.com

ILLINOIS

AMERICAN ACADEMY OF
  ANTI-AGING MEDICINE
1510 West Montana St.
Chicago, IL 60614
773-528-4333
www.worldhealth.net

LAURA BERMAN, PhD
Berman Center
211 East Ontario St.
Chicago, IL 60611
800-709-4709
www.bermancenter.com

DR. PAUL SAVAGE
BodyLogicMD
4753 N. Broadway Ave.,
  Suite 101
Chicago, IL 60640
866-535-BLMD
  (866-535-2563)
866-344-BLMD
  (866-344-2563) (fax)
www.bodylogicmd.com

Other locations may be
found on our website, in-
cluding Chicago, IL; Hart-
ford, CT; Ft. Lauderdale,
FL; Naples, FL; and Jack-
sonville, FL.

INDIANA

DR. TAMMY BORN
Crossroads Healing Arts
21764 Omega Ct.
Goshen, IN 46528
574-875-4227
www.bornclinic.com

DR. LINDA J. SPENCER
Complementary Family
  Medical Care of Indiana
3850 Shore Dr., Suite 205
Indianapolis, IN 46254
317-298-3850
www.complementaryfamily
  medicalcare.com

DR. CHARLIE TURNER
3554 Promenade Pkwy.,
  Suite H
Lafayette, IN 47909
765-471-1100
www.charlesturnermd.com

MASSACHUSETTS

DR. ALAN ALTMAN
55 Pond Ave.
Brookline, MA 02445
617-232-0202

MICHIGAN

DR. TAMMY BORN
3700 52nd St. SE
Grand Rapids, MI 49512
616-656-3700
www.bornclinic.com

DR. DAVID BROWNSTEIN
Center for Holistic Medicine
5821 W. Maple Rd.,
  Suite 192
West Bloomfield, MI 48322
248-851-1600
www.drbrownstein.com

NEW JERSEY

DR. ALLAN MAGAZINER
Magaziner Center for
  Wellness and Anti-Aging
  Medicine
1907 Greentree Rd.
Cherry Hill, NJ 08003
856-424-8222
www.DrMagaziner.com

DR. NEIL ROSEN
555 Shrewsbury Ave.
Shrewsbury, NJ
732-219-0895

NEW YORK

DR. KENNETH BOCK
DR. STEVEN BOCK
DR. MICHAEL COMPAIN
Rhinebeck Health Center
108 Montgomery St.
Rhinebeck, NY 12572
845-876-7082
www.rhinebeckhealth.com

Dr. Kenneth Bock
Dr. Steven Bock
Center for Progressive
  Medicine
Pinnacle Place, Suite 224
10 McKown Rd.
Albany, NY 12203
518-435-0082
www.rhinebeckhealth.com

Dr. Rashmi Gulati
31 East 28th St., 6th floor
New York, NY 10021
212-794-4466
www.patientsmedical.com
info@patientsmedical.com
  (E-mail)

Dr. Ronald Hoffman
The Hoffman Center
40 East 30th St.
New York, NY 10016
212-779-1744
www.drhoffman.com

Dr. Alexander N. Kulick
625 Madison Ave.
New York, NY 10022
212-838-8265
www.ostrow.medem.com

Dr. Richard Linchitz
Metropolitan Medical
  Healthcare and
  Wellness/Natural
  Horizons Wellness
45–51 East 25th St.,
  7th Floor
New York, NY 10010
212-252-1942 or
  516-759-4200
www.metropolitanwellness
  .com

Dr. Jeffrey A. Morrison
103 Fifth Ave., 6th floor
New York, NY 10003
212-989-9828
212-989-9827 (fax)
www.themorrisoncenter.com
drmorrison@themorrison
  center.com (E-mail)

Dr. John Salerno
14 W. 49th St., Suite 1401
New York, NY 10020
212-582-1700
www.salernocenter.com

Dr. Erika Schwartz
10 W. 74th St.
New York, NY
212-873-3420

NORTH CAROLINA

DR. LARRY WEBSTER
719 Green Valley Rd.,
  Suite 101
Greensboro, NC 27408
336-272-2030
866-266-8869
www.lwebster.com

TEXAS

DR. CLARK RIDLEY
2706 Fairmount St.
Dallas, TX 75201
214-303-1888
www.lifespanmedicine.com

UTAH

DR. GORDON REYNOLDS
Green Valley Spa
1871 W. Canyon View
St. George, UT 84770
435-628-8060

VERMONT

PAUL SCHULICK
New Chapter
99 Main St.
Brattleboro, VT 05301
802-257-9345
www.new-chapter.info

THE WILEY PROTOCOL

DR. YUN-CHING CHEN
720-A Capitola Ave.
Capitola, CA 95010
831-462-6013
831-462-4494 (fax)
www.emotrics.com

DR. ALLAN MAGAZINER
Magaziner Center for
  Wellness and Anti-Aging
  Medicine
1907 Greentree Rd.
Cherry Hill, NJ 08003
856-424-8222
www.DrMagaziner.com

DR. ROBERT MATHIS
9 E. Mission St.
Santa Barbara, CA 93101
805-569-7100
www.BaselineHealth.net

DR. CLARK RIDLEY
2706 Fairmount St.
Dallas, TX 75201
214-303-1888
www.lifespanmedicine.com

DR. JULIE TAGUCHI
317 West Pueblo Street
Santa Barbara, CA 93105
805-681-7500
drtaguchi@thewileyprotocol
  .com

DR. DUNCAN TURNER
219 Nogales Ave., Suite A
Santa Barbara, CA 93105
805-682-6340
www.duncanturner.com

CANADA

DR. CAROLINE HUH
DR. ELIZABETH HARTLEY
Menopause Health Clinic
1920 Yonge St., Suite 105
Toronto, Ontario M4S 3E2
416-322-9602
www.menopausehealth
  clinic.com
info@menopausehealth
  clinic.com (E-mail)

DR. NISHI DHAWAN
DR. BAL PAWA
DR. KARLA DIONNE
Westcoast Women's Clinic
1003 West King Edward
  Ave.
Vancouver, B.C. V6H 1Z3
604-738-9601
604-738-9605 (fax)
www.westcoastwomen-
  sclinic.com

OTHER HELPFUL WEBSITES

JULIE CARMEN
www.juliecarmenyoga.com
juliecarmenyoga@charter
  .net

DR. DIANA SCHWARZBEIN
www.schwarzbeinprinciple
  .com

SUZANNE SOMERS
www.suzannesomers.com

TESTING HORMONE LEVELS

AERON LIFECYCLES
1933 Davis St., Suite 310
San Leandro, CA 94577
800-631-7900
www.aeron.com

LIFE EXTENSION
1100 West Commercial
  Blvd.
Fort Lauderdale, FL 33309
800-208-3444
www.lef.org

Life Extension offers some
of the most comprehensive
and competitive hormone

testing in the country. They offer male and female hormone panels designed by their MDs as well as complete individual hormone tests. The service is available anywhere in the U.S.

SABRE SCIENCES, INC.
2233 Fairday Ave., Suite K
Carlsbad, CA 92008
www.sabresciences.com

PHARMACIES

www.angelfire.com/fl/endo
    hystnhrt/ pharmacy.html
This website lists compounding pharmacies by state.

APOTHÉCURE, INC.
4001 McEwen Rd.
Suite 100
Dallas, TX 75244
972-960-6601
800-969-6601
www.apothecure.com

BLUE RIDGE APOTHECARY
621-F Townside Rd.
Roanoke, VA 24014
Graham Stephens, RPh,
    PharmD
540-345-6480
540-345-6844 (fax)

COMPOUNDING PHARMACY
    OF BEVERLY HILLS
9629 West Olympic Blvd.
Beverly Hills, CA 90212
310-284-8675
888-799-0212
www.compounding-expert
    .com

CUSTOM PRESCRIPTION
    SHOPPE
42 Timber Lane
South Burlington, VT
    05403
800-928-1488
802-864-0812
Scott W. Brown, PD
scott@customrxshop.com
    (E-mail)

HEALTH PHARMACIES
2809 Fish Hatchery Rd.,
    Suite 103
Madison, WI 53713
800-373-6704

INTERNATIONAL ACADEMY
    OF COMPOUNDING
    PHARMACISTS
P.O. Box 1365
Sugar Land, TX 77478
800-927-4227
www.iacprx.org

You may call them or go to their website and enter your zip code for a referral to the closest compounding pharmacy in your area.

DR. ELEANOR KONG
3435 Ocean Park Blvd.,
  Suite 105B
Santa Monica, CA 90403
310-393-2755
Eleanor155@aol.com
  (E-mail)

KRONOS PHARMACY
  (FORMERLY MEDICAL
  CENTER PHARMACY)
3675 South Rainbow Blvd.
Las Vegas, NV 89103
800-723-7455

MEDICAL CENTER
  PHARMACY
Redondo Beach
Sue Decker
Pharmacist: Nilesh Bhakta
310-540-3312

PROFESSIONAL COMPOUND-
  ING CENTERS OF
  AMERICA
www.pccarx.com

SAN DIEGO COMPOUNDING
  PHARMACY
Jerry Greene, RPh, FACA
5395 Ruffin Road,
  Suite 104
San Diego, CA 92123
858-277-8884
866-413-2673
858-277-8889 (fax)

SOLUTIONS PHARMACY
4632 Highway 58 N.
Chattanooga, TN 37416
423-894-3222
800-523-1486
www.solutions-
  pharmacy.com

STEVEN'S PHARMACY
1525 Mesa Verde Dr. East
Costa Mesa, CA 92626
800-352-3784
www.stevensrx.com

MEDICINE SHOPPE
  PHARMACY
649 West High St.
Piqua, OH 45356
937-773-1778
888-723-5344
www.hormoneconnection
  .biz

Town Center Drugs and
  Compounding
  Pharmacy
72624-A El Paseo
Palm Desert, CA 92260
760-341-3984
877-340-5922

Village Green
  Apothecary
5415 W. Cedar Lane
Bethesda, MD 20814
Paul Garcia, marketing
  director
301-530-0800
240-644-1362 (fax)
www.myvillagegreen.com

Women's International
  Pharmacy
12012 N. 111th Ave.
Youngtown, AZ 85363
800-279-5708
www.womensinternational
  .com

SEXUAL AIDS

www.goodvibes.com
www.grandopening.com

NATURAL BEAUTY PRODUCTS

All active ingredients used
in Suzanne Somers' beauty
care line are naturally derived (plants, minerals,
herbs, flowers, wheat, fruits
and vegetables, sea algae,
and so on). We use high-
quality, effective, naturally
derived ingredients. We use
organic ingredients when
possible. Paraben-free preservative systems. Synthetic
fragrance–free in all facial
skin care products. Use natural oils and plant infusions.

FRESH FACIAL MASKS

Apple and Pectin Age
  Defying
Papaya and Pectin
  Exfoliating
Oat Milk and Honey
  Moisturizing
Cranberry Vitamin C
  Rejuvenating
Pumpkin Mineral Radiance
Pore Little Me Purifying
  Clay Facial Mask

Fit to Be Tight Firming
Body Treatment—AM
Natural Tint
Fit to Be Tight Firming
Body Treatment—PM
Hydra Lift Firming Serum
Soft as Silk Finishing Gel

BASIC SKIN CARE

Clean It Out Cleanser
Exfoliating Cleanser
Fresh Face Gentle Cleansing
Gel
Freshen Up Soothing Aloe
Vera Toner
State of Face SPF30 Daily
Moisturizer
Forty Winks Nightly Facial
Lotion
Eye Smile AM Eye Cream
Eye Sleep PM Treatment

COSMETICS

Spray On Makeup—
Professional Foundation
Spray On Primer—
Perfecting Base

FACEMASTER

800-770-2521
www.facemaster.com

BIBLIOGRAPHY

Bader, Myles H. **1001 All-Natural Secrets to a Pest-Free Property.** 2005. www.asseenontvnetwork.com/vcc/allstar/pestfreeproperty/209715/

Berman, Jennifer, and Laura Berman. **For Women Only: A Revolutionary Guide to Reclaiming Your Sex Life.** New York: Warner Books, 2001.

Berman, Laura. **The Passion Prescription: Ten Weeks to Your Best Sex—Ever.** New York: Hyperion, 2006.

Braverman, Eric R. **The Edge Effect: Achieve Total Health and Longevity with the Balanced Brain Advantage.** New York: Sterling, 2005.

Brownstein, Art. **Extraordinary Healing: The Amazing Power of Your Body's Secret Healing System.** Gig Harbor, Wash.: Harbor Press, 2005.

Brownstein, David. **Iodine: Why You Need It, Why You Can't Live Without It.** 2nd ed. West Bloomfield, Mich.: Medical Alternatives Press, 2006.

Cass, Hyla, and Kathleen Barnes. **8 Weeks to Vibrant Health.** New York: McGraw-Hill, 2004.

Darrow, Marc. **Prolotherapy: Living Pain Free.** Los Angeles, Calif.: Protex Press, 2003.

Emoto, Masaru. **The Hidden Messages in Water.** New York: Atria, 2005.

Gillson, George, and Tracy Marsden. **You've Hit Menopause, Now What?** Calgary, Canada: Rocky Mountain Analytical Corp., 2004.

Greene, Robert, and Leah Feldon. **Perfect Balance: Dr. Robert Greene's Breakthrough Program for Finding the Lifelong Hormonal Health You Deserve.** New York: Clarkson Potter, 2005.

Hemmes, Hilde. **Detox and Live.** Australia: Australian School of Herbal Medicine, 1999.

Hendel, Barbara, and Peter Ferreira. **Water & Salt: The Essence of Life.** Natural Resources, Inc., 2003.

Hotze, Stephen F., and Kelly Griffin. **Hormones, Health, and Happiness: A Natural Medical Formula for Rediscovering Youth with Bioidentical Hormones.** Houston, Tex.: Forrest Publishing, 2005.

Kakkis, Joyce A. **Confession of an Estrogen Evangelist: Setting the Record Straight on Estrogen Replacement Therapy.** Long Beach, Calif.: Joyce Kakkis, 2001.

Klatz, Ronald. **Grow Young with HGH: The Amazing Medically Proven Plan to Reverse Aging.** New York: Collins, 1998.

————. **Infection Protection: How to Fight the Germs That Make You Sick.** New York: Collins, 2002.

Kurzweil, Ray, and Terry Grossman. **Fantastic Voyage: Live Long Enough to Live Forever.** Emmaus, Pa.: Rodale, 2004.

Lee, John R., and Virginia Hopkins. **What Your Doctor May Not Tell You About Menopause: The Breakthrough Book on Natural Progesterone.** New York: Warner Books, 1996.

Levy, Thomas E. **Vitamin C, Infectious Diseases, and Toxins: Curing the Incurable.** Philadelphia: Xlibris Corporation, 2002.

Life Extension Foundation. **Disease Prevention and Treatment,** expanded 4th ed. Hollywood, Fla.: Life Extension Media, 2003.

Lipton, Bruce H. **The Biology of Belief: Unleashing the Power of Consciousness, Matter and Miracles.** Santa Rosa, Calif.: Mountain of Love, 2005.

London, Gary. **Thank You, Suzanne Somers: A Simple Guide to Youthful Beauty, Better Sex, and a Healthier Life.** Los Angeles, Calif.: City View Books, 2006

Miller, Philip Lee, and Monica Reinagel. **The Life Extension Revolution: The New Science of Growing Older Without Aging.** New York: Bantam, 2005.

Mulhall, Douglas, and Katja Hansen. **The Calcium Bomb: The Nanobacteria Link to Heart Disease & Cancer.** Cranston, R.I.: Writers' Collective, 2004.

Myss, Caroline, and C. Norman Shealy. **The Creation of Health: The Emotional, Psychological, and Spiritual Responses That Promote Health and Healing.** New York: Three Rivers Press, 1998.

Plourde, Elizabeth. **Your Guide to Hysterectomy, Ovary Removal, & Hormone Replacement: What All Women Need to Know.** Irvine, Calif.: New Voice Publications, 2001.

Randolph, C. W., and Genie James. **From Hormone Hell to Hormone Well: Discover Human-Identical Hormones as a Safe & Effective Treatment for PMS, Perimenopause, Menopause or Hysterectomy.** Jacksonville, Fla.: Natural Hormone Institute of America, 2004.

Rogers, Sherry A. **Detoxify or Die.** Sarasota, Fla.: Prestige Pubs, 2002.

Rothenberg, Ron, and Kathleen Becker. **Forever Ageless.** Encinitas, Calif.: California HealthSpan Institute, 2001.

Schwartz, Erika. **The Hormone Solution: Naturally Alleviate Symptoms of Hormone Imbalance from Adolescence Through Menopause.** New York: Warner Books, 2002.

——. **The 30-Day Natural Hormone Plan: Look and Feel Young Again—Without Synthetic HRT.** New York: Warner Books, 2005.

Schwarzbein, Diana, and Nancy Deville. **The Schwarzbein Principle: The Truth About Losing Weight, Being Healthy and Feeling Younger.** Deerfield Beach, Fla.: HCI, 1999.

Shames, Karilee, and Richard Shames. **Feeling Fat, Fuzzy or Frazzled?: A 3-Step Program to: Beat Hormone Havoc, Restore Thyroid, Adrenal, and Reproductive Balance, and Feel Better Fast!** New York: Hudson Street Press, 2005.

Sher, Bob, Bob Goldman, and Ronald Klatz. **The Anti-Ageing Diet: How to Look and Feel 20 Years Younger No Matter What Your Age.** Australia: Redwood Publishing, 2000.

Shippen, Eugene, and William Fryer. **The Testosterone Syndrome: The Critical Factor for Energy, Health, and Sexuality—Reversing the Male Menopause.** New York: M. Evans and Company, Inc., 2001.

Smith, Roy, and Michael O. Thorner (eds.). **Human Growth Hormone Research and Clinical Practice.** Totowa, N.J.: Humana Press, 2000.

Starr, Mark. **Hypothyroidism Type 2: The Epidemic.** Irvine, Calif.: New Voice Publications, 2005.

Streicher, Lauren F. **The Essential Guide to Hysterectomy: Complete Advice from a Gynecologist on Your Choices Before, During, and After Surgery—Including the Latest Treatment Options and Alternatives.** New York: M. Evans & Co., 2004.

Thomas, John. **Young Again!: How to Reverse the Aging Process.** Medford, N.J.: Plexus Press, 2002.

Vliet, Elizabeth Lee. **It's My Ovaries, Stupid.** New York: Scribner, 2003.

————. **Screaming to Be Heard: Hormone Connections Women Suspect . . . and Doctors Still Ignore.** New York: M. Evans & Co., 2001.

Wiley, T. S., and Bent Formby. **Lights Out: Sleep, Sugar, and Survival.** New York: Atria, 2001.

Wiley, T. S., Julie Taguchi, and Bent Formby. **Sex, Lies, and Menopause: The Shocking Truth About Synthetic Hormones and the Benefits of Natural Alternatives.** New York: Perennial Currents, 2004.

INDEX

ABOUT THE AUTHOR

SUZANNE SOMERS is the author of sixteen books, including the **New York Times** bestsellers **Keeping Secrets,** five Somersize titles, and **The Sexy Years**. The former star of the hit television programs **Three's Company** and **Step by Step,** Suzanne is one of the most trusted and respected brand names in the world, representing cosmetics and skin care products, apparel, jewelry, a computerized facial fitness system, fitness products, and an extensive food line. She was named Entertainer of the Year in Las Vegas in 1987 and debuted her one-woman Broadway show in 2005. Suzanne received an honorary doctorate of humane letters from National University and is a highly sought-after commencement speaker. She lives in California with her husband and family. For more information, go to SuzanneSomers.com.

I am always interested in your reactions to this new information and what you have uncovered independent of this book. Please contact me with this information at suzannesomers.com.

Thank you,

LIKE WHAT YOU'VE SEEN?

If you enjoyed this large print edition of AGELESS, look for other books by Suzanne Somers available from Random House Large Print.

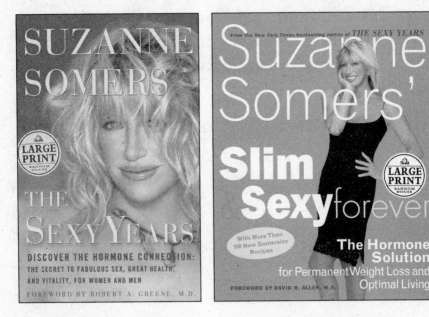

THE SEXY YEARS
(hardcover)
0-375-43296-5
$27.00/$41.00C

SUZANNE SOMERS' SLIM AND SEXY FOR-EVER
(hardcover)
0-375-43480-1
$25.95/$35.95C

Large print books are available wherever books are sold and at many local libraries.

All prices are subject to change. Check with your local retailer for current pricing and availability.
For more information on these and other large print titles,
visit www.randomlargeprint.com